The Wholesome Child

A NUTRITIONAL GUIDE WITH MORE THAN 140 FAMILY-FRIENDLY RECIPES

MANDY SACHER

FOREWORD BY DR. PAUL SACHER

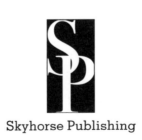

Skyhorse Publishing

Visit our website at www.skyhorsepublishing.com.

10 9 8 7 6 5 4 3 2 1

Library of Congress Cataloging-in-Publication Data is available on file.

Cover design by Kerry Alice
Cover photo credit: Cath Muscat

Print ISBN: 978-1-5107-3685-6
Ebook ISBN: 978-1-5107-3687-0

Printed in China

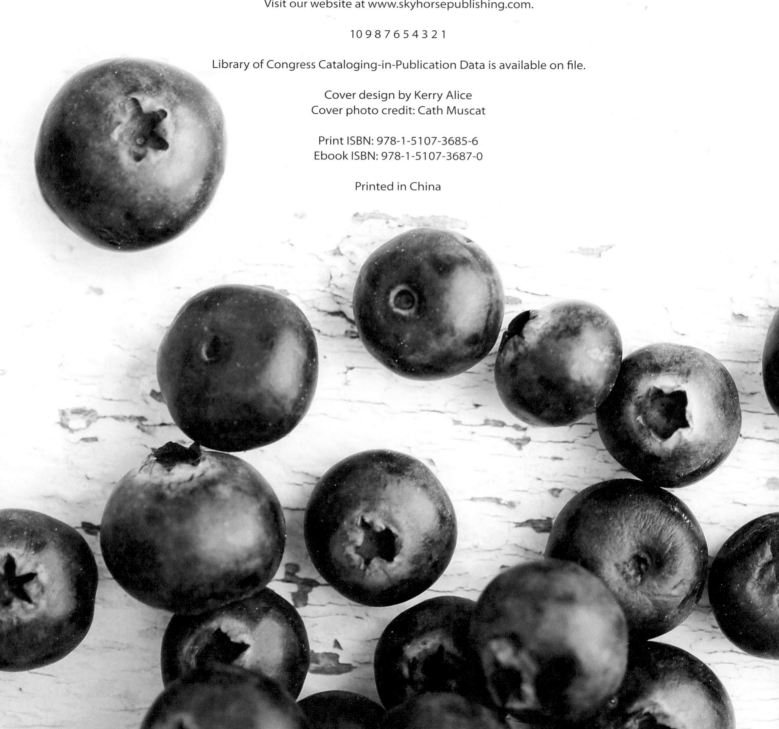

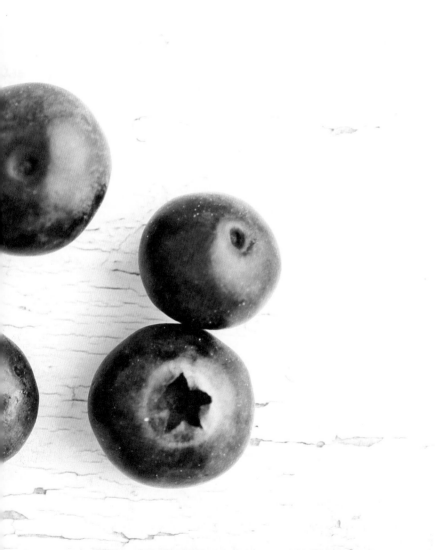

For Aaron and Summer.

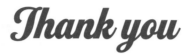

Thank you

To my husband Neil, for his commitment, unwavering support and belief in Wholesome Child and in this book. My darling children, Aaron and Summer: you guys are the reason for everything and have taught me the true meaning of love. My amazing parents, I am forever grateful for your unconditional love and guidance and for being such incredible grandparents to my children. My brother Paul for his mentorship and guidance and for writing the foreword. My brother Ivan, my Aunty Elaine, Uncle Earle, cousin Wallis, and my special grandmother Bella for believing in me.

My incredibly dedicated team: my literary agent Nadine Rubin Nathan who shared my vision and helped bring this book to life; my editor Nicole Frail, who helped get this edition ready for the US market, talented art director Kerry Alice, and recipe developer and fellow nutritionist Sandra Bendersky. Daisy Stockbridge, Jody Moses, and Sarah Fitzpatrick, who lent their sub-editing and fact-checking skills to the book. Food stylist Sally Parker and photographer Cath Muscat for the cover image and most of the delicious images inside that I hope will inspire you to get cooking. Photographer Justine Perl and stylist Nicola Landau Tkachenko for my portrait on the back cover. Photographers Grace Alyssa Kyo and Effie White and stylist Yael Barkhan for their valuable contributions. Also, to Shula Endry-Walder and Suzy Moss who provided their beautiful homes for photo shoots.

I am honored to have had the input of experts including pediatrician and lactation consultant Dr. Leila Masson, clinical and developmental psychologist Romy Kunitz, speech and pediatric feeding therapist Mandy-Lee Adno, and clinical neuropsychologist Dr Roy Sugarman. Thank you also to dietitian Maria Kolotourou for her advice and assistance.

Naturopath and lecturer Fran Music-Innes, Dr. Jeff Jankelson who has been an incredible support and mentor, and to my special friends who mean the world to me and who have been extremely patient when I have not been around. You all know who you are.

My clients—children and their parents—who have taught me so much and inspired me to go that extra mile to find the best solutions for an array of eating challenges.

Melissa Cavenagh and all the recipe testers—busy moms who signed up to test recipes over and over again. Your commitment and hours in the kitchen really helped us to perfect the recipes in this book.

Finally, this book would never have become what it is if it wasn't for my loyal supporters who contributed to and widely shared the Kickstarter campaign that ultimately funded this book and allowed us to take it to the next level creatively. I am forever grateful to you for sharing my dream. An extra special mention to Apurva Chiranewala.

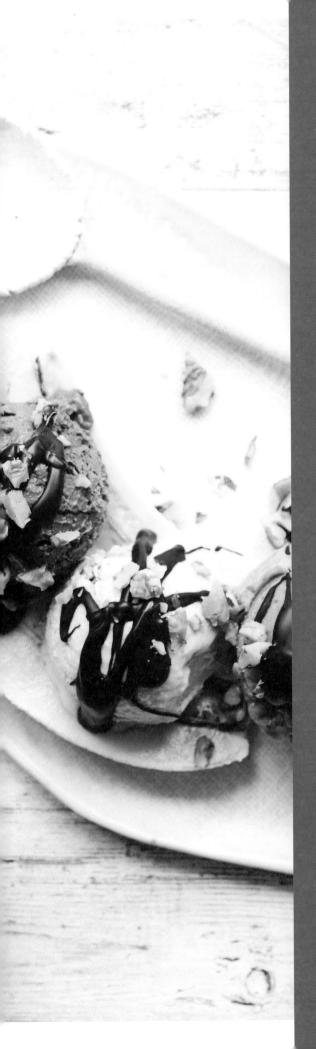

CONTENTS

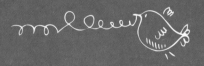

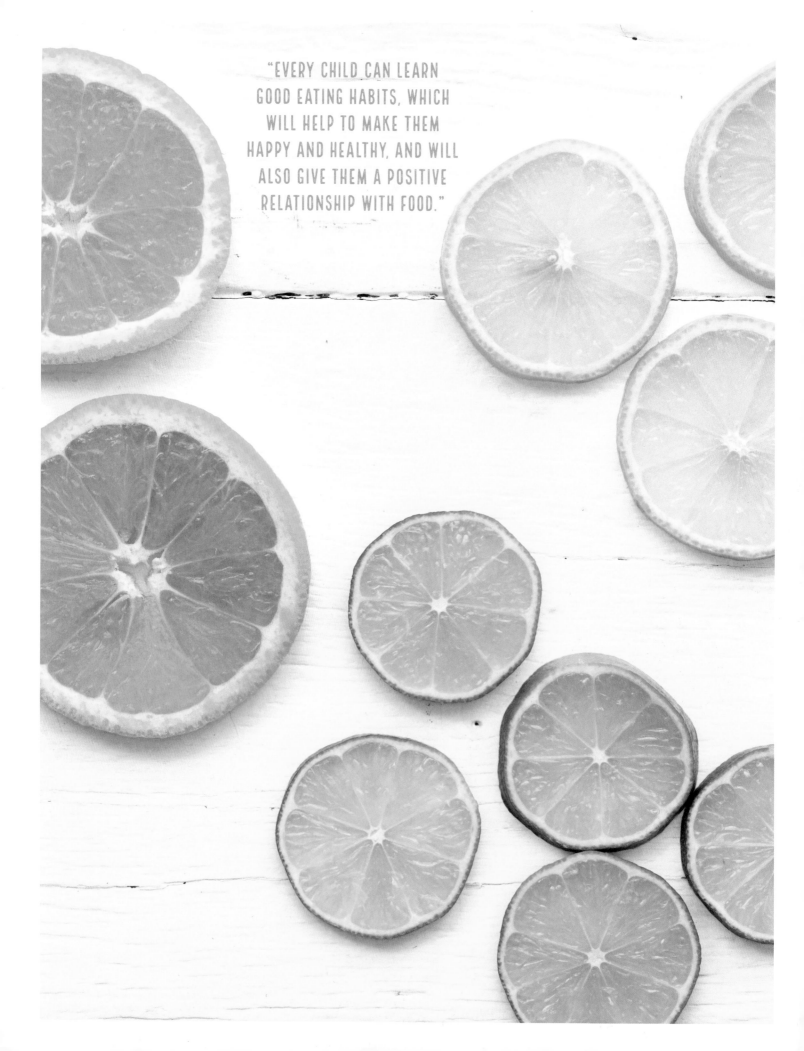

"EVERY CHILD CAN LEARN GOOD EATING HABITS, WHICH WILL HELP TO MAKE THEM HAPPY AND HEALTHY, AND WILL ALSO GIVE THEM A POSITIVE RELATIONSHIP WITH FOOD."

I have been deeply passionate about children's health for the past twenty-one years as a specialist pediatric dietician and nutritionist. Worryingly, around one in three children in developed countries are affected by overweight or obesity. Even in healthy weight children, we are now seeing cases of kids consuming poor quality diets, containing high levels of fat and sugar, with insufficient vitamins, minerals, and trace elements essential for healthy growth and development. Providing children with good nutrition is essential for their growth and development. It is also a fundamental health right. Now, more than ever, feeding children healthily is an international priority.

Every parent wants their child to have the best start in life, yet unhealthy diets in childhood are now associated with unprecedented levels of serious medical conditions in children, including dental cavities, gastrointestinal problems, and even insulin resistance. It is more important than ever to encourage children to develop a lifelong love for healthy and nutritious foods.

You may have noticed Mandy and I share a surname. Mandy is my sister and, along with a matching last name, we have shared a common interest in nutrition and health since our teenage years. We're both qualified pediatric nutritionists, dedicated to raising healthy, happy children. Both of our approaches have at their core the premise that the healthiest, most affordable way to feed your family is to cook from fresh. We also believe in empowering families with the skills to understand nutrition labels so they can make healthier choices.

Mandy supported me for many years, both in writing my third book *From Kid to Superkid* (Vermilion) as well as working closely with me on the development of the first ever Mind, Exercise, Nutrition…Do it! (MEND) program, specifically developed for children who are above a healthy weight. MEND is now the largest healthy lifestyle program for children above a healthy weight and their parents, internationally. It is available in five countries and has the largest amount of scientific research supporting benefits of the program.

Young children learn by copying those around them. In the early years, children learn most by imitating their parents. "Do as I do" and not "as I say" has been scientifically shown to be an effective method for changing children's behavior around eating. Therefore, I cannot emphasize enough the importance of parents committing to being good role models when it comes to food. I have seen first-hand over the years working in the UK, Australia, USA, Canada, and the Netherlands, how the way that parents raise and feed their children is a product of their own upbringing, education, values, and perceptions of right and wrong. Certainly, raising healthy, happy children is not easy—and parenting, like any complex skill, needs to be learned. Feeding your child should not be a cause of anxiety for either child or parent and common nutrition concerns can often be solved with practical and simple advice like that found in the *Wholesome Child* book.

With the right approach and emphasis, every child can learn good eating habits, which will help to make them happy and healthy and give them a positive relationship with food for life. I've worked with Annabel Karmel on her book *Superfoods for Babies and Children*, consulted with Jamie Oliver on *Return to Jamie's School Dinners*, and regularly appeared on the BBC TV family health makeover show, *Honey, We're Killing the Kids*. Like those projects, Mandy's *Wholesome Child* book is a great resource to address many of the most common child nutrition issues—and provides easy-to-follow ideas in the form of delicious recipes.

The Wholesome Child reflects the fact that there is no one-size-fits-all solution to feeding children healthily. Mandy breaks through the confusing media messages, which are constantly changing and often not based on any robust science. Her book is filled with up-to-date nutrition advice and experience gained in her practice working with children from the time they start eating solids and through Mandy's experience feeding her own children, my nephew Aaron and niece Summer.

I have the utmost admiration for Mandy and her knowledge, experience, drive, and passion to write and self-publish this book, to bring her extraordinary approach to child nutrition and cooking to you. I am very proud of my little sister and truly hope you benefit from the wealth of knowledge and experience packed into this book.

Stick to *Wholesome Child's* advice wherever it works for you and feel comforted that you are giving your child the best start in life.

Dr. Paul Sacher

Dr. Paul Sacher is a specialist pediatric dietician, scientist and leading child health expert. Dr. Sacher has been an invited speaker at over forty-eight international scientific conferences. He has published three books, and was awarded the British Dietetic Association's most prestigious award for 2011.

As every parent knows, having a baby turns your world upside down, but for me giving birth to my son was a total game-changer. For the first time in my life I understood true unconditional love, and more importantly the lengths a mother will go to for the wellbeing of her child.

I loved breastfeeding my son. Blame it on oxytocin, but those serene moments with my baby were some of the most joyous of my life. However, as he approached five months of age I started reading up about introducing solids and my euphoria began to dissolve. I spoke to a few health care professionals and found myself balking at some of their suggestions.

With my background as a nutritionist and in-depth knowledge of food labels, there was no way I was going to offer my newborn pureed porridge made from refined white rice, processed fruit pouches, teething rusks full of sugar or yogurts packed with fruit concentrate, sugar, and preservatives. So I set out to make my own homemade, preservative-free, and organic baby food.

There were many raised eyebrows from family, friends and some other mothers, and admittedly I did spend a lot of time in my kitchen—something I was luckily able to do as I worked from home—but to me it was worth it. One of my dearest friends, Nanda, shared my passion and together we would create menus for the week and slow-cook large quantities of lamb or chicken with vegetables and share what we had made. This way we saved time and increased variety. I truly believed I was giving my child the best start in life and it showed. He rarely got sick and he loved his food—especially his vegetables.

When my son was eighteen months old, Nanda opened Pear Tree House Family Day Care in my hometown of Sydney, Australia, and I helped design the menu, which is comprised of organic, homemade meals. Around this time I also began to focus solely on prenatal and pediatric nutrition, and established my private practice.

> "I WROTE THIS BOOK TO PROVIDE ANSWERS TO THE MANY QUESTIONS PARENTS HAVE AROUND KIDS' NUTRITION, WHILE OFFERING STRATEGIES THAT REALLY WORK."

Just before my son turned three, we welcomed his baby sister and this time things were a lot easier. I was more confident as a mom, firmer in my choices, and less concerned about being judged. (Plus, I'd thankfully learned many more time-saving tricks, which I've shared throughout this book.)

When my daughter was fifteen months old, my friend Tali suggested I create a back-to-school lunch box workshop. This was the inspiration for the Wholesome Child Workshop Series.

The workshops proved very popular and really helped Wholesome Child to flourish, with over a thousand participants having attended to date. In April 2014, I launched my website www.wholesomechild.com.au, an online destination for parents and caregivers to access relevant, practical feeding advice.

And as my private nutrition practice grew, I would regularly have mothers coming to see me in floods of tears after being given impossible-to-implement dietary advice from well-meaning health practitioners. I could see that there was a vast lack of information out there on how to support dietary changes, such as going dairy free, when all some children are prepared to eat is yogurt and string cheese. The same kind of challenges faced these mothers when they were told to eliminate gluten, but their kids refused to eat anything but sandwiches made from white supermarket bread.

Drawing on my experience as a qualified nutritionist, SOS feeding specialist, health writer, and co-developer of the MEND childhood obesity program (which runs in the US), I combined my in-depth knowledge of whole foods with behavioral advice and developed easy-to-follow, practical steps to guide parents on how to encourage healthy changes in their children's diets.

The feedback I was getting from my clients and workshop participants was very positive, and I soon realized I was helping parents feel okay with where they were at. The practical and incremental steps I suggested parents make to their children's diets were achieving amazing

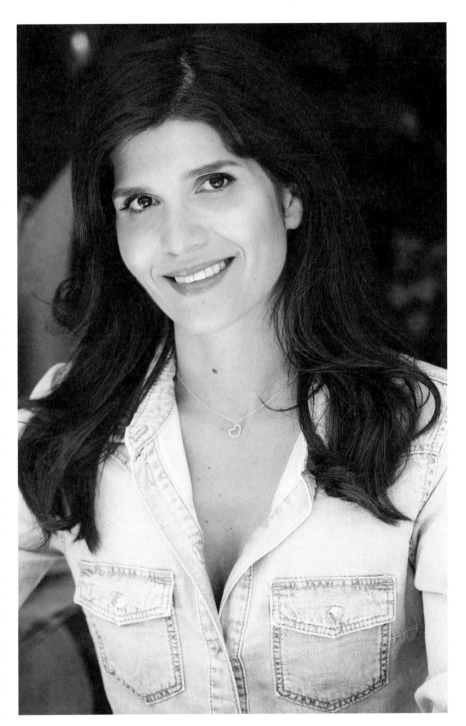

results. I also realized that although there are many so-called "bibles" out there on children's sleep, behavior, and parenting, when it came to nutrition and food, there were none. My decision to write *The Wholesome Child* was based on the knowledge that not one comprehensive book was available which provided answers to the many questions parents have around kids' nutrition, while also offering basic strategies that really work, as well as simple, family-friendly recipes to back them up.

To raise the funds needed to self-publish such a book, I made the crazy decision to run a Kickstarter campaign, and after a month of intense emotional anguish raised $45,000 and over four hundred copies of the book were pre-ordered. Determined to ensure the people who believed in me would receive a fantastic product that exceeded expectations, for the next six months the writing and production of this book took over my life and became my sole focus. I put my consultations and workshops on hold and with the help of my amazing and talented team, dedicated every working hour to ensure my vision came to life.

Creating *The Wholesome Child* has been an incredible learning curve for me as a mom and nutritionist. So many challenges presented themselves along the way, and to overcome them required grit, stamina, and a resourcefulness I did not know I had. The intensive research needed for the topics covered in this book has taken my own knowledge to a deeper level. I also had the privilege of working with experts in their fields, people I have long respected, as well as mentors who have inspired me to keep going at all costs. Of course when it comes to feeding my kids, I too am still learning. I don't get it right all the time—and I don't expect to either.

My goal for *The Wholesome Child* was to answer the questions I am asked repeatedly at workshops, in parenting social forums and by clients and friends. I have tried to remain a voice of reason and provide a balanced point of view, interjected with up-to-date nutrition information and real anecdotes. I also share the lessons I've learned from my experiences feeding my young children, as well as twenty-two years in the health and wellness industry, and the insights gained from my practice as a pediatric nutritionist.

I hope you find the answers you are seeking within these pages, and that this book will help you to grow as you continue on your family's health journey . . . creating delicious, nutritious, and wholesome meals that everyone can enjoy.

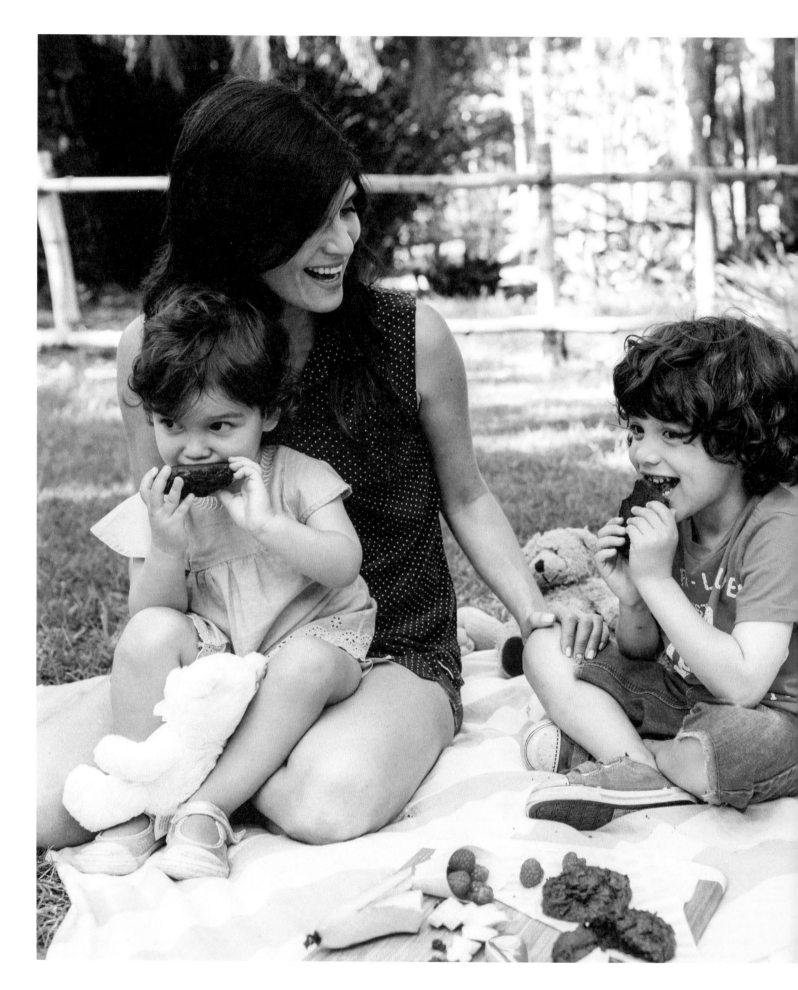

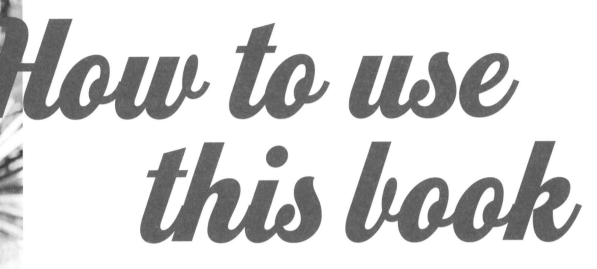

How to use this book

When it comes to trying new or different foods, I have learned through experience that young children respond best to incremental changes introduced slowly using careful, patient repetition. I designed the Wholesome Child 8-step guide in this book to provide a clear, simple, easy-to-follow plan for parents wanting to maximize their child's nutrition. It focuses on children between the ages of one and six, though older children will also benefit from the advice and enjoy the recipes. In fact, they're all designed to make perfect family meals.

You've probably noticed how food science is constantly changing. There's always a new fad diet or way of eating that's the latest trend. The problem is these don't necessarily work for children. Low-fat diets, carb-free diets, sugar-free diets, and vegan diets may be necessary for certain kids with medical conditions, allergies, special needs or for religious or philosophical reasons, but not all these eliminations are healthy for most children.

In the same way, it's not necessarily ideal for children to follow a Paleo diet loaded with protein or go gluten-free or dairy-free without supervision. Unfortunately, in our modern age, most children's diets are compromised by the inclusion of additives, processed foods and Genetically Modified (GM) ingredients. Children who eat a balanced diet of mostly clean foods have the best chance at good health.

At the beginning of each step, we present the facts based on up-to-date nutrition science. Then we share practical tips to help you take control of your child's health journey. But far from dictating how this should look, this book is about giving you all the options and tools, leaving you

to choose what is most relevant for your family.

Following on from the advice are recipes built around the theme of each step. We haven't categorized these according to breakfast, lunch, and dinner. When it comes to feeding children, eggs are a perfect breakfast, lunch, or dinner meal. Porridge, boosted with protein and added pumpkin is an acceptable dinner; mango chia pudding is an ideal breakfast, snack, or dessert option. Healthy sausage rolls are an ideal party food, but can also work in the lunch box, be offered for dinner or as an after-school snack. Mini salmon quiches are a perfect breakfast or dinner dish as are the veggie muffins ... you get the idea. The recipes have been categorized, instead, according to their nutritional benefits and to showcase different uses for certain ingredients which boost the nutrient value of typical dishes favored by kids.

This book will help you make important changes such as switching to whole grains (and broadening your child's nutrient spectrum while cutting down on gluten in the process), increasing protein, ensuring enough healthy fats exist in the diet, and decreasing sugar. I explain the reasons behind each suggested change to help you, the parent or caregiver, understand why these changes are considered a healthier option.

I have provided recipes for meals, snacks, party food, condiments, and marinades so that you can feed your children whole food that is free of additives, preservatives, food coloring and flavoring. The amount of time you have will obviously dictate the degree to which you follow these recipes.

Whether you're able to cook everything from

scratch or you blend homemade meals with store-bought options, there are plenty of choices. Our practical tips and advice will help you make more informed choices when shopping for ingredients or store-bought staples so you can still go about making healthy changes to your child's diet successfully. The most important thing is that you have the facts laid out in front of you and you get to choose what works for your family.

When it comes to healthy eating, children and adults differ greatly. Often, if an adult wants to change or believes that something in their diet is harmful, they will make the change knowing that it is beneficial for their health. But when it comes to children, the reasons for their food refusal and unwillingness to try new things is often complex and we need to employ positive behavior strategies and advice to guide them through these changes. There may be medical conditions that prevent some children from eating new foods. In the Fussy Eating chapter I try to help you get a clearer understanding of the many reasons behind refusal to eat. Even if you are struggling to feed a fussy eater anything other than their firm favorites, there are many beneficial tips throughout this book to guide you on how to broaden their repertoire. Perhaps you won't get your child to eat shepherd's pie with mashed cauliflower and parsnip, but you may be able to get them to eat the meat separated from the mash, or even simply improve on the bread you choose for your family. If time is an issue and cooking at this stage of your journey is difficult, then follow our time-saving tips and use our healthy swap guides to choose healthier store-bought options.

Always bear in mind that it's unrealistic to change everything all at once. My hope is that after reading this book you will feel empowered to make meaningful changes wherever you can.

SERVING SIZES

Examples of serving sizes have been listed in each of the 8 Steps. These are to be used as a guide only. It's very important to not restrict or limit a young child's natural appetite, especially when he or she is eating nutritious and wholesome foods. Children have different metabolisms, activity levels, shapes, and sizes. There is not a one-size-fits-all model. Serving sizes can be useful for parents who want the extra reassurance that their children are eating close to the required amounts, but it's not advisable to use the guides to restrict a child's healthy food intake.

If your child is asking for food at times when they are not hungry, look for triggers such as boredom and try to offer activity-based distractions (see Goal 3 on page 149). As a parent, it's important to offer an appropriate amount of food, but allow the child to decide how much they will actually eat. I once saw a nine-month-old boy who was in the first percentile for weight and not sleeping. When I visited the family home, I learned that his mother was measuring out his meals according to a book she had, and the portions were too small for him. Once I gave her the advice she needed to allow her son to eat until he was full, things changed almost overnight.

THE 8 STEPS

Unlike most guides, the Wholesome Child 8 Steps can be followed at whatever pace is most

My stance on sugar

We do not use refined sugar in any of our recipes. If your child is following a sugar-free diet or your family is following a sugar-free lifestyle then it's perfectly okay to leave out added sugar (which is often optional in the recipes) or follow the advice in the sugar chapter for ways to reduce and cut down on sweeteners. You're ultimately aiming to reduce your child's sweet tooth.

"THIS DELICIOUS WATERMELON CAKE IS A GREAT ALTERNATIVE TO SUGAR-FILLED CAKES. WE SERVED THIS AT MY DAUGHTER'S DAYCARE FOR HER BIRTHDAY AND EVERYONE LOVED IT!"

Watermelon Cake (see recipe on page 219)

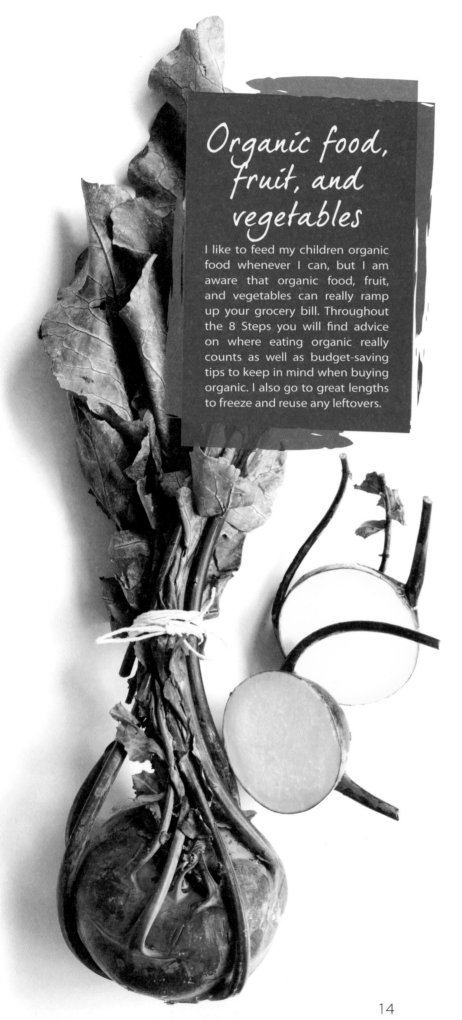

Organic food, fruit, and vegetables

I like to feed my children organic food whenever I can, but I am aware that organic food, fruit, and vegetables can really ramp up your grocery bill. Throughout the 8 Steps you will find advice on where eating organic really counts as well as budget-saving tips to keep in mind when buying organic. I also go to great lengths to freeze and reuse any leftovers.

comfortable or necessary for both you and your child and in whatever order works best.

To introduce new foods or tweak existing favorites, we always suggest setting your child up for success by choosing the meal or snack where he or she is usually most relaxed and interested in eating. It may be breakfast on a weekend or a snack after school. Setting parents up for success is just as important, especially since the food you've lovingly prepared may be rejected numerous times (some experts say you have to try a new food 10–15 times before a child will eat it).

It's crucial that the breakfast (or lunch or dinner) table is a calm space and not filled with family drama or power struggles, so identify how you feel at each meal and then choose to implement changes accordingly. If you're unable to try at weekday breakfasts because mornings are too rushed and stressful, try a weekend breakfast instead or tackle lunch (or the lunch box). Breathe. Remain calm. See the big picture.

THE GOALS

Each of the 8 Steps is matched with a Goal that will help you to make more subtle behavioral changes to support the dietary changes. These Goals are practical tools that I have learned over the years, during my time tackling childhood obesity with MEND and the numerous feeding courses I have completed.

The psychology of food has as much impact on children's food choices as the food being presented to them. These practical behavioral suggestions are techniques I have implemented in my private practice over the past five years and I have seen excellent results. It is common practice for parents to see numerous health care practitioners and to walk away with a list of forbidden foods, but once parents are home it becomes impossible to get the child to adhere to the changes. If we combine nutritional advice with behavior change techniques to support healthy eating then there is a far higher chance of success.

The most memorable result I've experienced was with a patient who was four years old and still struggling with cibophobia (the fear of food). Her parents had taken her to see numerous experts to no avail. From just one meeting with her it was clear to me that a previous experience with gagging and choking had made her incredibly anxious and, because of that, she only felt confident eating if her mother was present. Instead of focusing on her diet, I worked on the dynamics within the family and we implemented family meals, changing the focus from how we were going to get the child to eat, to focusing on fun at mealtimes and allowing her father to get more involved with meal preparation and creating a safe space. The results were dramatic and her parents thanked me for not only helping their daughter to overcome her reluctance to eat, but for making the whole experience vastly more enjoyable for the whole family.

THE RECIPES

For readers not wanting to follow the 8 Steps, *Wholesome Child* works just as well as a recipe book. Simply pick and choose the recipes you like most to make delicious, nutrient-packed meals, snacks, and treats for the whole family to enjoy. I've also created easy-to-follow Menu Planners that use the recipes found throughout the book in a more uniform breakfast, snack, lunch, and dinner sequence. And of course, with so much focus on reducing sugar in our diets, I've tackled party food too.

A WORD ABOUT PROBIOTICS

There are many probiotic-rich foods that can contribute to the health of your family such as yogurt, kefir, fermented vegetables, and kombucha. However, many children's diets—especially fussy eaters—lack these nutrients.

While it is the ideal for kids to get their daily nutritional requirements from food, when it comes to supplementation there is one exception: Lactobacillus and Bifidobacterium probiotics. A child's gastrointestinal tract is colonized by billions of friendly bacteria that help digest food, process toxins, and manufacture vitamins and metabolites that are beneficial to their wellbeing. Alongside the beneficial bacteria, however, are harmful and benign bacteria.

When an imbalance between beneficial and harmful bacteria occurs, a child's health is compromised, and this can affect their physical and mental wellbeing. The gut-brain connection is not one to take lightly. Mounting research shows supplementing from birth with probiotics can play a major role in maintaining a strong immune system and overall good health. Colic, allergies, IBS, constipation, diarrhea, eczema, obesity, behavioral problems, depression, anxiety, and autism spectrum disorders are just some of the medical conditions and disorders that may

Top five ways to increase friendly gut bacteria

1. Breastfeed for at least twelve months if you can.

2. Reduce sugar in the diet.

3. Use antibiotics only if necessary (antibiotics kill all of the friendly bacteria)

   and always give them with a probiotic supplement.

4. Supplement with the right strains for their age and stage.

5. Introduce probiotic-rich foods into the daily diet.

benefit from supplementation with probiotics. To choose the right probiotic for your child, speak to a trained health practitioner.

NUTRIENTS VS SUPPLEMENTS

For protein, healthy fats, and important minerals and vitamins, a child's requirements far exceed an adult's in terms of the amount needed per kilogram of body weight. I had the privilege of working with pediatrician and lactation consultant Dr. Leila Masson, the author of *Children's Health A to Z for New Zealand Parents*. Dr. Masson specializes in ADHD, autism spectrum disorders, behavior problems, recurrent infections, breastfeeding, and allergies and has helped thousands of children become healthier and happier. Like me, she believes that "real" nutrition is the cornerstone of a strong immune system and a healthy childhood and advises getting all the minerals and vitamins your child needs from his diet. However, if your child is deficient in a certain nutrient she recommends offering more foods that contain that specific nutrient and, if necessary, combining with the correct supplements. If your child's diet is limited and you're worried that he is lacking essential nutrients, have him assessed by a pediatrician, dietitian, or nutritionist before using supplements. Together, we compiled the list on the next page, outlining key minerals and vitamins needed to ensure healthy growth and development in childhood. The recommended food sources are a combination of Dr. Leila Masson's wholefood plant-based approach and my approach, which includes animal protein.

For more information on probiotics and the gut-brain axis visit www.wholesomechild.com.au

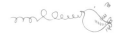

Essential Vitamins and Minerals

Name	RDI (1-8yrs)*	Function	Food sources
Vitamin A	300–400mcg	Healthy immune function, vision, promotes bone and tooth growth.	Apricots, butter, carrots, egg yolk, cod liver oil, green leafy vegetables, liver, spinach, sweet potatoes.
Vitamin B6	0.5–0.6 mg	Promotes healthy serotonin levels, aids in fatty acid and protein metabolism, necessary for zinc absorption.	Grass-fed meat, wild-caught fish, poultry, potatoes, legumes, egg yolk, oats, peanuts, sunflower seeds, walnuts.
Vitamin B12	0.9–1.2mcg	Necessary for brain and nervous system function, red blood cell formation and energy production. Works as a co-enzyme with folate.	Grass-fed meat, fish, chicken, turkey, milk, cheese, eggs, liver, nuts.
Vitamin C	25mg (for optimum health best to exceed this amount)	Strengthens collagen in bones, cartilage, muscles and blood vessels, promotes wound healing and a healthy immune system. Aids in absorption of iron and promotes healthy teeth and gums.	Citrus fruits, cabbage, bell peppers, broccoli, melon, strawberries, tomatoes, sweet potatoes, papayas, mangoes.
Vitamin D	15mcg	Important for healthy bones and teeth, immune function, growth and development.	Sunlight is the main source but also found in butter, egg yolks, oily fish.
Vitamin E	6–7 mg	Essential for a healthy immune system, Vitamin E is a potent antioxidant that protects cell membranes and protects against lipid peroxidation of polyunsaturated fats.	Almonds, grass-fed beef, leafy greens, egg yolk, hazelnuts, sunflower seeds.
Calcium	700–1000mg	Creates healthy bones and teeth, aids in muscle contractions and relaxations, promotes a healthy nervous system.	Almonds, berries, dairy products, beans, cabbages, dark leafy greens, leek, mandarin, seaweed, sesame seeds, salmon with bones, sardines with bones, broccoli, lentils, liver, organ meats, eggs.
Chromium	11–15mcg	Enhances insulin action and helps stabilize blood sugar levels.	Grass-fed beef, whole grains, nutritional yeast (brewer's yeast).
Folate (folic acid)	150–200mcg	Forms red blood cells and is especially important in pregnancy, when it helps to ensure proper development of a baby's nervous system, as well as healthy DNA production and cell growth.	Leafy green vegetables, beans, chickpeas, lentils, liver, organ meats, eggs, whole grains
Iodine	90mcg	Necessary for healthy thyroid function, physical and mental development and a healthy metabolism.	Asparagus, cod, dairy products, garlic, seaweed, mackerel, mushrooms, salmon, iodized salt.
Iron	7mg–10mg	Iron assists red blood cells to carry oxygen to the body, brain and muscle function. A lack of iron in the blood can lead to iron-deficiency anemia, a common nutritional deficiency in children.	Almonds, apricots, avocado, blackstrap molasses, clams, grass-fed red meat, lentils, liver, pumpkin seeds, parsley, spinach, walnuts.
Magnesium	80mg–130mg	Helps to reduce stress and aids in sleep, builds strong bones and balances blood sugar levels.	Almonds, bananas, cashews, cacao powder, figs, dark leafy greens, pumpkin seeds, sesame seeds, brown rice, quinoa.
Zinc	3mg–5mg	Promotes immune health, balances blood sugar levels, influences behavior and learning, aids wound healing, important for taste perception, prevents oxidative stress and DNA damage.	Grass-fed beef and lamb, kidney beans, liver, salmon, tuna, pork, potato, poultry, egg yolk, peanut butter, pinto beans, pumpkin, sunflower seeds, sesame seeds.

* **Reference:** Dietary Reference Intakes (DRI) reports, Food and Nutrition Board, Institute of Medicine, National Academies.
http://www.nationalacademies.org/hmd/~/media/Files/Activity%20Files/Nutrition/DRI-Tables/2_%20RDA%20and%20AI%20Values_Vitamin%20and%20 Elements.pdf?la=en

Conversions

We've created in-depth comparisons of weights so that fans of food scales, Thermomix users, or anyone using imperial measurements can create the Wholesome Child recipes with confidence.

OVEN TEMPERATURES

Celsius (electric)	Celcius (fan forced)	Fahrenheit	Gas
120º	100º	250º	1
150º	130º	300º	2
160º	140º	325º	3
180º	160º	350º	4
190º	170º	375º	5
200º	180º	400º	6
230º	210º	450º	7
250º	230º	500º	9

The recipes in this book were tested in a conventional oven. If using a fan-forced oven, decrease the temperature by 20ºC/70ºF.

LIQUIDS

Metric	Cup	Imperial
30ml	1/8 cup	1 fl oz
60ml	1/4 cup	2 fl oz
80ml	1/3 cup	2 1/2 fl oz
100ml		3 1/2 fl oz
125ml	1/2 cup	4 fl oz
160ml	2/3 cup	5 fl oz
180ml	3/4 cup	6 fl oz
200ml		7 fl oz
250ml	1 cup	8 fl oz
310ml	1 1/4 cups	10 1/2 fl oz
375ml	1 1/2 cups	13 fl oz
430ml	1 3/4 cups	15 fl oz
475ml		16 fl oz
500ml	2 cups	17 fl oz
625ml	2 1/2 cups	21 1/2 fl oz
750ml	3 cups	26 fl oz
1L	4 cups	35 fl oz
1.25L	5 cups	44 fl oz
1.5L	6 cups	52 fl oz
2L	8 cups	70 fl oz
2.5L	10 cups	88 fl oz

INGREDIENTS

INGREDIENT	1 cup	1/2 cup	1/3 cup	1/4 cup
FLOUR				
Almond meal	120g/4.25oz	60g/2oz	40g/1.5oz	30g/1oz
Arrowroot	120g/4.25oz	60g/2oz	40g/1.5oz	30g/1oz
Bread crumbs	90g/3.25oz	45g/1.5oz	30g/1oz	20g/0.75oz
Buckwheat flour	140g/5oz	70g/2.5oz	45g/1.5oz	35g/1.25oz
Cacao/carob powder	100g/3.5oz	50g/1.75oz	30g/1oz	25g/1oz
Chickpea flour	120g/4.25oz	60g/2oz	40g/1.5oz	30g/1oz
Chocolate buds	100g/3.5oz	50g/1.75oz	35g/1.25oz	25g/1oz
Cocoa butter	120g/4.25oz	60g/2oz	40g/1.5oz	30g/1oz
Coconut, desiccated	80g/3oz	40g/1.5oz	25g/1oz	20g/0.75oz
Coconut flour	110g/4oz	55g/2oz	35g/1.25oz	25g/1oz
Coconut, shredded	75g/2.5oz	35g/1.25oz	25g/1oz	20g/0.75oz
Kamut flour	150g/5.25oz	75g/2.5oz	50g/1.75oz	35g/1.25oz
Millet flour	140g/5oz	70g/2.5oz	45g/1.5oz	35g/1.25oz
Oat meal	110g/4oz	55g/2oz	35g/1.25oz	30g/1oz
Psyllium husk powder	80g/3oz	40g/1.5oz	25g/1oz	20g/0.75oz
Rice flour	160g/5.5oz	80g/3oz	55g/2oz	40g/1.5oz
Seed meal (pumpkin, sunflower)	120g/4.25oz	60g/2oz	40g/1.5oz	30g/1oz
Teff flour, brown	170g/6oz	85g/3oz	55g/2oz	45g/1.5oz
WC gf-flour mix	130g/4.5oz	65g/2.25oz	45g/1.5oz	35g/1.25oz
White spelt flour	130g/4.5oz	65g/2.25oz	45g/1.5oz	35g/1.25oz
Whole Spelt Flour	140g/5oz	70g/2.5oz	45g/1.5oz	35g/1.25oz

INGREDIENT	1 cup	½ cup	⅓ cup	¼ cup
NUTS & SEEDS				
Almonds	160g/5.5oz	80g/3oz	55g/2oz	40g/1.5oz
Almonds, slivered	140g/5oz	70g/2.5oz	45g/1.5oz	35g/1.25oz
Almond butter	320g/11.5oz	160g/5.5oz	105g/3.75oz	80g/3oz
Brazil nuts	150g/5.25oz	75g/2.5oz	50g/1.75oz	40g/1.5oz
Cashews	160g/5.5oz	80g/3oz	55g/2oz	40g/1.5oz
Chia seeds	200g/7oz	100g/3.5oz	65g/2.25oz	50g/1.75oz
Dates, pitted	240g/8.5oz	120g/4.25oz	80g/3oz	60g/2oz
Flaxseeds	180g/6.5oz	90g/3.25oz	60g/2oz	45g/1.5oz
Goji berries	100g/3.5oz	50g/1.75oz	35g/1.25oz	25g/1oz
Hazelnuts	150g/5.25oz	75g/2.5oz	50g/1.75oz	40g/1.5oz
Macadamias	140g/5oz	70g/2.5oz	45g/1.5oz	35g/1.25oz
Peanut butter	280g/10oz	140g/5oz	95g/3.5oz	70g/2.5oz
Pecans	110g/4oz	55g/2oz	35g/1.25oz	30g/1oz
Pine nuts	160g/5.5oz	80g/3oz	55g/2oz	40g/1.5oz
Pistachios	140g/5oz	70g/2.5oz	45g/1.5oz	35g/1.25oz
Pumpkin seeds	160g/5.5oz	80g/3oz	55g/2oz	40g/1.5oz
Sesame seeds	160g/5.5oz	80g/3oz	55g/2oz	40g/1.5oz
Sunflower seeds	160g/5.5oz	80g/3oz	55g/2oz	40g/1.5oz
Tahini	270g/9.5oz	135g/4.75oz	90g/3.25oz	70g/2.5oz
Walnuts, crushed	140g/5oz	70g/2.5oz	45g/1.5oz	35g/1.25oz
Walnuts, whole	110g/4oz	55g/2oz	35g/1.25oz	30g/1oz

INGREDIENT	1 cup	½ cup	⅓ cup	¼ cup
GRAINS & LEGUMES				
Adzuki beans, cooked	180g/6.5oz	90g/3.25oz	60g/2oz	45g/1.5oz
Adzuki beans, dry	190g/6.75oz	95g/3.5oz	65g/2.25oz	50g/1.75oz
Black beans, cooked	180g/6.5oz	90g/3.25oz	60g/2oz	45g/1.5oz
Black beans, dry	190g/6.75oz	95g/3.5oz	65g/2.25oz	50g/1.75oz
fava beans, cooked	150g/5.25oz	75g/2.5oz	50g/1.75oz	40g/1.5oz
Brown rice, cooked	200g/7oz	100g/3.5oz	65g/2.25oz	50g/1.75oz
Brown rice, dry	210g/7.5oz	105g/3.75oz	70g/2.5oz	55g/2oz
Brown teff	200g/7oz	100g/3.5oz	65g/2.25oz	50g/1.75oz
Buckinis	160g/5.5oz	80g/3oz	55g/2oz	40g/1.5oz
Buckwheat, dry	190g/6.75oz	95g/3.5oz	65g/2.25oz	50g/1.75oz
lima beans, cooked	180g/6.5oz	90g/3.25oz	60g/2oz	45g/1.5oz
Cannellini beans, cooked	180g/6.5oz	90g/3.25oz	60g/2oz	45g/1.5oz
Chickpeas, cooked	180g/6.5oz	90g/3.25oz	60g/2oz	45g/1.5oz
Chickpeas, dry	190g/6.75oz	95g/3.5oz	65g/2.25oz	50g/1.75oz
Couscous, dry	180g/6.5oz	90g/3.25oz	60g/2oz	45g/1.5oz
Green beans, cooked	180g/6.5oz	90g/3.25oz	60g/2oz	45g/1.5oz
Kidney beans, dry	190g/6.75oz	95g/3.5oz	65g/2.25oz	50g/1.75oz
Kidney beans, cooked	180g/6.5oz	90g/3.25oz	60g/2oz	45g/1.5oz
Lentils, brown, dry	210g/7.5oz	105g/3.75oz	70g/2.5oz	55g/2oz
Lentils, red, split, dry	190g/6.75oz	95g/3.5oz	65g/2.25oz	50g/1.75oz
Millet, hulled, dry	190g/6.75oz	95g/3.5oz	65g/2.25oz	50g/1.75oz
Millet, cooked	180g/6.5oz	90g/3.25oz	60g/2oz	45g/1.5oz
Miso paste	270g/9.5oz	135g/4.75oz	90g/3.25oz	65g/2.25oz
Polenta, dry	150g/5.25oz	75g/2.5oz	50g/1.75oz	40g/1.5oz
Quinoa, cooked	160g/5.5oz	80g/3oz	55g/2oz	40g/1.5oz
Quinoa, dry	180g/6.5oz	90g/3.25oz	60g/2oz	45g/1.5oz
Quinoa, puffed	20g/0.75oz	10g/0.5oz	7g/0.25oz	5g/0.25oz
Quinoa flakes	100g/3.5oz	50g/1.75oz	35g/1.25oz	25g/1oz
Quick granola	90g/3.25oz	45g/1.5oz	30g/1oz	20g/0.75oz
Rice puffs	20g/0.75oz	10g/0.5oz	7g/0.25oz	5g/0.25oz
Rolled oats	120g/4.25oz	60g/2oz	40g/1.5oz	30g/1oz
Semolina, dry	180g/6.5oz	90g/3.25oz	60g/2oz	45g/1.5oz

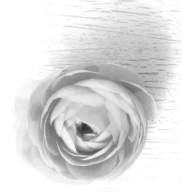

INGREDIENT	1 cup	½ cup	⅓ cup	¼ cup
DAIRY				
Butter, cold, cubed	150g/5.25oz	75g/2.5oz	50g/1.75oz	35g/1.25oz
Butter, softened	240g/8.5oz	120g/4.25oz	80g/3oz	60g/2oz
Coconut cream	250ml/8.5 fl oz	125ml/4.2 fl oz	85ml/3 fl oz	65ml/2.2 fl oz
Coconut yogurt	260g/9oz	130g/4.5oz	85g/3oz	65g/2.25oz
Cream cheese	250g/9oz	125g/4.5oz	85g/3oz	65g/2.25oz
Feta/goat cheese, crumbled	150g/5.25oz	75g/2.5oz	50g/1.75oz	35g/1.25oz
Ghee	240g/8.5oz	120g/4.25oz	80g/3oz	60g/2oz
Grated cheese	80g/3oz	40g/1.5oz	30g/1oz	20g/0.75oz
Mozzarella cheese, cubed	160g/5.5oz	80g/3oz	55g/2oz	40g/1.5oz
Natural yogurt	260g/9oz	130g/4.5oz	85g/3oz	65g/2.25oz
Parmesan, finely grated	80g/3oz	40g/1.5oz	25g/1oz	20g/0.75oz
Ricotta/quark	250g/9oz	125g/4.5oz	85g/3oz	65g/2.25oz
Sour cream	240g/8.5oz	120g/4.25oz	80g/3oz	60g/2oz
SUGAR/SWEETENERS				
Maple syrup	250ml/8.75 fl oz	125ml/4 fl oz	80ml/2.75 fl oz	65ml/2 fl oz
Coconut sugar	150g/5.25oz	75g/2.5oz	50g/1.75oz	35g/1.25oz
Raw honey	250ml/8.75 fl oz	125ml/4 fl oz	80ml/2.75 fl oz	65ml/2 fl oz
FRUIT				
Apple, pureed	270g/9.5oz	135g/4.75oz	90g/3.25oz	70g/2.5oz
Banana, mashed (3 bananas)	260g/9oz	130g/4.5oz	85g/3oz	65g/2.25oz
Blackberries, frozen	160g/5.5oz	80g/3oz	55g/2oz	40g/1.5oz
Blueberries	160g/5.5oz	80g/3oz	55g/2oz	40g/1.5oz
Cherries, frozen	160g/5.5oz	80g/3oz	55g/2oz	40g/1.5oz
Dried apricots	160g/5.5oz	80g/3oz	55g/2oz	40g/1.5oz
Mango, frozen	160g/5.5oz	80g/3oz	55g/2oz	40g/1.5oz
Pear, pureed	270g/9.5oz	135g/4.75oz	90g/3.25oz	70g/2.5oz
Pineapple, frozen	160g/5.5oz	80g/3oz	55g/2oz	40g/1.5oz
Pomegranate seeds	110g/4oz	55g/2oz	35g/1.25oz	30g/1oz
Raisins/golden raisins	150g/5.25oz	75g/2.5oz	50g/1.75oz	35g/1.25oz
Raspberries, frozen	160g/5.5oz	80g/3oz	55g/2oz	40g/1.5oz
Strawberries, frozen	160g/5.5oz	80g/3oz	55g/2oz	40g/1.5oz

INGREDIENT	1 cup	½ cup	⅓ cup	¼ cup
VEGETABLES				
Baby spinach	25g/1oz	15g/0.5oz	10g/0.5oz	5g/0.25oz
Beetroot, grated	160g/5.5oz	80g/3oz	55g/2oz	40g/1.5oz
Broccoli florets	80g/3oz	40g/1.5oz	25g/1oz	20g/0.75oz
Cabbage	80g/3oz	40g/1.5oz	25g/1oz	20g/0.75oz
Cabbage, chopped	80g/3oz	40g/1.5oz	25g/1oz	20g/0.75oz
Carrots, grated (2 carrots = 240g)	90g/3.25oz	45g/1.5oz	30g/1oz	25g/1oz
Carrot, cubed	150g/5.25oz	75g/2.5oz	50g/1.75oz	40g/1.5oz
Cauliflower florets	100g/3.5oz	50g/1.75oz	35g/1.25oz	25g/1oz
Cauliflower, steamed	250g/9oz	125g/4.5oz	85g/3oz	65g/2.25oz
Corn kernels	170g/6oz	85g/3oz	55g/2oz	40g/1.5oz
Fresh herbs (Basil, Parsley, etc)	25g/1oz	15g/0.5oz	10g/0.5oz	5g/0.25oz
Kalamata olives, pitted	200g/7oz	100g/3.5oz	65g/2.25oz	50g/1.75oz
Kale, shredded	30g/1oz	15g/0.5oz	10g/0.5oz	8g/0.25oz
Lettuce, shredded	75g/2.5oz	40g/1.5oz	25g/1oz	20g/0.75oz
Mushrooms, brown, chopped	100g/3.5oz	50g/1.75oz	35g/1.25oz	25g/1oz
Parsnip, raw, cubed	140g/5oz	70g/2.5oz	45g/1.5oz	35g/1.25oz
Parsnip, steamed	250g/9oz	125g/4.5oz	80g/3oz	60g/2oz
Peas, frozen	120g/4.25oz	60g/2oz	40g/1.5oz	30g/1oz
Pepper, chopped	140g/5oz	70g/2.5oz	45g/1.5oz	35g/1.25oz
Potato, raw	150g/5.25oz	75g/2.5oz	50g/1.75oz	40g/1.5oz
Pumpkin, cubed	140g/5oz	70g/2.5oz	45g/1.5oz	35g/1.25oz
Pumpkin, steamed	250g/9oz	125g/4.5oz	80g/3oz	60g/2oz
Rhubarb	120g/4.25oz	60g/2oz	40g/1.5oz	30g/1oz
Sweet potato, cubed	140g/5oz	70g/2.5oz	45g/1.5oz	35g/1.25oz
Sweet potato, steamed, mashed	250g/9oz	125g/4.5oz	80g/3oz	60g/2oz
Tomatoes, diced or pureed	250g/9oz	125g/4.5oz	85g/3oz	65g/2.25oz
Watercress sprigs	25g/1oz	15g/0.5oz	10g/0.5oz	5g/0.25oz
Zucchini, grated	180g/6.5oz	90g/3.25oz	60g/2oz	45g/1.5oz

Fussy Eating

WHAT EVERY PARENT NEEDS TO KNOW

If you have picked up this book in the hope that you can tempt your fussy eater (or eaters) to try new foods, you are not alone. Around 80 percent of the parents or caregivers I see in my practice are struggling to increase variety in their children's diets. There are many—often complex—reasons why children evolve into fussy eaters, and it can be quite common.

Around half of all toddlers can be classified as fussy eaters. Happily for most children, "fussy eating" is a stage that they will grow out of. They will become more adventurous eventually!

Unfortunately, the fussy eating period coincides with an important time in a child's development, so leaving children to eat a diet of only white bread and pasta, for example, for too long isn't a healthy option. The strategies we implement to deal with their food refusal, along with the food choices we offer them during this stage, can have a huge impact on how willing they are to try new foods and how their eating habits are ultimately shaped.

BANISH GUILT

The one thing that most parents are good at —especially moms—is feeling guilty. The last thing I want you to take away from reading this book is the feeling of guilt. None of this information is meant to overwhelm you or make you feel inadequate when it comes to feeding your child. There are countless reasons why children refuse their food and most of us are busy, time-poor parents trying to do the best we can for our children.

Each family situation is unique and success with mealtimes must be measured accordingly. Some of you may have children who are initially fussy at meal times, but with gentle encouragement, may end up eating most of their food. Or perhaps your child may have only two vegetables on their "like" list that they are happy to eat. If, after reading this chapter as well as the practical tips included in all eight steps, you learn ways to increase the number of veggies to four, find a new lunch box meal (other than their daily cheese sandwich) and manage to add one to three main meal recipes into your child's diet—consider that a great success.

Perhaps you have a child who refuses to go near a vegetable and will only eat peanut butter sandwiches and store-bought chicken nuggets. For you, the goal will be to gain a clearer understanding of what might be behind your child's fussiness. If you can make one change to their diet, even a small one, then that is also a great success. This may mean swapping their store-bought nuggets for homemade ones, changing their brand of peanut butter to one that is free from added sugars, and switching from white bread to sourdough.

Always keep in mind that change is a slow process when it comes to children, especially where fussy eating is concerned. It's important to always respect where you and your child are at and celebrate any changes you are able to make.

SO HOW DO CHILDREN'S TASTE PREFERENCES DEVELOP?

From the very first taste of food, we influence our baby's relationship with food and their preferences. A baby's food preferences begin in the mother's womb. Flavors pass through the placenta into the amniotic fluid, which fetuses swallow on a regular basis. Research shows that newborns are more accepting of flavors they have encountered during gestation, especially during the last trimester—which is a good thing, because by then, morning sickness has passed.

Numerous studies have also shown that breastfeeding mothers with a large range of nutrients are more likely to have infants who are more accepting of a wider range of foods when they begin eating solids. However, it does

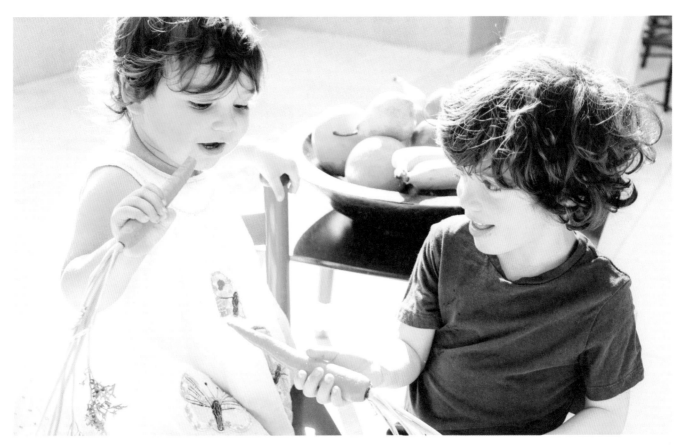

not all hang on the shoulders of parents. Nature also has a part to play as food preferences are often hereditary and affected by genes. And finally, some babies are simply born with more tastebuds than others and are superior tasters. These children will naturally be more sensitive to certain taste sensations and are more likely to reject sour or bitter. Others, without the same tastebud density, will not be as reactive to different flavors. Even though babies, and especially those with heightened taste perceptions, will naturally reject bitter tastes such as spinach, zucchini or even broccoli, they can, with repeated offerings, come to love sour and bitter foods.

HOW TO TRAIN TASTEBUDS RIGHT FROM THE START

The early years of a child's life are the most crucial in setting up long-lasting eating patterns and behaviors. If we train a young child's tastebuds to enjoy the natural flavors of foods without processed flavors and added sweeteners, we can avoid many problems later on. In the first two years of life, a child's immune system is largely dependent on the foods they eat. Given the right nutritional start in life they are more resilient to illnesses, infections, allergies and even

behavioral issues as their diet is strengthening the development of their immune system and their cognitive abilities too.

- It is far easier to make dietary changes while your kids are young. Repetition will pay off quickly at this stage. When I talk about exposing children to different tastes, I don't mean giving a particular food to your child once and then, if they reject it, deciding that they don't like it. For babies and young children it normally takes between six and sixteen experiences with a flavor before it will be accepted. Somewhere between six and 10 times is the most common. If your child rejects a food, please do not give up. Freeze the leftovers and try again and again and again. There is clear evidence that repeated offerings will, in most cases, lead to an acceptance of a new food.

- Once your child is two or older, it will most likely be more challenging for you, but with patience and persistence, changes can be made. Children learn through play and enjoyment and therefore mealtimes should remain an enjoyable and fun experience during which parents model positive behaviors. Often, the food groups that most parents struggle to get their child to eat are vegetables and protein—please refer to these chapters for lots of practical advice on making these foods more palatable.

DID YOU KNOW?

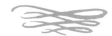

Studies show breastfed babies are more likely to be accepting of bitter vegetables, only if they are consumed regularly by their mothers during lactation.

21

Referenced from Dr Kay Toomey (PhD) SOS Approach to Feeding

A FUSSY EATER . . .	A PROBLEM FEEDER . . .
eats a decreased range of foods but will eat at least thirty types of foods.	eats less than twenty types of foods.
will eat the same peanut butter sandwich every day for months, then go off it and refuse to eat it. However, a few weeks later he/she will happily eat it again.	will demand a peanut butter sandwich every day for months, then tire of it and refuse to eat it again, even months later.
can tolerate new foods on their plate, touch new foods, may even (after lots of encouragement) taste a new food even if it's not swallowed.	will have a meltdown if a new food is placed on their plate; some children will refuse to sit at the table if certain foods are present, even if only on other family member's plates.
will eat foods from all the different food texture groups (e.g., crunchy, soft, hard).	will completely omit certain textures from their diet.
during mealtimes will be happy to sit with family as long as they are eating a food/meal they like. This will most likely be different to the rest of the family's meal but may include some components of the family meal (e.g., will eat corn or a meatball with no sauce).	will refuse to eat all components of the family's meal and demand a completely different meal to the family the majority of the time.
with lots of repetition, encouragement, and positive reinforcement from parents may slowly add new foods to their limited diet.	will refuse to taste new food no matter how much encouragement they receive.

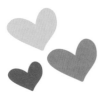

- If you are reading this with an older fussy child and wishing you had known this beforehand, then you are like many other parents. The most important thing you can do now is to continue to persevere in exposing your child to healthy food choices. As children grow up, and especially as they enter into their teens, their cognition takes over. It is far easier to speak to an older girl and explain that a healthy diet will make her skin glow, her hair shine, and her body strong for sports; and for boys, if they are into sport, explaining to them (or better yet, getting their coach or another male they respect and admire to speak to them) about the importance of eating nutritious foods.

FUSSY EATERS VS PROBLEM FEEDERS

Most children will go through fussy patches and there are many ways to ensure that this does not evolve into myriad unwanted behaviors. However, there is a small percentage of children who will require intervention as a result of physiological or psychological reasons for their ongoing food refusal such as oral motor delays, sensory issues, gastrointestinal disturbances or anxiety food-related disorders. These children may fall into the category of what is called 'problem feeders', and the sooner their issues are identified and treated, the more willing they will be to try new foods.

UNDERLYING CAUSES OF FUSSY EATING

A combination of occupational therapy (OT), speech pathology, nutritional therapy and medical supervision is often required to address the following conditions:

❶ DIGESTIVE ISSUES

There is a wide range of digestive disorders that can interfere with a child's ability to eat and enjoy their meals. This can range from hernias, constipation, reflux, and celiac disease to food allergies or intolerances and much more. The main thing to be aware of is that if your child is suffering from a gastrointestinal problem, it's likely they will not want to eat. The two most common issues I see in clinic are:

- **Reflux.** Most of the fussy eaters I see suffered from reflux as babies. These children have been wired to expect eating to be associated with pain and do not have a genuine love of food. For these children, it's essential to look for food allergies and eliminate any foods from the diet that may still be causing pain. Part of the treatment can be ongoing management for reflux, or healing the gut with nutritional supplements and probiotics to ensure the digestive tract is functioning well and nutrients are being absorbed.

- **Constipation.** This is a huge factor that can cause fussy eating and loss of appetite. If the bowels aren't being cleared daily then the appetite is more than likely switched off. One of the first things we do when treating children with eating difficulties is to heal their guts with probiotics and ensure they are evacuating all the contents of their bowels. Children with severe cases of constipation may initially need to be treated using a prescription laxative under medical supervision; however, as a nutritional therapist it's my aim to get them onto natural alternatives to support the body.

❷ SENSORY ISSUES

Children with sensory issues may get upset by things like the tags in their clothes, loud noises such as the vacuum cleaner, and certain smells or bright lights. One of the main sensory issues that leads to fussy eating is called oral defensiveness. A child with oral defensiveness shows unusual sensitivity to taste, smell, and texture.

Common signs that a child may be oral defensive is that they will easily gag, may not transition off purees onto finger foods, avoid messy tactile play (finger paints, sandpits, messy food), fuss when it's time to brush their teeth or wash their face as it creates an uncomfortable sensation, have repetitive diets and be picky about foods, and dislike eating in unfamiliar places such as friends' homes or restaurants. Sensory issues are very prevalent in children who have autism spectrum disorders and most of these children will need to seek help from experts such as occupational therapists, who specialize in this area. At the same time these children benefit from working with a trained nutritionist or dietitian to ensure the foods they are trying to integrate are beneficial.

❸ ORAL MOTOR DELAYS

These can begin with the inability to suck and swallow and include the inability to chew properly due to weak muscles. Many of these children are undiagnosed and for them it is easier to eat white bread, pasta, chocolate and foods that dissolve in the mouth and do not require excessive chewing. Hard vegetables and foods such as meat are avoided as they require skills these children do not possess. These children will need to be treated. Common signs that a baby or child may have oral motor delays is an inability to latch at the breast or suck at the bottle, an inability to bring their bottom lip down to suck food off a spoon, struggling to pick up food and bring it to the mouth, an inability to chew solid food without choking, frequently gagging because their gag reflex has not moved to the back of their tongue and every time they eat they feel like they are going to gag, choke or vomit. Older children may not have the ability to move food around their mouth using their tongues.

Other signs your baby or child may have an oral motor issue:
- drooling.
- gagging frequently on food.
- spitting up during and after meals.
- coughing and gagging while eating.
- difficulty chewing, difficulty keeping food in mouth during meals.

- refusal of foods, pocketing food and negative behaviors around mealtime.
- changes in voice during and after eating.
- recurring respiratory infections/pneumonia.
- poor weight gain/growth.

❹ LOW MUSCLE TONE

Children can be born with low muscle tone (hypotonic) or have low muscle tone due to a specific diagnosis such as Down syndrome, or they can acquire low muscle tone through "nutrient deprivation" or "cellular malnutrition." Children with low muscle tone:
- have reduced stamina.
- can have difficulty with maintaining positions like sitting for meals, hence the importance of correct highchairs and seating.
- become fatigued by chewing food.
- have trouble using their hands to self-feed.
- have trouble pushing with constipation due to muscle weakness.

NUTRITIONAL CAUSES OF FUSSY EATING

Common causes of fussy eating include zinc deficiencies, cravings for sugar or salt, as well as stressful mealtimes. Below are the main causes that I see in my practice:

1. Introducing sugary foods too early on.
If children are exposed to sugar too early, they will alter their sweet taste receptors. Research has also shown that sugar is highly addictive, and has a drug-like response in many children—the more a child eats it, the more he or she wants to eat it to feel the euphoric feelings associated with sweet foods. For fussy eaters, it's really important to balance their blood sugar levels and curb their cravings. (See more about the effects of too much sugar in children and how to manage it in the Reduce Sugar chapter).

2. Introducing too many commercially prepared foods. As a parent, you can't compete with processed foods that not only contain sugar and salt (two of the most highly addictive tastes that can interfere with children getting used to natural foods) but also contain flavor enhancers,

Consider this...

Research now shows that the most influential factor in determining children's taste preferences despite their genetic makeup (up to 85%) is due to the foods they are exposed to early on in life.

Goals and rewards are a very effective way for getting your children to eat foods they would prefer to avoid. See more about how to use this strategy on page 272.

artificial sweeteners, preservatives, and oils which have been cleverly designed by food chemists to create a perfect taste sensation—also known as the "bliss factor." These foods trick children's brains into believing that the foods they are eating are satisfying when, in fact, they are nutritionally empty. (See more about avoiding processed foods in the Avoid Nasties chapter).

3. **Too much salt in the diet.** Most packaged foods such as pizzas, ramen noodles and chicken nuggets contain a high amount of refined salt which can lead to salt cravings and a disruption of normal taste sensations. (See tips on how to lower sodium in the Avoid Nasties chapter).

4. **Iron and zinc deficiencies.** Many picky eaters do not have enough protein in their diets and this can lead to anemia (low iron) and low zinc levels. Low iron and low zinc levels can cause reduced appetites, and low zinc especially can cause homemade food to taste bland as this deficiency can interfere with taste receptors.

5. **Deficiencies in essential fats.** These are the healthy fats that are required for proper growth and development. Most junk food and packaged food is filled with unhealthy hydrogenated fat such as vegetable oils (canola, sunflower, soy or cottonseed oil) which may cause inflammation in the body. Many kids are deficient in healthy essential fats such as olives, avocado, fish oil, walnuts, almonds, chia seeds, grass-fed meats, and grass-fed butter. This imbalance causes them to crave fatty, deep-fried foods. The brain needs these essential fats to function properly. Research has shown that an increase in the beneficial fats in a child's diet can improve their cognition, their behavior, and result in lower mental health disorder rates. Practitioner-grade fish oil is a number one supplement, along with probiotics that I recommend to my

clients. It always amazes me how the fussiest of eaters will gobble up a fish gel capsule.

6. **Disguising food too early on.** Often we disguise food before our children have had a chance to try it. From the very start we add fruit to veggie purees, sweeten yogurts or add ketchup to spaghetti bolognaise in case they don't eat it. It's best to remain objective and give kids a chance to experience the true flavor of foods for themselves. Work to expand their range to include foods which do not fall into the salty and sweet categories. Little tastebuds are forever changing and, with repetition, what is not eaten today might become a firm favorite in the future.

7. **Too much junk food in plain view.** Keep veggies and healthy food in plain view in the fridge or pantry—what the eyes see, the tummy wants. Keep the junk food outside of the home and offer it as an occasional treat.

8. **Constantly cleaning, worrying, and commenting about mess.** How many of you remember your grandmother or mother spitting on a tissue to clean your face? I hated it. For some kids, having their mouths cleaned is really uncomfortable. Accept that there is always going to be an element of mess and it is actually beneficial for babies and toddlers to get messy while eating. Use appropriate language if an older child still struggles to use utensils due to lack of coordination.

9. **Forcing a child to eat when they are genuinely not hungry.** It's okay for a child not to eat their meal as long as you are firm and have consistent instructions. For example, "If you are not hungry, that's fine, but there will be no other snacks until the next meal." With older children this can be for the next two hours; for younger children and toddlers it can be anywhere between forty-five minutes to one hour. But try to ensure that when their hunger kicks in, they are not replacing their meal with a chocolate muffin. Offer the food that was refused earlier or another healthy alternative. If a child refuses to eat their dinner, review what they ate that day and decide whether they might be full. Remind them that there will be no more food or drink (other than water) available until breakfast.

Consider this...

You can encourage a fussy child to try new foods without extra work in the kitchen. Buy play foods and teach them the names of new foods and vegetables, or buy brightly colored books with food images. Stick pictures of disliked vegetables on the fridge—this makes new food and veggies a familiar everyday occurrence.

10 STRATEGIES FOR DEALING WITH FUSSY EATING

① DESENSITIZATION. Encourage your little ones to touch, smell, and engage with their food. This starts right from shopping for groceries. Can they help take items off the shelves? Encourage them to pick up a carrot, an apple, or a zucchini from the shelf and place it in the basket or shopping cart themselves—this begins the engagement with the new food. Can they put the dish or new veggie onto the table for the family? Don't be disappointed if they don't eat the new food the first time it's offered—stay positive, freeze what is not eaten, and offer it again.

② REPETITION. Make new foods familiar by repeatedly offering them in a calm, familial environment. A child will not go to a stranger the first time they meet them, but after a few visits they generally feel more comfortable to sit with them. The same goes for new foods. Repeated exposure aids the process of engaging with new tastes and flavors. You can also try offering these same foods in different ways—cut into fun shapes, laid out in color patterns, steamed veggies rather than raw.

③ MESSY PLAY. Allow your baby to reach for his food and feed himself. If your baby is being spoon fed, offer him his own spoon to attempt to feed himself or have two spoons at meal times, one for you and one for your child. If your little person refuses to be spoon fed, try offering finger foods but don't limit their choices to "appropriate finger foods." Offer porridge and make it thicker so it can be picked up in globs once it has cooled down, or offer bolognaise over spiral pasta shells so he can pick up shells covered in bolognaise sauce. Six months is an ideal age to start to encourage finger feeding with safe and appropriate choices.

Be creative and remember that enjoying food is a sensory experience. Children who are allowed to get messy with their food through exploration are often less fussy.

④ FAMILY MEALS. Make it a goal to eat together as a family as often as possible. See tips for making this a fun experience for all on page 46.

⑤ EDUCATE YOUR CHILD DAILY WITH INTERESTING, FUN-FILLED FOOD FACTS. Help them to make the connection that what we eat helps us to feel strong and healthy or will make them run faster or jump higher. For younger children, show images of carrots and let them know that carrots help us to see better. If they are sick give them an orange and say it has vitamin C to help to fight off the nasty bugs in their tummy. Go into greater detail for older children and show them books that explain that our health is dependent on the foods we eat.

⑥ WHEN TRYING TO OFFER NEW FOODS, WORK WITH THE TEXTURES THAT THEY LIKE. For instance if you really want to get your child to eat homemade French fries or sweet potato fries and you know they love crunchy food, its probably best not to make huge, fat wedge-shaped chips. Rather, using a peeler, grate the potatoes really finely and bake them for 25–30 minutes (avoid burning them). They will come out crispy and delicious. Once your child is happy to eat these you can offer it in a different form, maybe as a larger chip or as mashed potato. If your child is extremely fussy then it's important to show them how the potato can change shape—take one potato and make it thin and crispy and take another potato and make it thicker. One of the things we need to teach children, especially older children,

is that food can change shape but still taste the same.

⑦ OFFER CHOICE AT MEALTIMES. Children like to feel they have some control when it comes to food. Many moms do not want to become short order cooks or fall into the habit of making five different meals each evening. However, it is particularly important for fussy children to be given a choice between two healthy options. For example: "We can have fish fingers or lamb kofta for dinner—which would you like?" Vary the choices as the seasons change. For example: "So now we are heading into winter, would you like a soup or stew?" Give toddlers a choice of where they want to sit and ask them which plate they'd like. Give younger children a choice between two foods that you have already prepared. Take older children along to purchase ground beef and ask if they would prefer meatballs or bolognaise.

⑧ TRY TO SERVE A SMALL PORTION OF FOOD ON A LARGE PLATE. This way your child won't feel overwhelmed. If your child simply refuses to eat a particular food, do not let them see your frustration. Simply remove the food and continue to try another day. Children can often use food as a control mechanism if they see that you are getting upset.

⑨ MAKE MEALTIMES FUN. Sing songs, make pictures out of vegetable sticks and dips. The main thing is that young children should enjoy the whole sensorial experience, even if it means sticking their fingers into everything and eating with their hands.

⑩ PRAISE YOUR CHILD FOR EATING NEW FOODS. Children love praise, and if both parents praise a child for eating well it can have a long-lasting effect.

Shopping, cooking & kitchen essentials

Time is usually not something parents have in abundance. It's so easy to run out of ideas to feed the family and turn to take-away or processed convenience foods. Getting organized and making sure you have the right ingredients, makes planning healthy family meals a simple exercise. The secret to getting ahead is to schedule a weekly grocery shop followed by a cook-up. For some that may be once a week for two hours on a Sunday. For others, it may have to be one evening a week once the kids are asleep. If you are just beginning on your health journey and have fussy eaters (or a fussy partner) then you may want to start off slowly, introducing one new main meal, and one new snack food each week—remember to freeze what is not eaten and offer it again the following week, even if it was not a huge success the first time around. It can take time for new dishes to become accepted as part of the family's staple diet.

When choosing new recipes to try, work with your family's preferences. For example, if your child loves meat but not meat on the bone, go for shepherd's pie over lamb cutlets. For those who love cooking and have purchased this book for inspiration and new recipe ideas, get creative and get stuck in—but remember to be patient with your children and give them time to get used to the new recipes. Try to cook meals the whole family can enjoy so that you're only cooking one dish per meal. I've created a two-week meal planner in the Menu Planners section of this book on page 284, but you can create your own. To maximize time and minimize cooking, choose recipes where you can easily save leftovers for a second meal.

Make a shopping list so that you have all the ingredients on hand. There is no denying that healthy eating requires effort and time. Make grocery shopping and cooking a fun, shared activity rather than a chore for Mom or Dad. Kids can help make grocery lists, shop online with you, accompany you to the grocery store, unpack bags, and wash veggies. This way you can get ahead while still spending time together. Bonus: Your kids will be more inclined to try something new if they helped to make it.

HOW TO READ A NUTRITION LABEL

Before you head out to the shops, learn to understand food labels to help ensure you are informed about what your family is eating. Clever marketing means it's easy to miss a flavor enhancer such as MSG or an added sugar hiding behind another name. Add to that the fact a brand could be using potentially harmful preservatives in some products and not in others. It's easy to see why there is much confusion around making healthy choices.

Understanding nutrition labels will empower you to make the best decisions about what belongs in your shopping cart and what's best left on the supermarket shelf. By law, food labels need to contain both an ingredient list (all the nutritional ingredients included in a product) and a nutritional information table (a breakdown of the macro and micronutrients).

An ongoing area of debate is the need for genetically modified (GM) labeling. I believe we have the right to know whether the food we are eating or choosing to feed our families contains GM ingredients, regardless of whether they are safe or not. The real issue here is the right to be informed. At this stage the only way to ensure that there are no GM ingredients in a food product is to look for products labelled 100 percent organic or non-GMO or look for trusted organic institutions such as USDA, QAI, IFOAM and ACO.

THE INGREDIENT LIST

The ingredient list contains products listed in descending order of weight (the ingredient that contributes the most to a product is listed first and the ingredient that contributes the least is listed last). So for example, if you are purchasing a flavored yogurt and see sugar listed as the second ingredient you may choose to put it back on the shelf. How do you know if a food is low or high in a nutrient? Check the Daily Values (DV). In the % DV column, 5% DV or less is low and 20% DV or more is high. For nutrients you want to limit, such as added sugar, saturated fat and sodium, look for foods with less than 5% DV. For nutrients you want to get more of, such as fiber, calcium and iron, look for foods with 20% or more DV. For more information on reading sugar labels, see page 72 and for more information on sodium, see page 269.

NUTRITION FACTS

Nutrition Fact labels will differ from country to country. In the US, these panels highlight calories, total fat, cholesterol, sodium, total carbohydrate, sugars, protein, fiber, and vitamins and minerals (vitamin D, potassium, calcium, and iron). This panel has undergone quite a bit of change in recent years; by 2020, the FDA will require manufacturers to include calories and serving sizes that more accurately reflect how much consumers eat or drink in one sitting (note that this number is based on what people actually consume, not the amount they should be consuming), calories and servings sizes that are in larger bold print, and—perhaps most importantly—a separate line for added sugars to differentiate between the product's natural sugars and its added sugars. You can see these differences, as well as the revised footnote, in the panels on the left.

The panels on products that contain two to three servings but could be consumed in a single sitting will be required to carry a dual column label that lists the calories and nutrients per serving as well as per package or container. You'll find these on 24-ounce bottles of soda, or pints of ice cream. The dual-column label will make it easier for consumers to understand how many calories or nutrients they are getting if they eat or drink the entire container at one time.

Nutrition Facts

Serving Size 2/3 cup (55g)
Servings Per Container About 8

Amount Per Serving

Calories 230	Calories from Fat 72
	% Daily Value*
Total Fat 8g	**12%**
Saturated Fat 1g	**5%**
Trans Fat 0g	
Cholesterol 0mg	**0%**
Sodium 160mg	**7%**
Total Carbohydrate 37g	**12%**
Dietary Fiber 4g	**16%**
Sugars 1g	
Protein 3g	
Vitamin A	10%
Vitamin C	8%
Calcium	20%
Iron	45%

* Percent Daily Values are based on a 2,000 calorie diet. Your daily value may be higher or lower depending on your calorie needs.

		Calories:	2,000	2,500
Total Fat	Less than		65g	80g
Sat Fat	Less than		20g	25g
Cholesterol	Less than		300mg	300mg
Sodium	Less than		2,400mg	2,400mg
Total Carbohydrate			300g	375g
Dietary Fiber			25g	30g

Nutrition Facts

8 servings per container
Serving size   **2/3 cup (55g)**

Amount per serving

Calories   230

	% Daily Value*
Total Fat 8g	**10%**
Saturated Fat 1g	**5%**
Trans Fat 0g	
Cholesterol 0mg	**0%**
Sodium 160mg	**7%**
Total Carbohydrate 37g	**13%**
Dietary Fiber 4g	**14%**
Total Sugars 12g	
Includes 10g Added Sugars	**20%**
Protein 3g	
Vitamin D 2mcg	10%
Calcium 260mg	20%
Iron 8mg	45%
Potassium 235mg	6%

* The % Daily Value (DV) tells you how much a nutrient in a serving of food contributes to a daily diet. 2,000 calories a day is used for general nutrition advice.

NUTS, GRAINS AND LEGUMES

Throughout this book we use a combination of grains, nuts and legumes in our recipes. To boost their nutritional composition it's always best to soak them in water with a small amount of either salt or an acidic substance such as apple cider vinegar, lemon juice, whey or kefir, for a period of time. Why do we do this? Nuts and seeds, along with whole grains and legumes, contain small amounts of phytates, which can inhibit the digestion of minerals such as iron and influence enzymes, as well as reducing the digestibility of starches, proteins, and fats. The process of soaking and rinsing increases their nutritional value and makes them more beneficial to the body. This is especially important for young children who are still developing the enzymes to break down these plant foods. If you or your children prefer nuts and seeds to be crunchy, once activated, drain and dehydrate the nuts or seeds at a very low temperature in the oven, or preferably a dehydrator (a safer option) if you have one. This will give them a lovely crunchy texture and flavor.

HOW TO ACTIVATE YOUR NUTS AND SEEDS

- Dissolve 1–2 teaspoons of sea salt in enough filtered warm water to cover the amount of nuts/seeds you are activating. It is better to soak one variety at a time.
- Place your nuts or seeds of choice in a bowl and cover with salted water.
- Soak for the required number of hours (see below).
- Rinse under running water and strain.
- Spread onto a large baking tray and slowly dry out nuts and seeds in a dehydrator (if you have one) or on the lowest temperature in your oven (120–150°F) for around 6–24 hours.
- They are ready when they feel and taste dry and crunchy. It is important that nuts and seeds are really dry and crispy otherwise they can get moldy.
- Store in an airtight container in the fridge or freezer for up to three months.

Type of nut/seed	Soaking time (hours)
Almonds	12–14
Brazil nuts	8–12
Cashews	2–4
Hazelnuts (skinless)	7–12
Macadamia nuts	7–12
Peanuts	7–12
Pecans	4–6
Pine nuts	7–10
Pistachios	4–6
Pumpkin seeds	7–10
Sunflower seeds	2
Walnuts	4–8

(Continued on page 30)

PANTRY ESSENTIALS

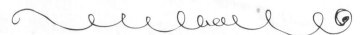

FRESH PRODUCE
Artichokes
Asparagus
Beetroot
Bok choy
Broccoli
Brussels sprouts
Cabbage (white, purple)
Carrot (orange, purple)
Cauliflower
Celeriac
Celery
Cucumber
Eggplant (aubergine)
Endive
Fennel
Garlic
Ginger
Green beans
Jerusalem artichoke
Jicama
Kale
Kohlrabi
Leeks
Lettuce
Mushrooms
Okra
Onion
Parsnip
Pepper (red, yellow, orange and green)
Pumpkin (Japanese, kent and butternut squash)
Radicchio
Radish
Rocket
Scallions
Seaweed (nori, dulse or kelp)
Silverbeet
Snow peas
Spinach
Spring onions
Squash
Sweet potato (orange, purple and white)
Taro
Tomatoes
Turnip
Water chestnut
Watercress
Yam
Zucchini

FRUIT
Apples (red and green)
Apricots
Avocados
Berries (frozen, fresh
Dried fruit, sugar- and sulphur-free (apricots, cranberries, dates, goji berries, figs)
Grapefruit
Guava
Kiwifruit
Lemons
Limes
Mangoes
Nectarines
Oranges
Papaya
Peaches
Pears
Pineapple
Plums
Pomegranate
Rhubarb

MEAT
(grass-fed where applicable and organic wherever possible)
Beef
Chicken
Duck
Ham
Lamb
Pork
Turkey

SEAFOOD
(wild-caught, low mercury)
Anchovy
Atlantic mackerel
Cod
Haddock
Perch, pacific freshwater
Sardines
Salmon (wild or organic)
Sole
Trout, freshwater
Tuna, skipjack (lowest in mercury)

EGGS
Organic where possible

DAIRY
(full-fat, organic where possible)
Milk, organic cow's, goat, or sheep
Butter, unsalted
Cream
Ghee
Goat's curd
Kefir
Unsweetened natural yogurt (cow, goat, sheep)
White cheese: Goat's cheese, mozzarella, quark, ricotta, Sheep's milk chevre, crème fraiche
Yellow cheese: Swiss, gouda, cheddar (preferably organic), Parmesan

MILK AND DAIRY ALTERNATIVES
(sugar-free, additive-free or make your own)
Almond milk
Coconut milk, yogurt and cream
Oat milk
Rice milk (use in baking in small quantities)

HERBS AND SPICES
(fresh, whole, ground)
Basil
Black pepper
Gardamom
Chives
Cinnamon
Cloves
Coriander (cilantro)
Cumin
Curry powder, mild
Dill
Fennel
Ginger
Mint
Oregano
Paprika
Parsley
Rosemary
Sage
Thyme
Turmeric

FATS AND OILS
Cold-pressed avocado oil
Cold-pressed extra virgin olive oil
Cold-pressed macadamia nut oil
Cold-pressed sesame oil
Flaxseed oil
Virgin coconut oil

SEEDS, NUTS AND NUT BUTTER
Note: Nuts are best stored in the fridge or freezer. Whole nuts are not recommended for children under three.
Almonds
Almond butter (no added sugar or oil, or make your own)
Brazil nuts
Cashew nut butter (no added sugar or oil, or make your own)
Cashew nuts
Chia seeds
Flaxseeds
Hazelnuts
Macadamia nuts
Peanut butter (no added sugar or oil, or make your own)
Pecans
Pine nuts
Pumpkin seeds
Sesame seeds
Sunflower seeds
Sunflower seed butter (no added sugar or oil, or make your own)

GRAINS (gluten-free)
Amaranth
Brown rice
Buckwheat
Millet
Polenta
Quinoa
Teff

GRAINS
(non-gluten free)
Barley
Kamut
Rye
Semolina
Spelt

BEANS AND LEGUMES
(dried or canned, look for BPA-free cans)
Adzuki beans
Black beans
Borlotti beans
fava beans
lima beans
Cannellini beans
Chickpeas
Green beans
Kidney beans
Lentils
Peas

CONDIMENTS
Apple cider vinegar
Balsamic vinegar (preservative free)
Celtic sea salt or Himalayan rock salt (use interchangeably in recipes)
Dijon mustard (sugar- and preservative-free)
Nutritional yeast
Tamari (wheat-free)
Tomato paste (sodium reduced)
tomato puree or pasta sauce, natural or mixed with herbs (choose bottled instead of canned, sugar-free and preservative-free)

FLOUR AND BAKING ESSENTIALS
Almond flour or meal
Arrowroot flour
Baking powder (gluten-free, additive- and aluminium-free)
Bicarbonate of soda (aluminium-free)
Brown rice flour
Brown rice puffs

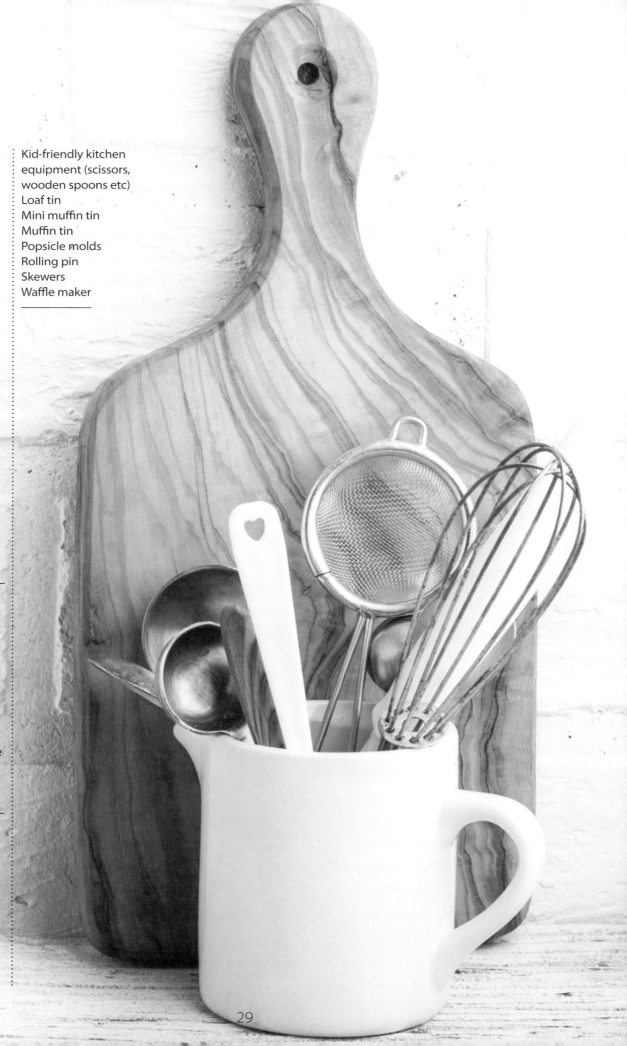

Buckwheat flour
Cacao powder
Carob powder
Coconut flakes
Coconut flour
Dark chocolate (60%-
85%), organic where
possible
Flax meal
Kamut flour
Millet flour
Oat flour
Quinoa flour
Rice paper wraps
Spelt flour, whole, and
white (only use white
while transitioning to
whole or if
stated in recipe—mix
half and half)
Sorghum flour
Tapioca flour
Teff flour
Pure vanilla bean
extract (alcohol-free),
vanilla powder, vanilla
paste or fresh vanilla
bean

SWEETENERS
Coconut sugar
Dates
Honey (organic,
raw, Manuka)
Molasses
Pure maple syrup
(Grade A, organic
where possible)
Stevia, unprocessed
green leaf or 100% pure
drops or powder (100%
natural not blended
with erythritol)

**EQUIPMENT
ESSENTIALS**
Baking paper
Baking trays
Cookie cutters
Doughnut tin
Hand-held blender
High-speed food
processor (we love the
Vitamix, but any one
will do)

Kid-friendly kitchen
equipment (scissors,
wooden spoons etc)
Loaf tin
Mini muffin tin
Muffin tin
Popsicle molds
Rolling pin
Skewers
Waffle maker

MONEY SAVERS

Leftover smoothies	→	Frozen popsicles are a nutritious replacement for ice cream and kids love them. If you don't have popsicle molds use everyday ice cube trays.
Fruit that is about to spoil	→	Freeze to add to smoothies. This will ensure you always have a good variety on hand.
Uneaten cooked veggies	→	Puree and freeze. Defrost at a later stage to add to muffins, cookies, sauces, and casseroles to boost the nutritional value.
Stale bread	→	Make your own bread crumbs. Use to coat homemade chicken or fish nuggets.
Meat approaching its best before date	→	Freeze for later or cook and then freeze. If you look out for specials at the supermarket on meat that is soon approaching the best before date, you can save a lot on your grocery bill. Cook on the same day and then freeze.

SOAKING GRAINS AND LEGUMES

Use filtered warm water and an acidic medium such as yogurt, buttermilk, whey, milk kefir, coconut kefir, apple cider vinegar, or lemon juice. The acid medium is essential as it serves as a catalyst to initiate the culturing/fermenting process that enables phytase (an enzyme that helps to release beneficial nutrients, making them more digestible).

HOW TO SOAK GRAINS

- Place grains in a bowl and cover completely with filtered warm water.
- Add acidic medium of choice. For every cup of liquid you will need one tablespoon of acidic medium.
- Cover tightly, place in a warm spot in the kitchen, and soak overnight or for the required number of hours.
- Drain and rinse under running water.

HOW TO SOAK BEANS/LEGUMES

The traditional method for preparing beans is to soak them in hot water for at least 12–24 hours, changing the soaking water at least once during this time, followed by a thorough rinsing and then cooking process.

- Place beans/legumes in a bowl and cover completely with hot filtered water.
- Add ½ tsp baking soda if you're soaking larger beans (optional).
- Cover and allow to sit in a warm kitchen spot for required number of hours, changing the water once or twice.
- For larger beans such as kidney beans, you can add ¹/₂ tsp of baking soda to reduce cooking time but do not use for smaller beans such as adzuki beans, lentils or navy beans as they will cook too fast and become mushy.
- Drain and rinse under running water and cook on low heat until desired consistency is achieved.

SOAKING TIMES

Type of grain/legume	Soaking time (hours)
Adzuki beans	8–12
Black beans	8–12
Brown rice	8–12
Buckwheat	6
Chickpeas	12–24
Lentils	8
Millet	5
Oats	8
Quinoa	3–4

BATCH COOKING

One of my biggest time-saving tips is to start batch cooking. My kids love black bean brownies and salmon millet rissoles, for example, so I always double the batch and freeze some for later. Make double quantities of any recipes that you know your family loves and enjoys and you will be well on your way to having a freezer full of healthy, homemade "convenience" food.

The same can be said for vegetables. I advise using plenty of veggies in your child's daily diet. If you are chopping carrots or celery into veggie sticks for the lunch box or a snack, chop extra. They will last 2–3 days in an airtight container in the fridge. If you are roasting pumpkin or steaming cauliflower, make extra for the next night's dinner or to use in a sweet potato or cauliflower pizza or in vanilla cupcakes.

The best way to batch cook is to choose two recipes on a weekly basis to double batch, for example tuna lasagne and spaghetti bolognaise. If you do this every week for a couple of weeks, the freezer will begin to fill with wholesome emergency back-up plans for when cooking is not an option. Try to use similar ingredients in each cook-up session, for example asparagus tart, veggie muffins, and spinach and cheese slices; salmon rissoles, fish nuggets, and fish curry; or black bean brownies, chocolate chia bliss balls, raw slice, almond ganache cake and chocolate spread.

You can also prepare ahead with batches of cooked grains such as quinoa, brown rice, and even millet. Freeze and heat as needed.

SEVEN MORE IDEAS

1. Freeze preservative-free or homemade dips and spreads. Instead of always tossing them out half eaten, on day of opening decant half into another container and freeze.
2. Freeze milk too. My husband is the only member of the family who drinks milk and organic full cream milk is hard to find in small cartons. So instead of wasting the leftovers, we now pour out half into a separate container and freeze for later use.

How to bake with different flours

FLOUR	RATIO TO WHEAT FLOUR	BEST FOR	FLAVOR	NUTRITION	TIP
ALMOND	Replace only 25% of total flour with almond flour	Baking and crumbing	Nutty, rich and wholesome	High in fat with little saturated fat; low carbs and high protein.	Tends to burn easily, so be careful when using as crumbing.
ARROWROOT	½:1	Baking, thickening and coating	Relatively flavorless	High in carbs and protein, fat free and low in fiber.	Use as a replacement for corn flour or potato flour.
BUCKWHEAT	1:1 Replacing 50% of the total flour is best	Cookies, muffins, breads, pastry	Earthy, nutty and a little bitter	High in fiber and potassium.	Start by replacing only 25% of the total flour as the flavor can be strong.
CHIA	1:1	Baking	Nutty and wholesome	Low in carbs, high in fiber and protein; rich in omega 3 fatty acids and calcium.	Can be used as a binder.
COCONUT	¼-1 cup	Good for baking and thickening	Mild coconut flavor but easily overpowered	High in fiber, protein and saturated fat; low carbohydrate content.	Recipes without enough liquid can turn out dense as it absorbs a big amount of water.
MILLET	¾:1 Replacing 20% of total flour is best	Baking, thickening and coating	Mildly sweet, relatively flavorless	High in carbs and fiber. Very alkaline, making it more digestible.	Use for flatbreads, hotcakes etc.
QUINOA	¾:1	Baking and coating	Earthy, nutty and sometimes bitter	High in protein, low in carbs and rich in iron.	Toasting the flour can reduce the bitterness.
RICE	¾:1	Baking, thickening and coating	Brown rice has a nutty, wholesome taste; white rice is relatively flavorless	Slightly higher in carbs and lower in protein. Brown rice flour can be higher in fiber and contains iron, manganese and potassium.	Can give your baked goods a gritty texture.
SORGHUM	1:1	Baking, thickening and coating	Relatively flavorless	High in fiber and antioxidants.	Use for tortillas, flatbreads, cakes.
TAPIOCA	Should be combined with other flours	Thickening and baking	Sweet and starchy	High in carbs and protein, fiber and fat free.	Acts as a binding agent.
TEFF	1:1	Baking and thickening	Mild, sweet and earthy	Very high in calcium and higher in dietary fiber.	Use for breads and cakes.

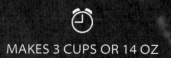

Wholesome Child Gluten-Free Flour Mix

INGREDIENTS

1 cup (5 oz) buckwheat flour

1 cup (5 oz) millet flour

1 cup (4 1/4 oz) arrowroot

INSTRUCTIONS

In a large bowl, add all ingredients and whisk until well combined.

Transfer to a glass jar and use as a gluten-free flour option for your favorite dishes.

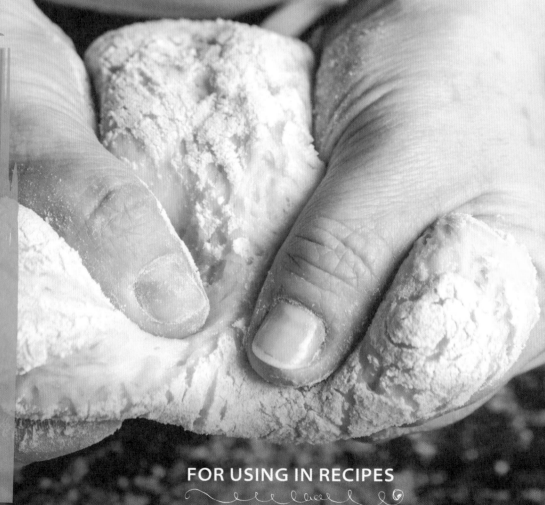

Baking tips and tricks

1. Don't forget to preheat oven first (this will save you time).

2. If you're dealing with dough that is too sticky, add a little more flour. You can also wet your hands with a little water.

3. The easiest way to roll out dough is in between two sheets of baking paper or cling wrap, otherwise make sure that the surface is floured and also flour the rolling pin and the top of the dough (pastry).

4. Working with the Wholesome Child gluten-free flour mix can be a bit tricky at first but we know it works and tastes great, so don't give up if you mess it up the first time. You'll get a better feeling for it the more you work with it.

FOR USING IN RECIPES

1 CUP = 4 OZ OF THE PRE-MADE WHOLESOME CHILD GLUTEN-FREE FLOUR MIX

½ CUP = 2 OZ WHOLESOME CHILD GLUTEN-FREE FLOUR MIX OR
³/₅ OZ BUCKWHEAT FLOUR, ³/₅ OZ MILLET FLOUR, ³/₅ OZ ARROWROOT.

3. Buy bulk vegetables when they are in season and freeze to use later in soups and casseroles.
4. Keep nuts and seeds in the fridge or freezer to prevent them from going rancid.
5. Save veggie peels, cut offs, and herb stalks and put in airtight containers in the freezer. Use to make vegetable stock/broth.
6. Use leftover roast chicken for chicken broth.
7. Be creative. If you don't have black beans on hand use adzuki beans or kidney beans instead, for making black bean brownies. Try different flours in your muffins.

PREPARE TO GO GLUTEN-FREE

If you are planning to try a gluten-free diet for your child, mix up a big batch of our Wholesome Child gluten-free flour mix. We use this in many of our gluten-free recipes so having a big batch on hand will save you having to prepare it each time you want to try a new recipe.

EGG SUBSTITUTES

Egg and dairy allergies are prevalent among young children. In most of our recipes we have offered substitutes for dairy, however many of our recipes contain egg. If your child has an egg allergy, replace the egg in baked items such as muffins, breads, squares, etc. with the following egg substitutes. Each of these suggestions are substitutes for one egg, so if a recipe calls for more, increase the quantities as needed.

- 1–2 tbs ground chia seeds (measured whole) and 3 tbs hot filtered water. Allow the mixture to sit for approximately 5–10 minutes.
- 1 tbs ground flaxseeds and 3 tbs water. It's important to refrigerate for at least 15 minutes before adding to the batter.
- 1/4 cup unsweetened applesauce and 1/2 tsp additional baking soda.

DAIRY-FREE SUBSTITUTES

- Coconut oil for butter
- Avocado puree for butter (best as a spread)
- Almond, coconut, rice, oat milk for cow's milk
- Coconut milk for evaporated milk
- Coconut cream for cream or ricotta cheese
- Coconut yogurt for yogurt

HEALTHY LUNCH BOX PREP

- **Plan ahead.** Leaving lunch box prep for the morning, just before school, can spell disaster. If your household is anything like mine, then mornings are not the time to be thinking about what to put in a healthy lunch box.
- **Focus on variety.** Purchase a bento-style lunch box with separate compartments to encourage variety on both your

and your child's part. It's easy to fall into the habit of sending the same thing every day but if there are a few compartments to fill we can increase variety even if some things remain the same. I am also a firm believer in getting rid of all packaging. To get children off processed foods, we first need to break the habit of kids expecting their food to arrive in brightly colored packaging. It's bad for the environment and bad for their health. The other thing is serving sizes—when we decant food into small compartments, we often reduce the serving size, automatically making it more appropriate for children. I love Planet Box and Lunchbots (all lunch boxes featured in this book are Lunchbots).

- **Ensure balance.** A healthy lunch box needs a good balance of protein and iron-rich foods, calcium-rich foods, healthy fats, slow-release carbohydrates (starchy veggies or grains), vegetables, and an optional piece of fresh fruit. (See our Lunch Box Menu Planner on page 287 for practical tips and inspiration.)

- **Avoid soggy sandwiches and discolored food.** If you are going to put something wet or runny into the lunch box, ensure that is does not seep onto the other food and also be mindful of what goes in a sandwich. To prepare a sandwich the night before, butter the bread and arrange the ingredients but layer the tomato, cucumbers and grated carrot in the morning. Remember to avoid store-bought cold cuts of meat, which can contain nasty preservatives and too much sodium—try roasting your own instead.

- **Hydration is essential.** Always send a stainless steel bottle filled with water. For something special, send a flask filled with a healthy smoothie or kombucha. Home-brewed iced tea is also a great sometime alternative. Use caffeine-free tea like rooibos and mix with a squeeze of lemon, and one teaspoon of raw or Manuka honey or stevia and lots of ice. Place a slice of lemon or orange or some mint into your child's water bottle to encourage drinking on hot days.

- **Rely on leftovers.** Use leftovers for school lunch boxes. Bean casseroles, bolognaise, leftover meatloaf, and grilled fish can all be used for delicious sandwich fillings. Or invest in a good quality thermos and fill with chicken stew, meatballs, mac 'n' cheese or lamb koftas. Don't stop at lunch boxes. Leftovers are great for breakfast too. Leftover veggies can easily be used in omelettes or added to smoothies, and leftover rice or quinoa can easily be made into porridge (mix with coconut milk, cinnamon, and slivered almonds). Save leftover roast meats for sandwich fillings, finely slice roast beef or lamb or shred leftover chicken and freeze into small portion sizes. Remove from freezer the night before and it will be ready to go into the sandwich in the morning.

Visit
www.wholesomechild.com.au
for ongoing lunch box ideas
and inspiration.

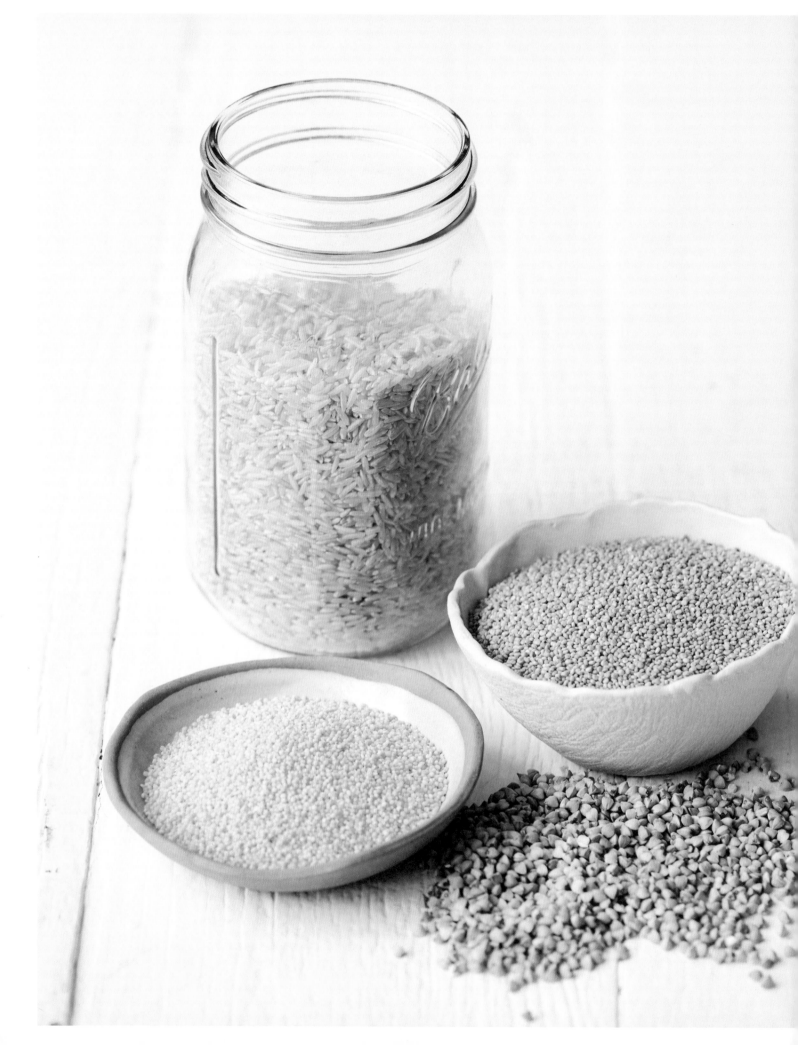

Swap to Whole Grains

REPLACE PROCESSED GRAINS
WITH WHOLE GRAINS AND
FOCUS ON VARIETY

Carbohydrates have been getting a bad rap; however, the fact is that for most children, carbs provide the best source of fuel for their growing muscles and active brains. Children can get carbohydrates from starchy vegetables and fruit, but a large portion of their intake tends to come from grains. That's why choosing the best quality grains is the first step toward improving the quality of your child's diet.

Many of the children I see in my practice won't eat anything other than processed or refined grains like white bread, white rice or pasta and their parents' attempts to offer alternatives are met with tight-lipped rejection. Making gradual changes within the framework of each child's favorite foods can lead to tremendous progress.

One young child I worked with literally lived on white rice before his family came to see me. Initially we tried mixing the white rice with basmati rice and, once we saw that he didn't resist that change, we slowly started adding brown rice to the mix. Now, whenever his family eat rice, they stick to brown rice.

Often parents are surprised at how easy it is when they slowly swap white rice for brown or white flour for a wholegrain version in recipes. Repetition is the secret to success. Start by swapping refined grains for different whole grains—one meal (or snack or even dessert) at a time. It's the single most important change that I encourage parents to make to their child's diet.

SO WHAT'S THE PROBLEM WITH REFINED GRAINS?

Processed or refined grains like white rice or white flour are simple or "empty" carbohydrates. All of the fiber, vitamins, and minerals your growing child needs have been stripped during processing. Unlike all whole grains, which contain three parts: the bran (the outer layer), endosperm (the middle layer), and germ (the inner layer), refined grains are left with only the endosperm, the least nutritious part composed of starchy carbohydrates and low in nutrients.

So instead of retaining all their natural goodness and satiating your child, they very quickly convert to sugar in the bloodstream. A rapid spike in blood sugar may give your child an instant energy hit, but very soon afterwards he will feel tired and struggle to concentrate.

Introducing complex carbohydrates in the form of whole grains, a change that can be as easy as swapping white bread for sourdough in your child's lunch box, won't create that insulin wobble. This one change alone also has the power to set the foundations for healthy eating, may even help to reduce blood cholesterol levels and lower heart disease risk later on in life.

Swapping to whole grains will:
- ✓ help stabilize blood sugar levels
- ✓ improve concentration
- ✓ steady mood swings
- ✓ reduce sugar cravings

REFINED GRAINS VS WHOLE GRAINS: WHAT'S THE DIFFERENCE?

While processed grains are stripped of the most important nutrients, whole grains (grains that are kept intact) contain:

- original phytonutrients and micronutrients.
- several B vitamins (thiamin, riboflavin, niacin, and folate) to unlock the energy found in carbohydrates.
- minerals (iron, magnesium, calcium, manganese, and selenium).
- dietary fiber essential for stabilizing blood sugar and eliminating constipation.

WHAT'S THE DIFFERENCE BETWEEN WHOLE WHEAT AND WHOLE GRAIN?

If wheat is left unprocessed it qualifies as a whole grain. How can you tell? When you read a nutrition label you want to see the word "whole" before "wheat," so it should read whole wheat (and not just wheat). But whole wheat is only one kind of whole grain. Read on to learn about the many other varieties to choose from.

Consider this...

The constant rise and fall of blood sugar levels that happens when we feed our children refined grains can predispose them to insulin resistance, type 2 diabetes, and obesity. In the US, type 2 diabetes is increasing at faster rates than type 1 diabetes among children. Main culprits include overconsumption of refined or processed grains, obesity, and being sedentary.

36

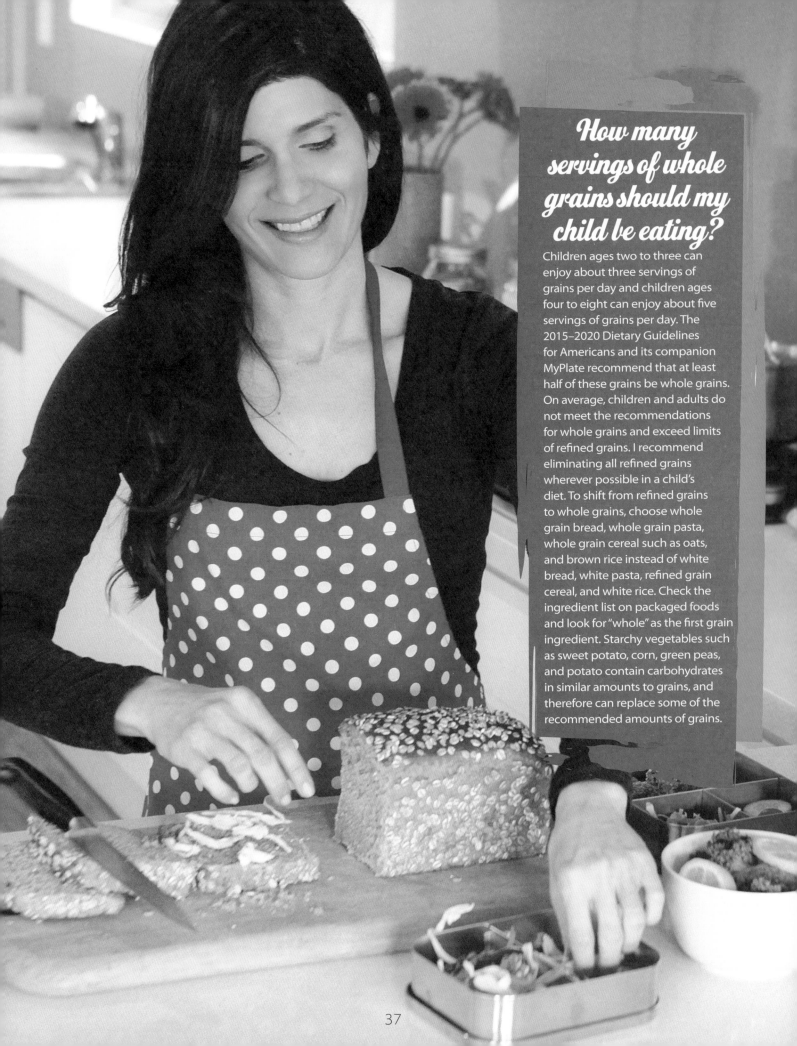

How many servings of whole grains should my child be eating?

Children ages two to three can enjoy about three servings of grains per day and children ages four to eight can enjoy about five servings of grains per day. The 2015–2020 Dietary Guidelines for Americans and its companion MyPlate recommend that at least half of these grains be whole grains. On average, children and adults do not meet the recommendations for whole grains and exceed limits of refined grains. I recommend eliminating all refined grains wherever possible in a child's diet. To shift from refined grains to whole grains, choose whole grain bread, whole grain pasta, whole grain cereal such as oats, and brown rice instead of white bread, white pasta, refined grain cereal, and white rice. Check the ingredient list on packaged foods and look for "whole" as the first grain ingredient. Starchy vegetables such as sweet potato, corn, green peas, and potato contain carbohydrates in similar amounts to grains, and therefore can replace some of the recommended amounts of grains.

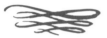
VARY AND ROTATE WHOLE GRAINS FOR THE BIGGEST NUTRITION PUNCH

Swapping from refined grains to whole grains will immediately boost your child's nutrition; however, by only offering whole grains that contain wheat and gluten, we are adding to an already overloaded situation. While the jury remains out on whether we are eating more wheat than our grandparents did, I think we can all agree that we are certainly consuming more gluten.

Gluten is a sticky protein found in wheat, barley and rye. Due to the abundance of wheat and wheat products in our diet—especially processed and refined varieties—there has been a rise in the number of people suffering from celiac disease, gluten intolerance, or an allergy to gluten.

Not only are we eating it in foods such as bread, muffins, cupcakes and cakes, gluten is also added as a filler and binding agent in many processed foods such as soy sauce, processed meats like sausages or cold cuts, anything crumbed, sugar that is not labelled "pure cane sugar," flavored milk, store-bought stews and soups, mustard, gravies, sauces, salad dressings, pastries, and even sweets. It's no surprise that the typical Western child's diet is overloaded with wheat and food products containing gluten.

Consider that a child may have toast or cereal for breakfast, crackers for morning tea, a sandwich in their lunch box, a muffin for afternoon tea, and stir-fry with noodles or pasta for dinner and it's easy to see how they could be eating wheat and gluten all day long. By increasing the variety of whole grains to include some that don't contain any wheat or gluten, you greatly reduce your child's risk of developing sensitivity to wheat or gluten (which is sometimes only diagnosed when a child is ten).

Alternative options could include oatmeal for breakfast, rice or quinoa crispbreads for morning tea, buckwheat pancakes for afternoon tea, and rice noodles for dinner. Variation and rotation of a variety of whole grains is the best strategy to ensure your child is getting the full spectrum of nutrients available. However, it's also important to note that children can thrive and survive without including grains at each meal.

ARE WE EATING THE SAME WHEAT AS OUR ANCESTORS?

While some experts say that the wheat seed hasn't been altered, others call out the hybridization (cross-breeding) of the wheat we eat today as a major culprit in the rise of celiac disease. In the mid-twentieth century, the American agronomist Norman Borlaug pioneered the development of a hybrid dwarf wheat strain, in order to create a greater crop yield and one that was more disease resistant. This created a wheat strain with a higher and different type of gluten content upon which a substantial portion of the world's population now depends for sustenance.

Along with hybridization, small studies have found that the breads we ate fifty years ago were not as immunogenic (able to provoke a response from our immune systems) as modern breads. This is the main reason why ancient wheat grains such as spelt and kamut have become increasingly popular. These grains have not undergone the same form of hybridization and therefore contain less gluten, which, for some, makes them easier to digest (see page 44 for more information on Ancient Grains).

WHAT ABOUT GENETICALLY MODIFIED (GM) WHEAT?

This is another major source for concern. There are ongoing trials of genetically modified wheat strains that have not yet tested safe for human or animal consumption. GM foods are produced from organisms that have been subjected to changes to their DNA using various methods of genetic engineering, as opposed to traditional cross breeding.

Health risks associated with GM foods may

WHAT DOES ONE SERVING OF WHOLE GRAINS LOOK LIKE?

WHOLE GRAIN	SERVE
Rice, quinoa, pasta, polenta, buckwheat, millet or noodles	½ cup
Oatmeal	½ cup
Bread	1 slice
1 waffle or pancake	About the size of a CD case
Dinner roll	half
Muesli	¼ cup
Wholegrain cereal	¾ cup
wholegrain crackers	3

include immune-related problems, faulty insulin regulation, infertility, and changes in major organs and the gastrointestinal system.

Add to that the fact that Monsanto's Roundup herbicide (active agent glyphosate), sprayed heavily on 85 percent of all GMO crops, has been declared a "probable carcinogen" by the World Health Organization (WHO). So for now:

- **Buy organic** Certified organic products do not intentionally include any GMO ingredients.
- **Look for non-GMO labels** These should be prominently displayed on packaging.
- **Avoid "at-risk" ingredients** Unless whole grain products are labelled organic or verified non-GMO, avoid those made with ingredients that might be derived from GMOs. These include corn, soybeans, canola, and cottonseed oil.

(See page 270 for more information about genetically modified foods).

Tip: If your child has celiac disease, gluten intolerance, or a wheat allergy or you just want to reduce the amount of gluten consumed each day, try almond meal, coconut flour, and buckwheat flour in place of wholegrain flour. Lettuce or cabbage leaves and nori sheets also make excellent replacements for wraps.

SO IS A GLUTEN-FREE DIET THE BEST WAY TO GO?

Gluten-free products are everywhere in answer to the growing number of people following a gluten-free lifestyle. But before you overhaul your pantry, it's important to know that many of these products are not necessarily 'healthy'. Most common gluten-free supermarket products are highly refined as their main ingredients include maize, potato starch, and cornstarch as well as added sugars and preservatives.

If your family is following a gluten-free lifestyle, make sure you choose whole food gluten-free options such as quinoa, amaranth, millet, brown rice, sorghum, teff, and buckwheat. Another thing to remember is to not only choose rice-based products; too much rice and rice-based products, even wholegrain rice, can contribute to arsenic in the diet. Inorganic arsenic is found in nearly all foods and drinks, but is usually only found in small amounts.

However, slightly higher levels can be found in rice and rice-based products such as rice milk, rice syrup, infant rice cereal and rice bran. Therefore, even for those following a whole food gluten-free diet, it is still best to rotate your grains. After all, each whole grain has something different to offer, from the calcium in teff to the protein in quinoa.

DID YOU KNOW?

Whole grains are an excellent source of fiber. Children aged 1 to 3 years need 19 grams of fiber per day. For children aged 4 to 8 years, that number rises to 25 grams per day.

CELIAC DISEASE **VS** GLUTEN INTOLERANCE **VS** WHEAT ALLERGY

CELIAC DISEASE	GLUTEN INTOLERANCE	WHEAT ALLERGY
Definition: Genetic, autoimmune disorder; gluten ingestion triggers damage to small intestine.	**Definition:** Intolerance to gluten or other wheat components without damage to small intestine.	**Definition:** Immune response to one or more of the proteins found in wheat (can include gluten).
Gastrointestinal symptoms: diarrhea, constipation, nausea, vomiting, flatulence, cramping, bloating, abdominal pain.	**Gastrointestinal symptoms:** Diarrhea, bloating, abdominal pain, constipation.	**Gastrointestinal symptoms:** Nausea, vomiting, diarrhea, bloating, constipation.
Other symptoms: Weight loss, malnutrition, iron deficiency, dental cavitiies, low bone density, skin issues, neurological disorders, liver dysfunction, joint pain, hair loss, fatigue.	**Other symptoms:** Brain fog, neurological disorders, joint pain, fatigue, mood and behavior disorders.	**Other symptoms:** Hives, rash, nasal congestion, eye irritation, difficulty breathing, irritation of mouth or throat, mood and behavior disorders.
Treatment: Strict adherence to a gluten-free lifestyle.	**Treatment:** Adherence to a wheat-free/gluten-free diet (level of adherence variable).	**Treatment:** Strict adherence to a wheat-free lifestyle.

Source: UCLA division of Digestive Diseases

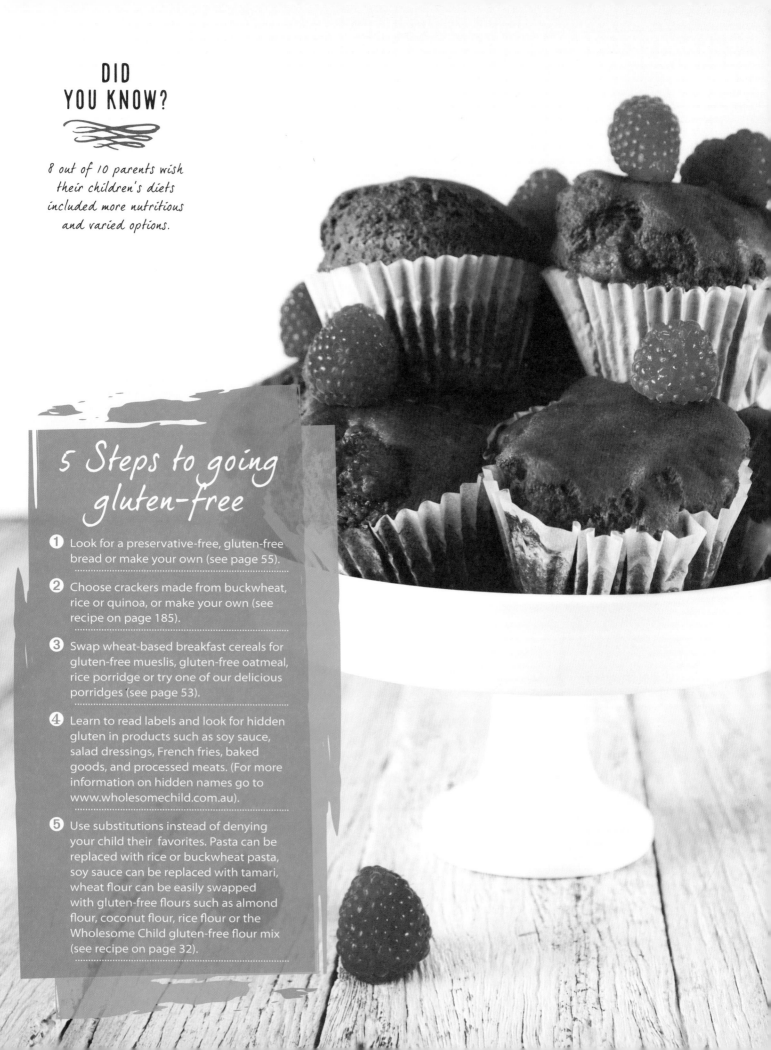

5 Steps to going gluten-free

❶ Look for a preservative-free, gluten-free bread or make your own (see page 55).

❷ Choose crackers made from buckwheat, rice or quinoa, or make your own (see recipe on page 185).

❸ Swap wheat-based breakfast cereals for gluten-free mueslis, gluten-free oatmeal, rice porridge or try one of our delicious porridges (see page 53).

❹ Learn to read labels and look for hidden gluten in products such as soy sauce, salad dressings, French fries, baked goods, and processed meats. (For more information on hidden names go to www.wholesomechild.com.au).

❺ Use substitutions instead of denying your child their favorites. Pasta can be replaced with rice or buckwheat pasta, soy sauce can be replaced with tamari, wheat flour can be easily swapped with gluten-free flours such as almond flour, coconut flour, rice flour or the Wholesome Child gluten-free flour mix (see recipe on page 32).

Top 7 gluten-free grain options for kids

Millet
Amaranth
Rice
Quinoa
Buckwheat
Teff
Sorghum

**Raspberry & Pear Muffins
(see recipe on page 49)**

Tip: While many children accept changes to staples like white bread, if they are extremely fussy eaters with sensory issues, do not tamper with their staples. Instead, offer whole grains in the form of muffins or aim for one sandwich-free day a week by using a preservative-free wrap in place of bread. Another great option is to send savory muffins, scrolls, wholegrain pasta, or homemade tortillas to school.

IS SOURDOUGH BREAD BETTER?

Supermarket breads are highly processed and do not follow traditional methods of bread making. Sourdough bread is higher in protein and minerals than white bread.

A sourdough loaf is also more easily digested than a standard loaf due to the fermentation process, which involves lactic acid breaking down the phytates and starches in the dough. As a result, once digested it enters into the bloodstream at a slower rate, avoiding blood sugar spikes.

While sourdough is not suitable for celiac sufferers or those with wheat allergy, people with gluten intolerance or sensitivities may be able to tolerate small amounts of spelt sourdough. However, it is important to look for an authentic spelt sourdough loaf, most commonly found in health food stores or artisan bakeries. These breads should only contain whole spelt flour, sourdough starter culture, salt, and water. Supermarket versions are becoming more readily available but they are often not true sourdough breads, containing yeast and other artificial ingredients, so always check the ingredients before purchasing.

DID YOU KNOW?

High in vitamin B and low GI, arrowroot powder is a healthier alternative than non-organic cornstarch (likely to contain GMOs). Try it as a thickener the next time you make mac 'n' cheese.

BEST GLUTEN SUBSTITUTES

TYPICAL GLUTEN CONTAINING DIET	DIET WITH ROTATED GRAINS
Toast or cereal for breakfast	Gluten-free oats for breakfast
Crackers for morning tea	Rice or quinoa crispbreads for morning tea
A sandwich in the lunch box	Gluten-free bread or hamburger bun with filling of choice (see recipe on page 51)
Muffin for afternoon tea	Buckwheat pancakes for afternoon tea
Stir-fry with noodles or pasta for dinner	Rice noodles for dinner

How to buy supermarket bread

- Whole wheat, wholewheat flour, whole spelt flour or another whole grain should be the first ingredient on the ingredients list.

- It should offer at least 1/12 oz of dietary fiber per serving.

- Avoid bread with added gluten (this is used to increase fluffiness), vegetable oil, sugar, and high levels of sodium (anything above 400mg per $3^1/_2$ oz).

- If the ingredient panel contains more than 4–6 ingredients, move on to the next loaf.

- Avoid likely GM additives such as canola oil and soy lecithin.

- Go for breads that are preservative-free. The main preservatives to avoid in bread are propionates 280–282 (including cultured dextrose or whey), potassium bromate, butylated hydroxyanisole (BHA) or butylated hydroxytoluene (BHT). See Step 8: Avoid Nasties.

SIMPLE SWAPS

No time to cook? Start swapping refined grains for whole grains at the supermarket.

Highly processed breakfast cereals	Wholegrain breakfast cereals
White bread	Wholegrain spelt sourdough
Refined crackers	Wholegrain crackers, quinoa crackers, or seed crackers
Instant oats	Rolled oats, brown rice flakes, quinoa flakes
White pasta	Whole wheat, whole spelt, buckwheat or brown rice
Whole wheat flour	Whole spelt, buckwheat, brown rice flour
Bread crumbs	Brown rice bread crumbs

42

Tip: When swapping to a whole grain or sourdough bread for a lunch box, change the bread first. You can introduce healthier spreads or toppings later on.

PASS THE PASTA . . .

If you are not ready to move on from wheat pasta, then focus on quality when it comes to buying pasta too. Good quality pasta is made from durum wheat, which is naturally higher in protein. This means that even white pasta will convert at a slower rate into sugar in the bloodstream.

HOW TO CHOOSE FLOUR

Avoid white flour when baking. It offers little nutritional value and is also bleached (unless it says unbleached) using harsh chemicals such as chlorine dioxide. Along with wholegrain wheat flour there are other flours that make excellent choices. Experiment with oat flour, spelt flour, quinoa flour, brown rice flour, and buckwheat flour.

My favorite flours for baking, especially for muffins, are buckwheat, millet flour or spelt. If you are following a recipe that calls for wholemeal spelt flour, you can substitute gram for gram with spelt, kamut or buckwheat. Or to pack an even bigger nutritional punch and avoid gluten entirely, mix it up. In a conventional muffin recipe, for example, replace 1 cup of wholegrain wheat flour with 1/3 cup rice flour, 1/3 cup almond meal and 1/3 cup coconut flour, or the Wholesome Child gluten-free flour mix (see page 32).

Note: If you use coconut flour, you may have to increase fluid or add an extra egg.

HOW TO CHOOSE CEREALS

Sugary cereals made from refined grains create insulin spikes that leave kids feeling irritable. An average serve of breakfast cereal can have between 3–5 tsp of sugar per serve. Mueslis containing dried fruit generally contain preservative 202 (sulphur dioxide) which can cause gastrointestinal disturbances, bloating, stomach pain, and diarrhea.

Look for whole grain cereals with no added sugar containing rolled oats and puffed, sugar-free grains like brown rice, quinoa or buckwheat. If you need to sweeten them to begin with, it's preferable if you are in charge of the quantity and type of sweetener you choose and over time you can reduce the amount.

Tip: Make your own muesli by mixing seeds such as pumpkin seeds, sunflower seeds, and chia seeds, nuts such as slivered almonds, cashews and pistachios, oats, toasted coconut, goji berries, and chopped dates (see recipe on page 199).

TIME-SAVING HACKS FOR BUSY PARENTS

If you can't find the time to cook grains from scratch during the weeknight dinner rush, later in the evening may be a more relaxed time to let a pot of whole grain goodness simmer so that it's ready for the following day.

- Once the kids are in bed and you've eaten dinner, toss together a cup of wild rice with some water, extra virgin olive oil, and a pinch of salt, and cook gently for fifty minutes. Once cooled, place in the fridge for the next day.
- Do the same with rolled oats for the following day's breakfast. Overnight oatmeal (or refrigerator oatmeal) is an effortless way to prep whole grains while you sleep. Combine 1 part rolled oats to 2 parts liquid (water, milk, kefir or non-dairy milk alternatives), fruit and desired seasonings like cinnamon, carob powder, nuts and seeds, and then soak overnight in the fridge so that it's ready to heat and eat the next morning. You can even make a large pot of oats on a Sunday night to last for 2–3 days in the fridge and just heat it up as needed.
- Bircher muesli is another great idea that can be made the night before. For variety, try any rolled whole grain—such as rolled quinoa flakes, rolled spelt flakes, rolled kamut flakes or rolled rye flakes—in place of rolled oats (see recipe on page 257).
- To cut twenty minutes off the cooking time for grains such as brown rice, quinoa, buckwheat or wild rice, soak overnight (learn how below).

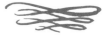
Consider this...

Varying whole grains is a great step towards addressing fussy eating. For example, alternate the type of pasta you prepare—try spelt, quinoa or buckwheat in differing shapes and they'll slowly start to accept that not all pasta looks the same.

Healthiest Whole Grains

QUINOA	AMARANTH	BARLEY	MILLET	OATS	RICE*
What is it? Quinoa, a gluten-free ancient grain and a complete protein is packed with iron, phosphorous, magnesium, and fiber. It is especially high in folate (perfect for pregnant and nursing mothers) and potassium, which helps control blood pressure.	**What is it?** An ancient grain that is also gluten-free, amaranth provides one of the highest grain sources of protein, calcium, and iron and is high in manganese, phosphorous and magnesium too. Amaranth's fiber content is triple that of wheat and it also contains essential amino acids.	**What is it?** Barley's high levels of soluble beta glucan fiber helps to reduce cholesterol, improve immunity and control blood sugar. It's also high in protein, manganese, thiamine, and selenium. Choose hulled barley and avoid pearl barley, which has undergone "polishing" and "pearling." Barley is significantly lower in gluten than other flours, but it's not 100 percent gluten-free.	**What is it?** A versatile gluten-free grain that is high in manganese, phosphorous, and magnesium. It's easy on your child's digestive system and has a delicious nutty flavor. Millet is also the most alkaline (non-acid forming) of all the grains, so it's a great choice for babies and young children (see the Wholesome Child gluten-free flour mix on page 32).	**What is it?** Oats almost never have their bran and germ removed in processing. Rich in soluble beta glucan fiber, they stabilize blood sugar levels, boost the immune system, prevent recurring childhood infections and even fight off cancer. Oats contain antioxidants that have strong anti-inflammatory and anti-itching properties. They do not contain gluten but may be contaminated with wheat.	**What is it?** Swapping white rice for brown rice, colored rice, or wild rice will increase your child's intake of fiber, vitamin B1, magnesium, phosphorous and manganese. Brown rice, a staple in most gluten-free diets, can also help boost serotonin, the feel-good hormone that can also help your child sleep better. * (Brown rice, colored rice, and wild rice)
How to use it • Popped or puffed quinoa can replace sugary breakfast cereals. • Add toasted quinoa to homemade muesli and use to make crispy treats or muesli bars. • Use quinoa flakes to make porridge—either alone or mix with rolled oats if you find the taste too earthy. • Use the quinoa in place of rice or couscous. Add to vegetable, chicken, or bone broth. • Cooked quinoa can also be added to muffin recipes to boost protein. • Quinoa flour is perfect for making bread. Toast the flour before using to remove its slightly sour flavor or use it in combination with other gluten-free flours such as rice flour, sorghum flour, or chickpea flour.	**How to use it** • Add amaranth flakes to rolled oats or quinoa flakes for a nutritious porridge. Amaranth tends to be sticky so it's best not to use it alone. • Offer popped or puffed amaranth as a replacement for sugary breakfast cereals. It can also be added to homemade muesli. • Toasted amaranth can be added to homemade granola, used to make crispy treats and muesli bars, or added as a topping to yogurt. • Replace 25 percent of your regular flour with amaranth flour or add to other gluten-free flours. • Use the cooked whole grain to thicken soups and stews.	**How to use it** • Use barley flakes or cracked barley to make porridge. • Add the cooked whole grain to stews and soups for extra heartiness, or to create a delicious pilaf. • Add barley flour to bread, muffins, or pancakes to replace white flour or wheat flour, however, it should not constitute more than 25 percent of the entire recipe for breads and muffins and no more than 50 percent for cookies and flat cookies that do not need to rise.	**How to use it** • Use millet flour for baking bread that is light, white, and quite similar in texture to wheat bread. For those wanting to avoid gluten, millet bread is the most palatable substitute. Try our Gluten-free Yogurt Bread on page 55. • Use traditional cracked millet to ensure that you are using it in its wholegrain form. Once cooked, its fluffy rice-like consistency is perfect as a replacement for rice or polenta in rissoles, patties or fritters. • To reach a creamy porridge-like consistency add more water and cook for longer. • Prepare a big batch of the Wholesome Child gluten-free flour mix and use in our gluten-free recipes (see page 32).	**How to use it** • Add 1/3 cup oats into pancake or muffin recipes. • Add rolled oats into a rice crumb and almond meal mixture for chicken nuggets or fish fingers. • Add oat flour to cookies, breads and pancakes. Since oat flour doesn't contain gluten, you will need to adjust your ingredients to make your baked items light and fluffy. When making recipes that require baking powder, add 2½ teaspoons baking powder per cup of oat flour. In cookie and bread recipes, replace up to ¼ cup of the wheat flour with oat flour.	**How to use it** • Use whole brown rice in sushi, meatballs, and hamburger patties. • Brown rice flakes make a delicious, gluten-free porridge. • Substitute rice crumbs for wheat bread crumbs to add a nutty, crunchy texture to any crumbed food. • Brown rice flour can be used as a standalone flour in baked goods such as cookies and muffins or in combination with other gluten-free flours. Be aware that many rice flours are made from white rice, so always look for a brown rice variety.

Wholesome Child's 12 favorite grains and how to serve them

BUCKWHEAT	RYE	SORGHUM	KAMUT	SPELT	TEFF

BUCKWHEAT

What is it?

Buckwheat contains higher levels of zinc, copper, manganese, potassium, and lysine than other cereal grains. Because of its high level of protein (second only to oats), buckwheat has a lower GI than rice, corn or wheat. And because it is gluten-free, it's far less likely to provoke an allergy, making it a perfect super food for babies.

How to use it

- Buckwheat groats, cooked like oats, make a delicious porridge (see recipes on page 53).
- Buckwheat pancakes have long been an Eastern European staple. Buckwheat flour can easily replace flour in a pancake recipe for children too.
- Use toasted buckwheat (kasha) to add crunch to homemade muesli, make chocolate crispy treats or sprinkle over yogurt.
- Popped buckwheat is great as a cereal.
- Buckwheat flour can be used to create delicious gluten-free bread.

RYE

What is it?

Rye has a low GI and is rich in fiber. It contains arabinoxylan, a type of fiber which is also known for its high antioxidant activity. To ensure you're eating the whole grain, make sure "whole rye" is listed in the ingredients. Be aware that most rye breads do contain wheat.

How to use it

- Make your favorite sandwiches on rye bread.
- Use the cooked whole grain as a replacement for rice, quinoa or couscous.
- Use rye flakes to make porridge.
- Substitute some rye flour for wheat flour in your favorite pancake, muffin or bread recipe. This is an especially good idea if your child suffers from constipation.

SORGHUM

What is it?

Gluten-free and low GI, sorghum doesn't have an inedible hull like some other whole grains so it's able to retain the majority of its nutrients. It's also grown from traditional hybrid seeds making it non-GMO. Some specialty sorghums are high in antioxidants. In addition, the wax surrounding the sorghum grain contains compounds called policosanols that may have the ability to lower cholesterol.

How to use it

- Sorghum can be substituted for wheat flour in a variety of baked goods including muffins, breads, pizza bases, cookies, cakes, and pies.
- Its neutral, sometimes sweet flavor and light color make it easily adaptable to a variety of dishes like casseroles.

KAMUT

What is it?

Kamut only has twenty-eight chromosomes, while most modern wheats have forty-two. It is essentially a durum wheat that dates back to biblical times and is unusually high in lipids giving it a buttery taste. It is nutritionally superior to common wheat in trace minerals too.

How to use it

- Look out for kamut breakfast cereals, pasta and baked goods, including bread.
- It's also available in wholegrain form to cook and use instead of rice.
- Kamut flour is great for creating delicious tortillas or wraps (see recipe on page 63).

SPELT

What is it?

Another ancient form of wheat, spelt is higher in protein than common wheat. It is highly water soluble, which means your child can easily absorb its nutrients.

How to use it

- Spelt flour is best for baking bread. Substitute whole meal spelt flour cup for cup for all-purpose or bread flour.
- Spelt sourdough breads are the best non gluten-free option to replace processed, store-bought breads.
- Spelt flour can be used to make muffins, cookies and pancakes.
- Spelt puffs are a great alternative to wheat puffs for a breakfast cereal.

TEFF

What is it?

Teff boasts more than twice the iron of other grains, and three times the calcium. All varieties of teff are whole grain, because the kernel is too small to mill easily. White or ivory teff has the mildest flavor, with darker varieties having an earthier taste.

How to use it

- Use teff flour in pancakes, breads and crackers (see recipe on page 62).
- The cooked grain has the texture of poppy seeds that's great for sprinkling on vegetables or for adding to soups. Wholegrain teff porridge is a delicious alternative to oatmeal (see recipe on page 53).

DID YOU KNOW?

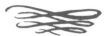

Amaranth, quinoa, and buckwheat are technically "pseudo-grains" but they're included with true cereal grains because they offer similar nutritional value. Pseudograins are the starchy seeds of broad-leafed plants (compared to grains which are the fruits or seeds of grasses).

Consider this...

My shared belief of feeding expert Ellyn Satter, pioneer of the Satter Feeding Dynamics Model, is that parents decide what, when, and where their child will eat. And children learn to regulate their own appetite by being responsible for how much they eat.

TAKE IT TO THE NEXT LEVEL . . .

Once your child is eating a wide variety of whole grains, consider soaking your grains before cooking them. Grains contain anti-nutrients like gluten, lectin and phytic acid. Soaking them in water with an acidic medium, such as lemon juice or vinegar, and then rinsing before cooking, can remove these anti-nutrients giving your child an even better boost of nutrients. Soaking also significantly reduces the cooking time of most grains (for tips on soaking grains, see page 30).

GOAL 1: REGULAR FAMILY MEALS

Studies show that regular family meals can improve a child's vocabulary, mood, academic success, and outlook on the future. I am a firm believer that family meals are also the cornerstone of healthy eating, so every night I sit down with my children. Often it is too early for me to eat a full dinner, so I eat a fresh salad and part of what they are eating. Sometimes it's one meatball, a piece of fish, a small portion of pasta or an egg.

I have always put a large salad bowl in the middle of the table with child-sized tongs and side plates for them to explore and pick out what they want. They now each fill their bowls with salad and their favorite dressing—extra virgin olive oil and balsamic vinegar.

Sitting down to meals as a family is the ideal opportunity for children to benefit from positive role modeling. But in order for it to be truly beneficial, the main focus of the experience must also be pleasant and engaging.

More than anything, family meals should be about enjoying quality time together as a family. In this manner, your child can start to relax and, when he does, his whole sensory system will calm down. Over time he may even be more likely to explore new foods.

Tip: If you notice that your child is anxious or stressed as dinner approaches change up the routine. Try dancing or doing some yoga, then run a bubble bath before dinner. Anxiety tends to negatively affect appetite because once our fight or flight instinct kicks in it switches off our digestive systems.

A MOMENT OF MINDFULNESS FOR PARENTS

Your state of mind and your attitude can help your child self regulate his emotions. If you find yourself getting anxious or worked up as dinner approaches, then your child will feed off this energy. Shift your focus from the fact your beloved quiche may end up in the bin again and try to offer meals that work within his framework of food preferences to ensure that he can eat some aspect of the meal you've made.

Dinner can often be the most difficult meal of the day as everyone is tired, which means it's not always the best meal to introduce new or tricky foods. Relax if your child is not an enthusiastic dinner eater. The focus should be on getting him to sit at the table and enjoy the time with his family. (Do ensure that his breakfast and lunch are more nutritious). By the same token, if children see their parents arguing at the table, they are more likely to become distressed. The real value of a family meal is its ability to help develop strong bonds.

Don't feel guilty about being unable to find the time for regular family meals if your family is able to relate well through other activities. Start by having family meals on the weekends when it's more manageable. Even though this takes the burden off parents to force children to eat dinner, it also makes sense to take your child's sensory preferences into consideration to give them the best chance of getting the nutrition they need at each meal.

The aim is to only cook one meal for a family dinner, but if you have a fussy eater who does not want any of his food to touch or who prefers sauces to be put on the side then it makes sense to plan that meal around his preferences. For example, if you are making hamburgers, before you add all the ingredients together, separate the patty, lettuce, cucumber, tomato and the bread roll for your fussy eater. The same can easily be done with shepherd's pie or fried rice. Being sensitive to each family member's sensory food preferences can help make mealtimes more enjoyable and successful for everyone.

Eating a healthy breakfast leads to improved cognition and memory, helps reduce sick days off school, and generally improves mood. A 2008 study in the journal *Pediatrics* found that teenagers who ate breakfast regularly had a lower body-mass index than those who did not. If you can't make regular family dinners, try instead to eat breakfast together as often as possible.

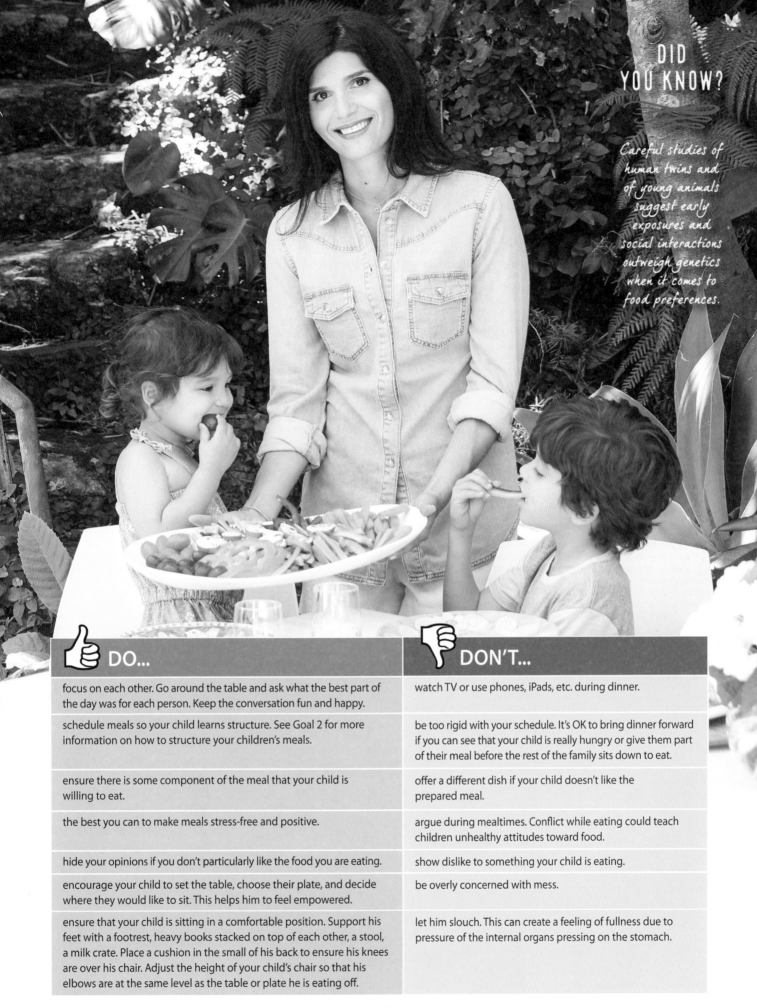

👍 DO...	👎 DON'T...
focus on each other. Go around the table and ask what the best part of the day was for each person. Keep the conversation fun and happy.	watch TV or use phones, iPads, etc. during dinner.
schedule meals so your child learns structure. See Goal 2 for more information on how to structure your children's meals.	be too rigid with your schedule. It's OK to bring dinner forward if you can see that your child is really hungry or give them part of their meal before the rest of the family sits down to eat.
ensure there is some component of the meal that your child is willing to eat.	offer a different dish if your child doesn't like the prepared meal.
the best you can to make meals stress-free and positive.	argue during mealtimes. Conflict while eating could teach children unhealthy attitudes toward food.
hide your opinions if you don't particularly like the food you are eating.	show dislike to something your child is eating.
encourage your child to set the table, choose their plate, and decide where they would like to sit. This helps him to feel empowered.	be overly concerned with mess.
ensure that your child is sitting in a comfortable position. Support his feet with a footrest, heavy books stacked on top of each other, a stool, a milk crate. Place a cushion in the small of his back to ensure his knees are over his chair. Adjust the height of your child's chair so that his elbows are at the same level as the table or plate he is eating off.	let him slouch. This can create a feeling of fullness due to pressure of the internal organs pressing on the stomach.

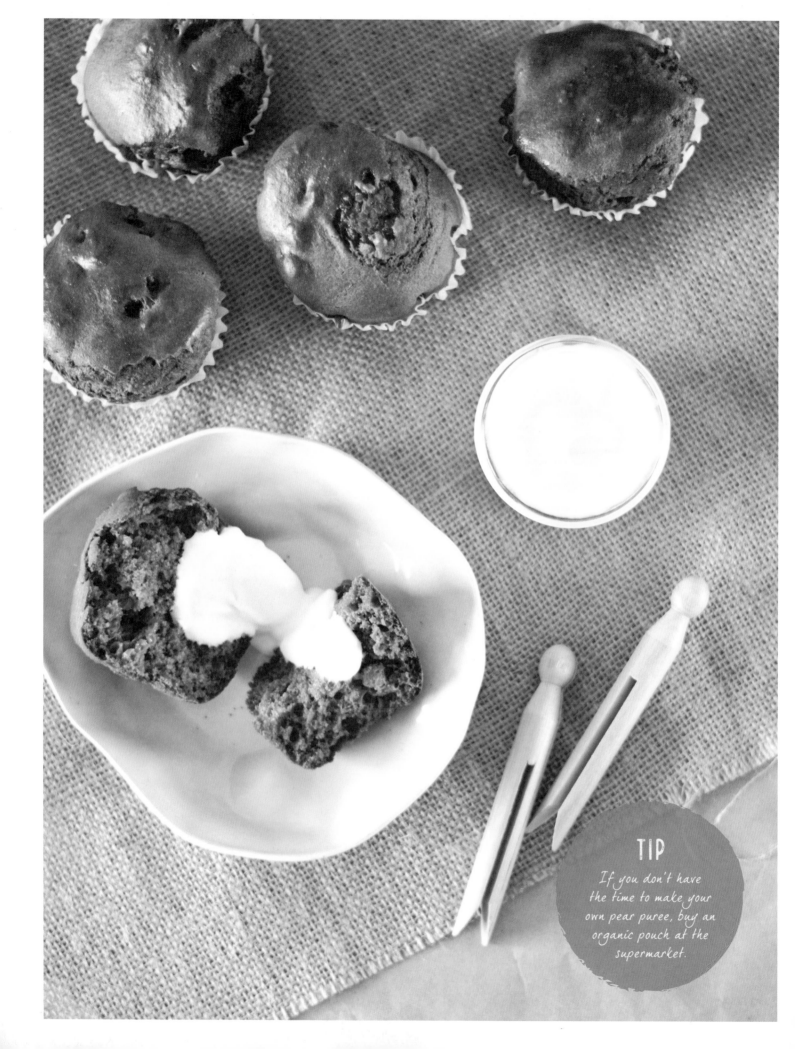

TIP

If you don't have the time to make your own pear puree, buy an organic pouch at the supermarket.

VEG — Vegetarian
Gluten Free
Dairy Free
Nut Free

Prep time: 15 mins
Cooking time: 20 mins
Makes: 36 mini muffins

Raspberry & Pear Muffins

This recipe was created for my daughter's first birthday party, and we used a coconut cream frosting. Try it with whole spelt flour for a non gluten-free option.

INGREDIENTS

1 cup (5³/₅ oz) brown rice flour

¹/₄ cup (⁷/₈ oz) coconut flour

¹/₂ tsp baking powder

1 tsp baking soda

³/₄ cup (3³/₄ oz) coconut sugar

pinch sea salt

3 eggs

¹/₂ cup coconut cream

1 tsp pure vanilla extract

2 tbs coconut oil, melted

¹/₃ cup (3¹/₅ oz) pureed pear

1 cup (5¹/₂ oz) raspberries

EQUIPMENT

high-speed food processor

INSTRUCTIONS

Preheat the oven to 350°F.

Place paper inserts into a mini muffin tray and grease with coconut oil (some paper inserts do not require greasing).

Place dry ingredients in a high-speed food processor. Process on low speed.

Slowly add eggs, coconut cream, vanilla extract, and coconut oil to the mixture and process on medium-high speed until smooth consistency is reached.

Next, add the pear puree to the mixture and process until smooth.

Place your mixture in a bowl and gently stir in the berries.

Spoon 1–2 tbs of batter into mini muffin trays and bake for 20 mins or until a cake tester comes out clear.

Serving and storing leftovers: Serve immediately, store in the fridge for up to 4 days or freeze for up to 4 months.

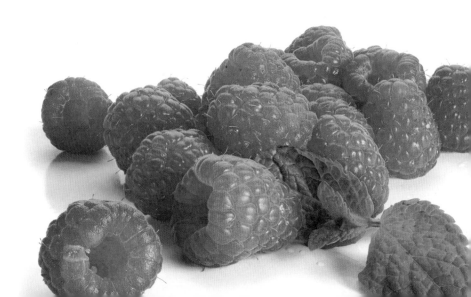

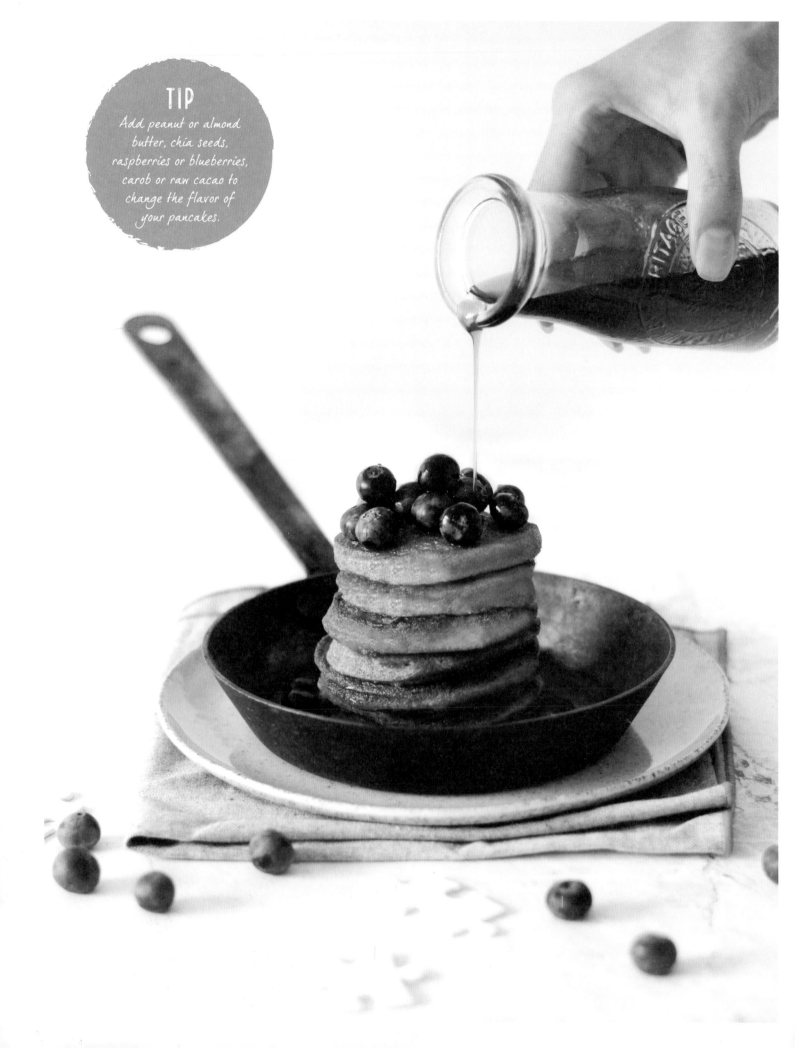

TIP

Add peanut or almond butter, chia seeds, raspberries or blueberries, carob or raw cacao to change the flavor of your pancakes.

VEG Vegetarian | Gluten Free | Dairy Free

Prep time: 5 mins
Cooking time: 15 mins
Makes: 20 small pancakes

Almond & Buckwheat Pancakes

These delicious, nutty pancakes are a real hit with my children. If your child doesn't mind texture, skip the food processor and mix by hand.

INGREDIENTS

¾ cup (3¹/₅ oz) almond flour or meal

½ cup (2½ oz) buckwheat flour

½ cup coconut milk

2 eggs

pinch Himalayan salt

¼ tsp baking powder

⅛ tsp baking soda

¼ tsp ground

cinnamon

¼ tsp pure vanilla extract

coconut oil (optional)

EQUIPMENT
high-speed food processor

INSTRUCTIONS

Place all the ingredients in a high-speed food processor and process until smooth.

Place a large pan over medium heat and coat with coconut oil.

For mini pancakes use 2 tbs of batter, for larger pancakes use ¼ cup of batter.

Cook pancakes for approximately 1–2 mins each side or until bubbles begin to appear.

Serve with maple syrup or toppings of your choice (optional).

Serving and storing leftovers: Serve immediately, store in the fridge for 4 days or freeze for up to 4 months.

VEG Vegetarian | Gluten Free | Dairy Free

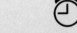
Prep time: 10 mins
Cooking time: 40–45 mins
Makes: 8

Gluten-free Hamburger Buns

INGREDIENTS

1 cup (4¼ oz) Wholesome Child gluten-free flour mix

1 cup (4¼ oz) almond flour or meal

⅓ cup (7/8 oz) psyllium husks

1 tbs baking powder

½–1 tsp sea salt

1 egg

1½ cups almond milk

2 tbs sesame seeds

INSTRUCTIONS

Preheat oven to 355°F and line a baking tray with baking paper.

In a large bowl, combine gluten-free flour mix, almond flour, psyllium husks, baking powder and salt.

In a smaller bowl, combine egg and almond milk.

Pour egg mixture into flour mixture and stir until well combined. Leave to sit for 20 mins.

Divide and shape dough into 8 equal-sized buns and place on baking tray. Sprinkle some sesame seeds on top and bake in the oven for 40–45 mins.

Allow to cool slightly before serving.

Serving and storing leftovers: Serve immediately, store in an airtight container for up to 3 days or freeze for up to 6 months.

For a school-friendly version, simply replace almond meal with seed meal.

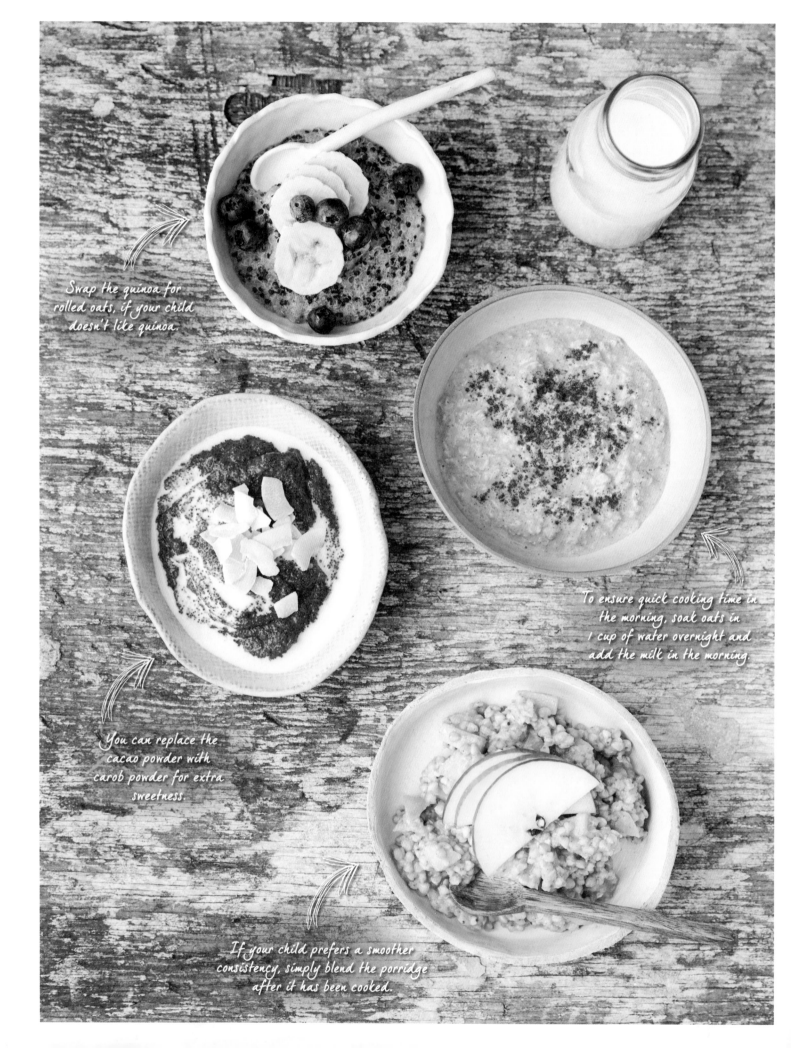

Swap the quinoa for rolled oats, if your child doesn't like quinoa.

You can replace the cacao powder with carob powder for extra sweetness.

To ensure quick cooking time in the morning, soak oats in 1 cup of water overnight and add the milk in the morning.

If your child prefers a smoother consistency, simply blend the porridge after it has been cooked.

Apple Buckini Porridge

INGREDIENTS

1 cup (5³/₅ oz) buckinis (activated buckwheat groats)

1 cup filtered water

1 cup coconut milk or mik of choice

1 tbs flaxseed meal

2 apples, peeled and grated

½–1 tsp ground cinnamon

1 tbs maple syrup or raw honey (optional)

INSTRUCTIONS

In a small saucepan, add buckinis and water and bring to a boil.

Turn heat down and simmer for 5 mins.

Add coconut milk, flaxseed meal, apples, cinnamon and maple syrup and simmer for another 5 mins.

Allow to cool slightly before serving.

Serving and storing leftovers: Serve immediately, store in the fridge for up to 4 days or freeze for up to 4 months.

Choc Coconut Porridge

INGREDIENTS

½ cup (3½ oz) brown teff grain

1½ cup almond milk

1 cup filtered water

1 tbs maple syrup (optional)

1 tbs raw cacao powder

1 tbs carob powder

pinch sea salt

½ banana, mashed

½ banana, sliced

¼ cup (1¼ oz) flaked almonds

extra milk for serving

INSTRUCTIONS

Place brown teff grain, milk, and water into a pot and cook for 15–20 mins with the lid on. Stir regularly until mixture is creamy.

Add maple syrup, cacao, carob, salt, and mashed banana and stir to combine.

Serve warm in bowls topped with sliced banana, flaked almonds, and extra milk on top.

Serving and storing leftovers: Serve immediately or store in an airtight container in the fridge for up to 4 days.

Gluten Free

Egg Free

Vegan

Quinoa Blueberry Porridge

INGREDIENTS

1 cup (6¹/₃ oz) quinoa, rinsed and drained

2 cups filtered water

1 tbs chia seeds

1 tsp pure vanilla extract

½ tsp ground cinnamon or 1 cinnamon stick

1 cup coconut milk or milk of choice

1–2 tbs coconut flour

1 tbs maple syrup or raw honey (optional)

1 ripe banana, mashed

½ cup (2⁴/₅ oz) blueberries, frozen or fresh

INSTRUCTIONS

Place quinoa, water, chia seeds, vanilla, and cinnamon in a medium-sized saucepan and bring to the boil. Reduce heat and simmer for 15 mins or until all liquid is absorbed, stirring occasionally.

Add coconut milk, coconut flour, and maple syrup and simmer for another 5 mins.

Fold in mashed banana and blueberries.

Serve warm in bowls.

Serving and storing leftovers: Serve immediately, store in the fridge for up to 4 days or freeze for up to 4 months.

Pumpkin Porridge

INGREDIENTS

1 cup (4¼ oz) gluten-free rolled oats

1 cup almond milk or milk of choice

1 cup filtered water

¹/₃ cup (2⁴/₅ oz) butternut squash, peeled, steamed and pureed

1 tsp ground cinnamon

1 tbs maple syrup (optional)

½ tsp pure vanilla extract

½ tbs coconut oil, ghee or butter

INSTRUCTIONS

Place oats, almond milk and water in a medium-sized saucepan and bring to a boil. Reduce heat and simmer for about 5 mins until thick and creamy.

Add squash puree, cinnamon, maple syrup, and vanilla and stir to combine. Simmer on low heat for another 2 mins.

Remove from heat, add coconut oil, and stir through.

Allow to cool a little before serving.

Serving and storing leftovers: Serve immediately, store in the fridge for up to 4 days or freeze for up to 4 months.

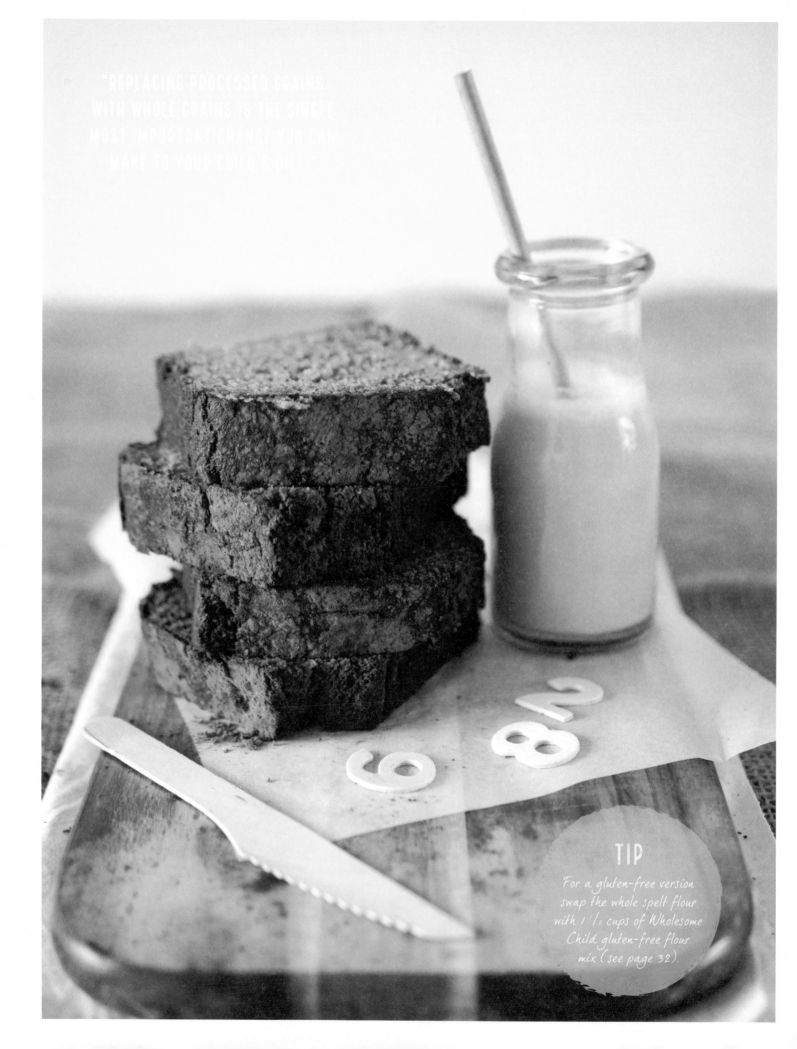

"REPLACING PROCESSED GRAINS WITH WHOLE GRAINS IS THE SINGLE MOST IMPORTANT CHANGE YOU CAN MAKE TO YOUR CHILD'S DIET."

TIP

For a gluten-free version, swap the whole spelt flour with 1 ½ cups of Wholesome Child gluten-free flour mix (see page 32).

Dairy Free | Nut Free | Vegetarian

Prep time: 15 mins
Cooking time: 55 mins
Makes: 1 loaf

Banana Bread

Store-bought banana breads are often overloaded with processed flours, sugars, and unhealthy fats. This far healthier version contains wholegrain spelt flour, a reduced amount of unprocessed sugar, coconut oil, and chia seeds.

INGREDIENTS

2 large ripe bananas

3 large eggs

½ cup coconut milk

4–6 Medjool dates, pitted

1 tbs chia seeds

½ cup coconut oil, melted

1½ cups (7²/₅ oz) whole spelt flour

⅓ cup–½ cup (2–2³/₅ oz) coconut sugar

1 tsp pure vanilla extract

1 tsp ground cinnamon

1 tsp baking powder

½ tsp baking soda

pinch sea salt

EQUIPMENT

high-speed food processor

INSTRUCTIONS

Preheat oven to 355°F and line a medium-sized loaf tin with baking paper.

Place bananas, eggs, milk, dates, chia seeds, and coconut oil in a high-speed blender and process for approximately 1 min or until it reaches a smooth consistency.

In a separate bowl whisk together spelt flour, coconut sugar, vanilla, cinnamon, baking powder, baking soda, and salt.

Slowly add dry ingredients into wet mixture and mix together on a medium speed.

Pour mixture into the loaf tin and sprinkle extra cinnamon on top.

Bake for approximately 45–55 mins or until a cake tester or knife comes out clean.

Allow to cool completely before cutting.

Serving and storing leftovers: Serve immediately, store in an airtight container in the fridge for up to a week or freeze for up to 4 months.

Vegetarian | Gluten Free | Nut Free

Prep time: 10 mins
Cooking time: 45–50 mins
Makes: 1 loaf

Gluten-free Yogurt Bread

INGREDIENTS

2½ cups (11½ oz) Wholesome Child gluten-free flour mix (see page 32)

1 tbs baking powder

1 tsp sea salt

1 tsp coconut sugar

1 tbs psyllium husks

1 tbs extra virgin olive oil

2 eggs

1 cup (9 1/6 oz) natural yogurt or coconut yogurt

1 cup (6 2/5 oz) zucchini, peeled and grated (optional)

EQUIPMENT

high-speed food processor

INSTRUCTIONS

Preheat oven to 375°F and flour a bread loaf tin (10" x 5").

Place all dry ingredients into a food processor and process until combined.

Add oil, eggs, and yogurt and process until it resembles homogenous dough.

Fold in grated zucchini, if using, and place mixture in the loaf tin.

Sprinkle some extra flour on top (about 1 tbs).

Bake for 45–50 mins. Leave to cool in loaf tin.

Serving and storing leftovers: Serve immediately, store in a paper bag for up to 4 days or in the fridge for up to a week, or freeze for up to 4 months.

Substitute the gluten-free flour with spelt flour. If your child doesn't eat green foods, leave out zucchini or replace with 1 cup grated carrot.

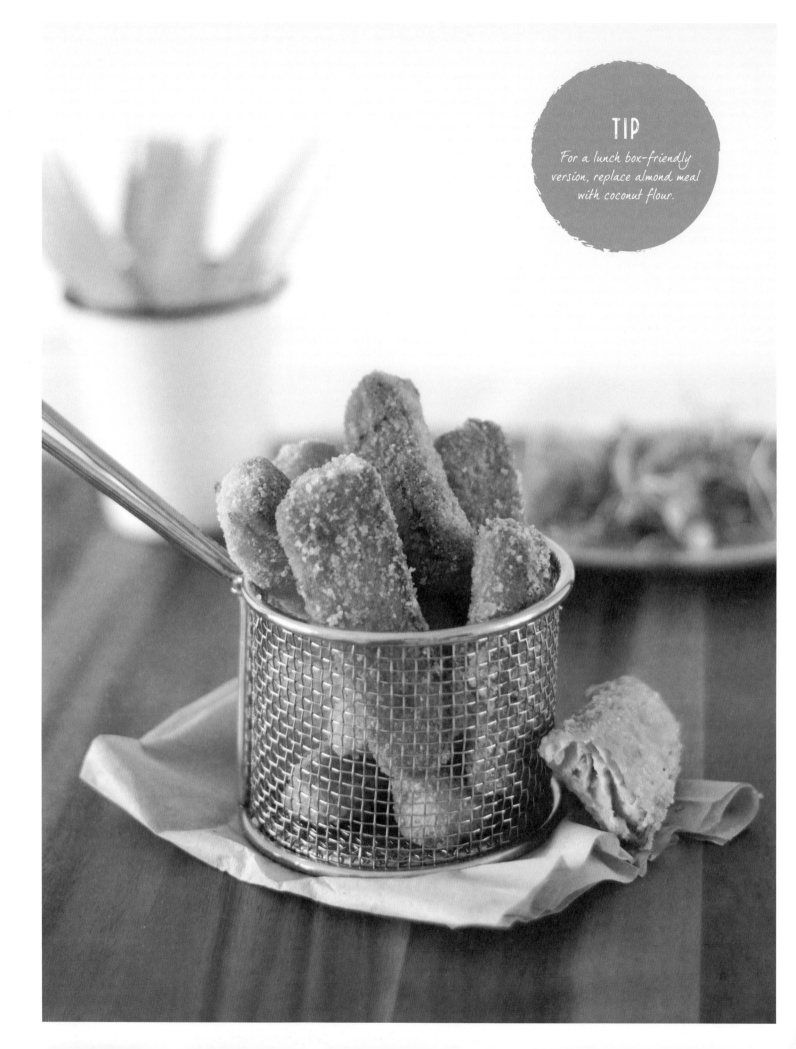

TIP

For a lunch box–friendly
version, replace almond meal
with coconut flour.

Gluten Free

Dairy Free

Prep time: 15 mins
Cooking time: 10 mins
Serves: 5–6

Fish Fingers

I tried for some time to create homemade fish fingers that can wean even the fussiest of eaters off the store-bought versions. So many of my clients with fussy eaters have had success with this recipe.

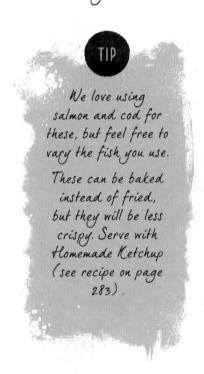

TIP

We love using salmon and cod for these, but feel free to vary the fish you use.

These can be baked instead of fried, but they will be less crispy. Serve with Homemade Ketchup (see recipe on page 283).

INGREDIENTS

1 cup (3¼ oz) rice bread crumbs

½ cup (2⅕ oz) almond meal

½ tsp Himalayan rock salt

½ cup (2⅕ oz) arrowroot powder or ½ cup organic cornstarch

1–2 tbs milk of choice

3 large eggs, lightly beaten

1 lb salmon or cod cut into finger-sized pieces (about the size of a dessert spoon)

1–2 tbs coconut oil

EQUIPMENT

high-speed food processor

INSTRUCTIONS

In a medium-sized bowl, combine the bread crumbs, almond meal, and a sprinkle of the salt and mix together.

In a separate bowl place the arrowroot or organic cornstarch.

In a shallow bowl, combine the milk and egg and whisk together using a fork.

Place the pieces of fish on a large plate and sprinkle with salt.

Dip each chunk separately into the arrowroot, then into the egg mix and finally into the bread crumbs. Press down firmly to ensure that each fish finger has a thick coating of the breadcrumb mix.

Coat a large frying pan with 1–2 tbs coconut oil and set over medium heat.

Place the fish fingers (as many as you can fit) to a single layer. Make sure that the fingers are not touching each other and that there is enough room to turn them over.

Cook for approximately 3–4 mins on each side or until golden brown.

Season with remaining salt if necessary.

Serving and storing leftovers: Serve warm. Once cooked, can be stored in the fridge for up to 3 days or frozen cooked for up to 4 months.

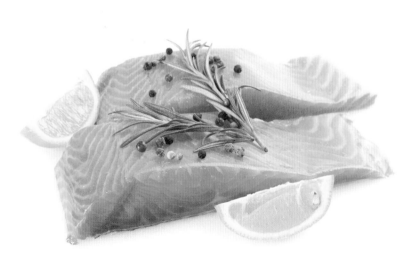

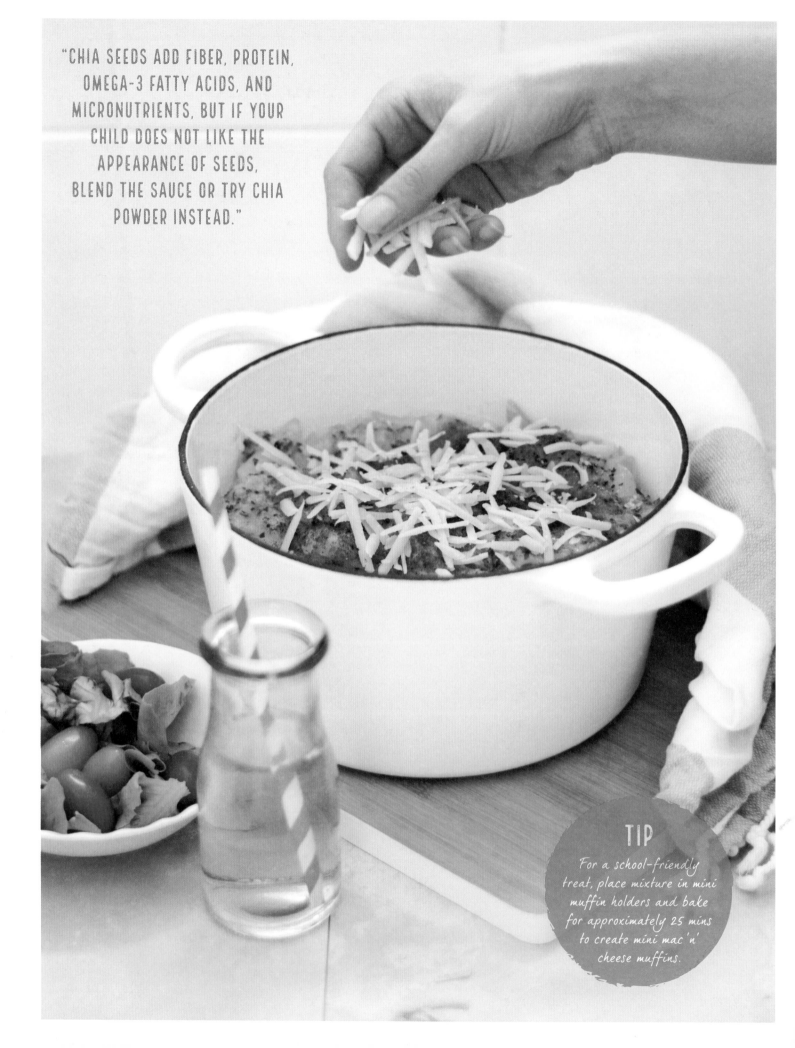

"CHIA SEEDS ADD FIBER, PROTEIN, OMEGA-3 FATTY ACIDS, AND MICRONUTRIENTS, BUT IF YOUR CHILD DOES NOT LIKE THE APPEARANCE OF SEEDS, BLEND THE SAUCE OR TRY CHIA POWDER INSTEAD."

TIP
For a school-friendly treat, place mixture in mini muffin holders and bake for approximately 25 mins to create mini mac 'n' cheese muffins.

VEG
Vegetarian

Gluten Free

Egg Free

Nut Free

Prep time: 30 mins
Cooking time: 30 mins
Serves: 4

Mac 'n' Cheese

Quality ingredients like preservative-free cheese, wholegrain pasta, vegetables, and chia seeds turn this dinner staple into a nutritious choice. I often send leftovers to school in the lunch box.

INGREDIENTS

2 cups (7 oz) brown rice penne

1 cup (7 oz) cauliflower florets

1 cup (7 oz) zucchini, peeled and shredded

1–2 tbs coconut oil

3/4 cup milk of choice

1 tbs tapioca flour

1 1/2 cup (4 1/4 oz) cheddar cheese, shredded

1 tbs chia seeds

sea salt and pepper, to taste

1 tsp paprika powder

EQUIPMENT

high-speed food processor

INSTRUCTIONS

Preheat oven to 355°F.

Cook the pasta until al dente. Drain and set aside.

Place cauliflower in a food processor and process until it reaches a rice-like consistency.

Heat oil in a large frying pan and sauté cauliflower and zucchini for about 5 mins.

In a saucepan, warm 1/2 cup of milk.

In a small bowl, whisk together the remaining milk and the flour until there are no lumps. Then whisk this mixture into the warm milk. Continue whisking gently until milk thickens to the consistency of heavy cream.

Mix cheese, chia seeds, sautéed cauliflower and zucchini into the milk-flour mixture and season with salt and pepper. For a smoother consistency you can process using a hand held blender.

Place the pasta in a casserole dish and pour the cheese and veggie sauce over it. Sprinkle with paprika powder and grated cheese (optional) and bake in the oven for 30 mins until the top is golden.

Serving and storing leftovers: Serve immediately, store in the fridge for up to 4 days or freeze for up to 4 months.

Egg Free

Gluten Free

Nut Free

Prep time: 30 mins
Cooking time: 55 mins
Makes: 15 small balls

Quinoa & Brown Rice Chicken Balls

INGREDIENTS

1 tbs extra virgin olive oil or avocado oil, for greasing tin

1 chicken breast

1 quart filtered water, chicken or vegetable stock

1–2 tbs extra virgin olive oil, or avocado oil

1/2 medium leek, finely sliced

1–2 cloves garlic, crushed

1 tsp fresh mixed herbs or cilantro

1 cup (5 oz) butternut squash or sweet

potato, peeled and diced

1/2 cup (1/2 oz) baby spinach, chopped

1 cup (7 oz) cooked brown rice

1 cup (5 2/3 oz) cooked quinoa

sea salt, to taste

1/2 cup (2 4/5 oz) mozzarella, cubed

1/3 cup (1 oz) rice crumbs

EQUIPMENT

hand-held blender

INSTRUCTIONS

Preheat oven to 390°F and grease three mini muffin trays with some oil. You can also place balls on a baking tray lined with baking paper.

In a medium-sized saucepan, poach the chicken breast in water or stock for around 20 mins. Allow to cool and cut into fine strips (shred).

In a small frying pan, heat oil over medium heat, add leek, garlic, and herbs and sauté for approximately 3 mins, or until leek is glassy.

Add butternut, cover with lid, and allow to cook for approximately 10 mins or until soft. You may need to add more oil or 1/2 to 1 cup of filtered water to prevent burning.

Add spinach and cook for another 2 mins then transfer cooked veggies to a bowl and, using a hand held blender, process until smooth.

In a large bowl, combine chicken, rice, quinoa, vegetable mix, and salt.

Take 1/4 cup of the mixture and wrap around one cheese cube to form a little ball. Continue until the rice mix is finished.

Place rice crumbs on a plate and roll each ball in the crumbs until covered.

Place balls in muffin trays or on baking tray. Bake for 15–20 mins or until golden brown and crispy on top.

Serving and storing leftovers: Serve immediately, store in the fridge for up to 3 days or freeze for up to 3 months.

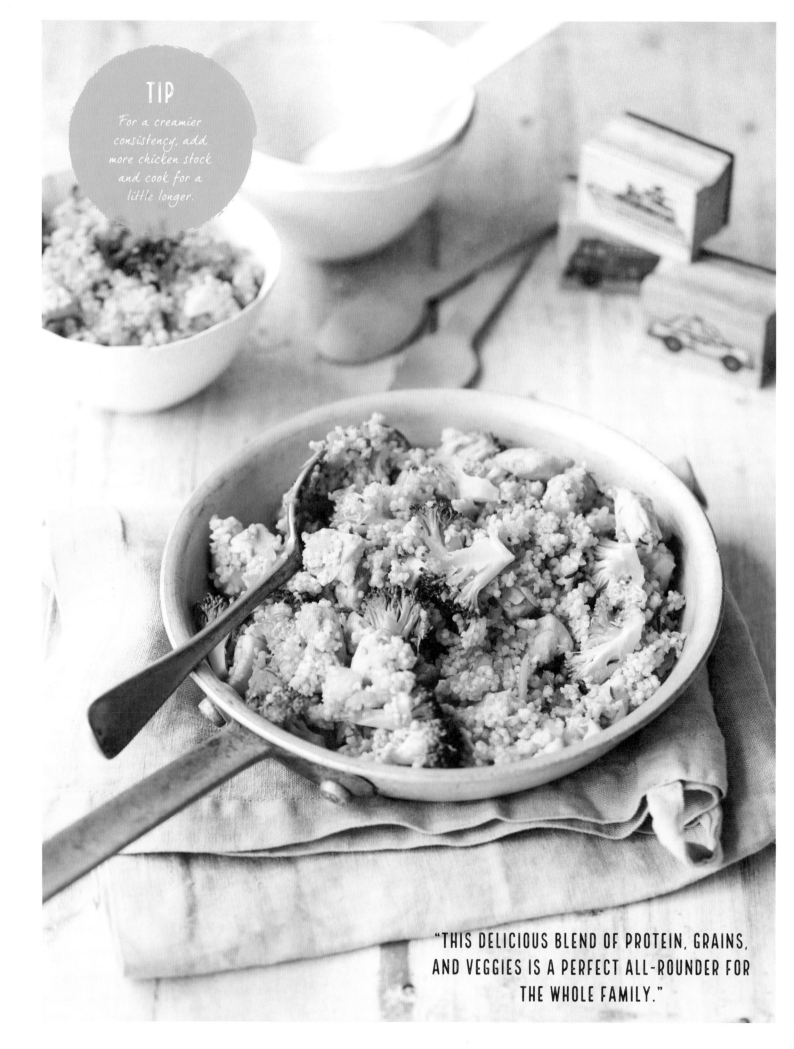

TIP

For a creamier consistency, add more chicken stock and cook for a little longer.

"THIS DELICIOUS BLEND OF PROTEIN, GRAINS, AND VEGGIES IS A PERFECT ALL-ROUNDER FOR THE WHOLE FAMILY."

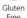

Gluten Free · Egg Free

Prep time: 15 mins
Cooking time: 15 mins
Serves: 2

Chicken Millet Pilaf

Millet, one of the most alkaline grains rich in B vitamins, calcium, and magnesium, is often overlooked as a supergrain. It has a nutty flavor and is a perfect, gluten-free replacement for couscous.

INGREDIENTS

1 tbs extra virgin olive oil

1 yellow onion, finely diced

2 cloves garlic, finely diced

1 chicken breast, cubed

1 medium carrot, peeled and grated

1 medium zucchini, peeled and grated

2 tbs sundried tomatoes, diced

1 cup (6¾ oz) millet

2 cups chicken stock or filtered water

half head broccoli, cut into florets

juice of ½ lemon

2 tbs fresh basil or cilantro

sea salt and pepper, to taste

4 tbs natural yogurt (to serve)

INSTRUCTIONS

Heat oil over medium heat in a medium-sized pot. Add onion and garlic and sauté for 2 mins.

Add chicken and cook until lightly browned.

Add carrot, zucchini, and sundried tomatoes and sauté for another minute.

Add millet and chicken stock and bring to the boil. Simmer on low heat for approximately 5 mins, stirring occasionally.

Add broccoli and cook for a further 5 mins, stirring occasionally, until the stock has evaporated.

Season with lemon juice, basil, and salt and pepper.

Spoon into bowls and drizzle with yogurt.

Serving and storing leftovers: Serve immediately. Store in an airtight container in the fridge for up to 3 days or freeze for up to 4 months.

 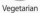

VEG · Vegetarian · Gluten Free · Dairy Free · Nut Free

Prep time: 15 mins
Cooking time: 15–20 mins
Serves: 3–4

Quinoa Fried Rice with Vegetables

INGREDIENTS

1 cup (6 2/5 oz) quinoa, rinsed and drained

pinch mild curry powder

2 cups vegetable stock or filtered water

1 tbs extra virgin olive oil, or coconut oil

½ yellow onion, finely diced

1–2 cloves garlic, crushed

1 zucchini, diced

1 cup (3½ oz) cauliflower florets, diced

½ cup (2⅕ oz) peas

squeeze of lemon

sea salt and pepper, to taste

2 eggs, lightly whisked

INSTRUCTIONS

Add quinoa and curry powder to a medium-sized pot and place on medium heat. Toast for 2 mins, stirring occasionally. Add vegetable stock, put a lid on top and simmer until all stock has evaporated.

Heat oil in a frying pan over medium heat. Add onion and garlic and cook until lightly browned.

Add zucchini, cauliflower, and peas and sauté for 5–10 mins or until cooked.

Combine vegetable mixture with quinoa and add a squeeze of lemon juice and salt and pepper.

Add eggs and stir until heated through.

Serving and storing leftovers: Serve immediately, store in an airtight container in the fridge for up to 4 days or freeze for up to 4 months.

If you prefer to make fried rice the traditional way you can also fry the eggs separately, chop them up and combine them with the quinoa mixture as a last step.

Egg Free | Gluten Free | Dairy Free

Prep time: 30 mins (+ 30 mins marinating time)
Makes: 20 rolls

Asian-style Rice Paper Rolls

INGREDIENTS

2 chicken breasts, cut into strips

20 rice paper wraps

MARINADE
⅓ cup tamari

2 garlic cloves, crushed

½ tsp ground ginger

2 tbs raw honey

½ tsp cold-pressed sesame oil

2–3 tbs extra virgin olive oil or coconut oil

2 tbs fresh cilantro, finely chopped

squeeze of lemon

RICE PAPER WRAPS
vermicelli rice noodles (2 oz)

1 large carrot, cut into fine strips

1 medium-sized cucumber, cut into fine strips

1 large avocado, sliced

fresh cilantro leaves

INSTRUCTIONS

For the marinade, place all the marinade ingredients into a medium-sized bowl and mix together. Place chicken strips in bowl and mix together ensuring that the chicken is completely coated. Cover and place in fridge for 30 mins to 1 hr.

Place rice noodles in a medium-sized bowl and cover with boiling water. Let sit for 10 mins. Drain and set aside.

Put a medium-sized frying pan on high heat and cook the marinated chicken strips for approximately 2–3 mins on each side, or until cooked through. Set aside and allow to cool.

Half-fill a large, shallow bowl with hot water. Dip 1 rice paper wrapper in water. Soak for 10 to 20 seconds or until it starts to soften. Remove, allowing excess water to drain. Place on a large plate.

Place 1–2 chicken strips, 2 carrot strips, 2 cucumber strips, slice of avocado, a few rice noodles and cilantro on one edge of rice paper, leaving ¾" at each end (don't overfill or wrapper will split). Fold edges in and roll up to enclose filling. Place roll, seam side down, on a plate. Continue with remaining ingredients.

Serving and storing leftovers:
Serve immediately or store in the fridge for up to 2 days.

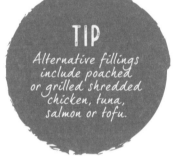

TIP
Alternative fillings include poached or grilled shredded chicken, tuna, salmon or tofu.

Egg Free | Gluten Free | Nut Free | VEG Vegetarian

Prep time: 15 mins
Cooking time: 20–25 mins
Makes: 50 crackers

Teff & Parmesan Crackers

INGREDIENTS

½ cup (3 oz) brown teff flour

½ cup (2⅕ oz) arrowroot

⅓ cup (25g) Parmesan, grated (optional)

½ tsp sea salt

2 tbs ghee or coconut oil, melted

¼ cup + 2 tbs filtered water

TOPPINGS (optional):
chia seeds, sesame seeds, poppy seeds, flaxseeds

INSTRUCTIONS

Preheat oven to 350°F. Grease and line two baking trays.

Combine teff flour, arrowroot, Parmesan and salt in a medium-sized bowl.

Add ghee and water and form a dough, using your hands. Knead until well combined.

Divide dough into 2 batches and place one half in between 2 sheets of baking paper. Using a rolling pin, roll out dough to about ⅛" thick.

Take top baking sheet off and using a pizza cutter, cut dough into 1½" x 1½" squares.

Brush top with some water and sprinkle with some seeds if desired.

Transfer to a baking tray. Repeat with other half of the dough and place on a second baking tray. Bake for 20–25 mins or until golden. It will crisp up once it cools down.

Leave to cool on a wire rack.

Serving and storing leftovers:
Serve immediately, store in an airtight container for up to 2 weeks or in the fridge for up to 1 month.

Replace the teff flour and arrowroot with 1 cup of Wholesome Child gluten-free flour mix or 1 cup whole spelt flour. For a dairy-free version leave out Parmesan cheese.

Nut Free Egg Free Gluten Free

Prep time: 15 mins
Cooking time: 35–40 mins
Serves: 4

Tuna, Vegetables & Chia Lasagne

INGREDIENTS

1 tbs coconut oil or extra virgin olive oil

1 large yellow onion, finely diced

2 garlic cloves, finely diced

1 medium carrot, grated

1 medium zucchini, grated

2 cups (7 oz) button mushrooms, diced

3 cups (1³⁄₄ lbs) tomato puree or pasta sauce

¹⁄₄ cup fresh parsley, finely chopped

15 oz canned tuna

sea salt and pepper, to taste

6–8 rice lasagne sheets (or spelt for a non gluten-free version)

BÉCHAMEL SAUCE

3 tbs unsalted butter

¹⁄₃ cup (1¹⁄₃ oz) arrowroot

3 cups coconut milk or milk of choice

1 cup to 1¹⁄₂ cups (2⁴⁄₅ oz to 4¹⁄₄ oz) cheddar cheese, grated

sea salt, to taste

1 tbs chia seeds

INSTRUCTIONS

Preheat oven to 355°F.

Heat oil in a large saucepan and sauté onion and garlic for 2–3 mins or until soft.

Add carrot, zucchini, mushroom, tomato puree, tuna, and parsley and cook, covered, over low heat for approximately 15 mins, stirring occasionally. Season with sea salt and pepper.

In a medium-sized saucepan, melt the butter over medium heat.

Add arrowroot and whisk quickly to combine, then add milk, one cup at a time, and cook until it thickens, whisking regularly.

Stir in grated cheese, season with sea salt, and set aside.

In a medium-sized casserole dish, place the lasagne sheets, then the tomato and tuna mix, then béchamel sauce. Continue layering in this way with the rest of the sheets and finish with a layer of béchamel sauce.

Sprinkle chia seeds over the top layer. and bake in the oven for 30–45 mins.

Serving and storing leftovers: Serve immediately, store in the fridge for up to 3 days or freeze for up to 4 months.

If you want to use fresh fish, simply cook the fish with the onions until browned on both sides, then continue with recipe.

V Vegan Nut Free

Prep time: 15–20 mins
Cooking time: 16 mins
Makes: 8 tortilla wraps

Wholesome Kamut Tortilla Wraps

INGREDIENTS

³⁄₄ cup (3³⁄₄ oz) wholegrain kamut flour

¹⁄₄ cup (1 oz) tapioca flour

¹⁄₂ tsp sea salt

¹⁄₄ cup extra virgin olive oil

¹⁄₃ cup filtered warm water

INSTRUCTIONS

Place flours and salt in a medium-sized bowl and whisk to combine.

Stir in olive oil and warm water.

Turn mixture onto a floured surface and knead for 2 mins, adding a little flour or water if needed to achieve a smooth dough. Let rest for 10 mins.

Divide dough into eight portions. On a lightly floured surface, roll each portion into a 5¹⁄₂" circle.

In a large non-stick skillet cook tortillas over medium heat for 1 min on each side or until lightly browned. Keep warm.

Serving and storing leftovers: Serve immediately, store in the fridge for up to 4 days.

For a gluten-free version try our Arrowroot Tortillas (see recipe on page 153).

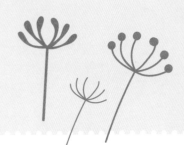

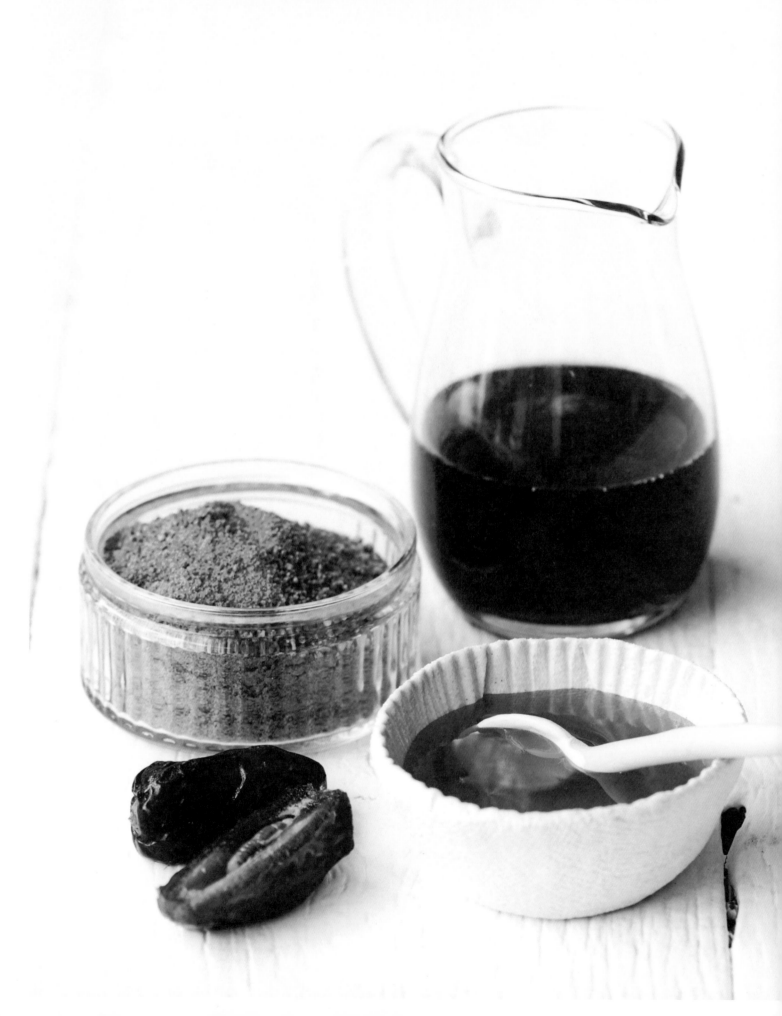

STEP 2

Reduce Sugar

SET HEALTHY LIMITS AND CREATE STRUCTURE

I am genuinely passionate and interested in all things nutrition-related. Sugar, in particular, is the area that I get questioned about the most.

Refined sugar regularly receives bad press, but despite what you may have read or heard, I believe there is nothing wrong with a little bit of sweetness in your child's diet. With a few simple tweaks to some of your favorite recipes, your family can still enjoy these types of foods in moderation.

As with so many things, moderation and balance is key. I am all for encouraging a diet that is largely free of refined sugars, but I'm also a mother and a realist and I know that the occasional sweet treat is not going to cause any long-term damage.

Before I get to the recommended sugar intake and which sweeteners are most nutrient-dense for children, let's first get a clearer understanding of why sugar has become so demonized.

The short answer is this—as our food supply has changed, we've unknowingly begun to consume too much sugar that is often hidden in processed foods once considered healthy. Things like vegetable soups, pasta sauce, yogurt, bagels or muesli all have significant quantities of hidden refined sugar.

Nutrition information panels on packaged foods don't always help us to navigate the sugar minefield, as different types of sugars are usually disguised or listed together as one component under the label "sugar." Because of this, it's important to look closely at the ingredients list to understand what type of sugar is in your child's favorite foods, identify its many hidden names, and look for non-processed healthier alternatives.

WHY WORRY ABOUT ADDED SUGAR?

1. Diabetes. Type 2 diabetes most often occurs in adults, usually after the age of thirty. Just fifteen years ago it was unheard of for children or teenagers to develop the disease. These days, increasing numbers of teenagers and children are developing type 2 diabetes or the pre-diabetic condition known as impaired glucose tolerance, which occurs when the glucose (sugar) in your child's blood is higher than normal, but not high enough to be called diabetes.

Both prediabetes and type 2 diabetes can result when the body becomes less sensitive to insulin (a hormone that helps regulate blood sugar levels), and both are associated with a variety of serious health problems, including heart disease and even infertility. To make matters worse, type 2 diabetes advances with complications more rapidly in children than in adults.

Endocrinologists warn that a high-sugar diet raises the risk of type 2 diabetes and impaired glucose tolerance directly, by overworking the pancreas, the organ that produces insulin.

According to the CDC, by the year 2050, one in three people will have diabetes. Please replace this sentence with:

More than 5,000 new cases of type-2 diabetes are estimated to be diagnosed among US youth younger than 20 years each year. So how can we make sure our children avoid this? Help your child to maintain a healthy, low-sugar diet and an active lifestyle.

2. Obesity. One in three US children is overweight or obese. According to the 2015–2016 NHANES data, about 20 percent of school-aged children (ages six to nineteen) are obese; about 14 percent of children ages two to five are obese. The percentage of children with obesity in the US has more than tripled since the 1970s. Children with obesity are bullied and teased more than their normal weight peers, and are more likely to suffer from social isolation,

Consider this…

Sugar alone doesn't make kids overweight or obese. Children gain too much weight when they take in more calories than they burn. Sugary drinks and treats that go down very quickly supply calories above and beyond what kids need. According to the American Academy of Pediatrics (AAP) drinking even one sugary drink a day, such as fruit juice, may increase the risk of obesity in children.

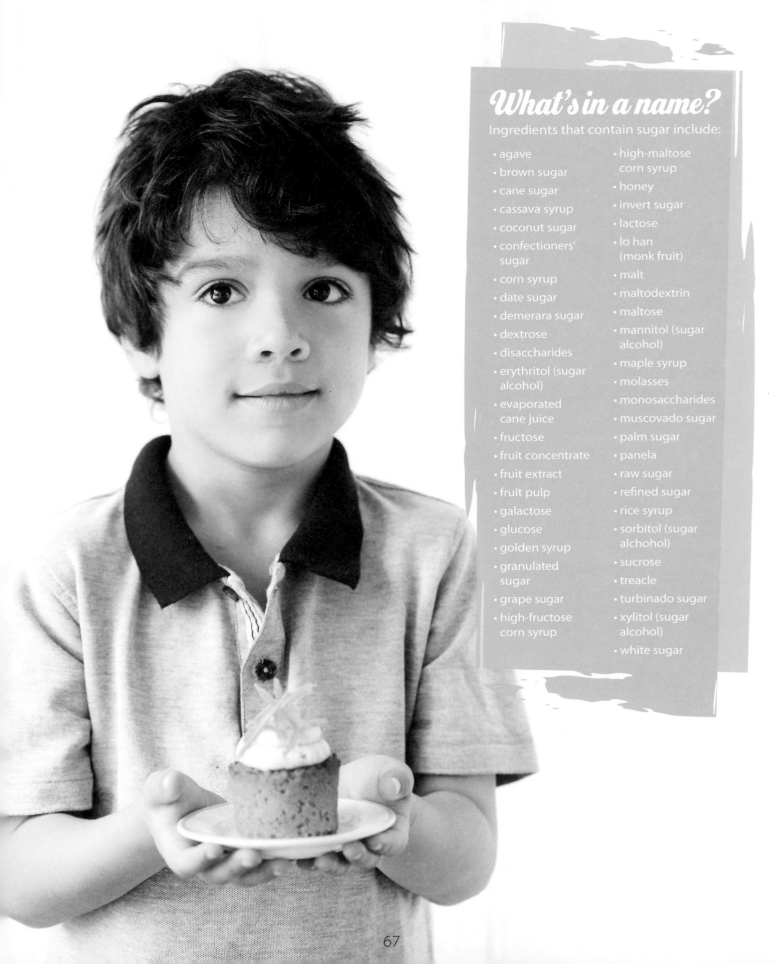

What's in a name?

Ingredients that contain sugar include:

- agave
- brown sugar
- cane sugar
- cassava syrup
- coconut sugar
- confectioners' sugar
- corn syrup
- date sugar
- demerara sugar
- dextrose
- disaccharides
- erythritol (sugar alcohol)
- evaporated cane juice
- fructose
- fruit concentrate
- fruit extract
- fruit pulp
- galactose
- glucose
- golden syrup
- granulated sugar
- grape sugar
- high-fructose corn syrup
- high-maltose corn syrup
- honey
- invert sugar
- lactose
- lo han (monk fruit)
- malt
- maltodextrin
- maltose
- mannitol (sugar alcohol)
- maple syrup
- molasses
- monosaccharides
- muscovado sugar
- palm sugar
- panela
- raw sugar
- refined sugar
- rice syrup
- sorbitol (sugar alchohol)
- sucrose
- treacle
- turbinado sugar
- xylitol (sugar alcohol)
- white sugar

DID YOU KNOW?

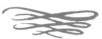

Children or teens with type 1 or 2 diabetes often feel no symptoms at all. However it's important to be aware of some common symptoms: Increased thirst, hunger even after eating, frequent or nighttime urination, blurry vision, unusual fatigue.

depression, and lower self-esteem. Children who become obese are also likely to stay obese into adulthood, placing them at greater risk of suffering from obesity-related chronic diseases such as diabetes, cardiovascular disease, certain cancers and other complications.

3. Immune function. When sweet sugary foods start to replace nutritious foods in the diet, deficiencies can occur such as reduced zinc intake. Adequate zinc levels are essential to maintaining a healthy immune system and proper growth and development in childhood. Low zinc levels are associated with recurrent childhood infections such as pneumonia and the common cold. Low zinc not only affects the immune system, it also dulls the sense of taste and smell, causing children to become less able to recognize new and unique flavors and they only want to eat foods that have been sweetened. Research also shows children with Attention Deficit Disorder (ADHD) have lowered levels of zinc in their blood. Improving zinc levels in children with ADHD has been shown to reduce symptoms of hyperactivity, impulsivity, and impaired socialization. Good sources include spinach, sunflower seeds, almonds, and beef.

4. Cavities. Sugar alone doesn't cause cavities, but it fuels the growth of the bacteria that do. That's why dentists advise against offering fruit juice over water or feeding your child raisins and other dried fruit that tends to stick to the teeth. An average 1½ oz box of raisins contains nearly six spoonfuls of sugar. Even smaller ½ oz boxes contain up to three teaspoons of sugar.

TOO MUCH SUGAR:

✓ increases the risk of type 2 diabetes.
✓ increases the likelihood of being overweight or obese.
✓ increases the risk of certain cancers.
✓ depletes the immune system.
✓ contributes to learning and concentration difficulties.
✓ contributes to anxiety, depression, and mood swings.
✓ increases the chance of fungal infections such as candida.
✓ disrupts the balance of beneficial and harmful bacteria in children's guts leading to chronic conditions such as eczema, allergies, leaky gut, and food sensitivities.
✓ causes imbalances in blood sugar levels —sugar highs followed by shaky sugar lows.
✓ is linked to tooth decay and cavities.
✓ is highly addictive, and has a drug-like

response. The more sugar a child eats, the more he or she wants.

ADDED VS NATURAL SUGARS: WHAT'S THE DIFFERENCE?

When it comes to sugar, you are specifically looking to monitor the amount of added sugars in packaged foods. These are any sugars that are added to a product, including refined or processed sugars such as cane sugar, high fructose corn syrup, sucrose, glucose as well as natural sweeteners like honey, maple syrup, coconut sugar, brown rice syrup, and molasses.

Natural or intrinsic sugars are those sugars that occur naturally in foods, like lactose in milk and fructose in whole fruit. Natural sugars are not limited like added sugars are because they are naturally occurring and accompanied by a host of other valuable nutrients like protein and calcium (in milk) or fiber and vitamins (in fruit). To reduce the added sugar in your child's diet, choose fresh or minimally processed foods, and always check the ingredients list of any packaged food to ensure that no added sugars have been included.

SUGAR VS SUGAR ALCOHOLS

When scanning ingredients, keep in mind that anything ending in the letters "ose" is a form of sugar, while anything ending in "ol" is a form of sugar alcohol. Sugar alcohols deliver fewer calories than sugar and have less of an effect on blood-sugar levels. Unfortunately, they're also void of any nutrients, often derived from genetically modified (GM) corn, and can cause significant tummy upsets. For these reasons I don't recommend them for children.

HOW MUCH SUGAR CAN CHILDREN EAT?

A study conducted by the American Heart Association (AHA), found children as young as 1-3 years of age typically consume around 12 teaspoons of sugar per day. Between the ages of four and eight years old, average sugar consumption skyrockets to around 21 teaspoons a day!

Ever since 1989, the World Health Organization (WHO) has recommended we eat no more than 12 1/2 teaspoons of added sugar per day (50grams), no matter what our age, to significantly reduce our risk of being overweight or obese, and to prevent tooth decay. Research shows that children with the highest intake of sugar-sweetened drinks are more likely to be overweight or obese than children with a low intake of these drinks. Numerous studies have also shown a link between diets that are high in added sugars, and conditions leading to cardiovascular disease. The AHA recommends that children eat less than 6 teaspoons (25 grams) of added sugar per day, to lower the risk of obesity and other risk factors for heart disease. This is in line with the 2015–2020 Dietary Guidelines for Americans, which recommends that children and adults consume less than 10 percent of their daily calories from added sugars.

As recently as 2015, the WHO revised its guidelines recommending we reduce our daily intake of added sugars to below 5%, roughly 3 teaspoons (12.5 grams) for young children per day, to achieve greater health benefits. Meeting these added sugar guidelines, as any parent can attest, can be challenging when sugar in our food and drink can add up so quickly. For example, a child who eats a half of a sliced turkey sandwich with two small chocolate chip cookies and a can of soda gets about 12 teaspoons (48 grams) of added sugar—more than a day's worth of sugar—at lunch alone. A whole grain turkey sandwich with a handful of grapes, carrot sticks and a glass of water is a more nutritious and filling choice.

The AHA also recommends that children under age two should not consume any added sugars at all given that their calorie needs are less than older children, leaving little room for sugary foods or drinks that provide little nutrition. Instead, serve mostly nutrient-rich foods such as vegetables, fruit, whole grains, healthy fats, protein and dairy, which are good for growing children's brains and bodies. At that age, a home-baked muffin sweetened with banana alone will suffice as a treat.

WHAT IS GLYCEMIC INDEX?

The Glycemic Index (GI) of a food measures how much the given food affects blood-sugar levels. A high GI rating means blood-sugar levels are increased quickly and the pancreas is stimulated to release insulin to keep blood sugar at a constant and safe level. Over time, this can lead to insulin resistance (a pre-diabetic condition) or diabetes. Sucrose has a GI of 58 to 65 and raw or Manuka honey has a GI of 35 to 55. The lower the GI rating, the slower the absorption and digestion of sugar.

HOW MUCH SUGAR DOES IT HAVE?

The amount of sugar listed on the nutrition labels of packaged foods, includes all types of sugar, whether naturally occurring intrinsic sugar from fruit (fructose) and milk (lactose), or added sugar, in the form of cane sugar, high-fructose corn syrup, honey or agave. Even seemingly healthy foods can contain as much as 50 grams of sugar (12½ teaspoons). The key is to always read nutrition labels carefully, even if the package says "100% juice" or "25% less sugar."

4 GRAMS OF SUGAR = ONE TEASPOON

PRODUCT	AMOUNT OF SUGAR	EQUIVALENT
1 cup soft drink (e.g., lemonade or cola)	39g	10 tsp
1 milk chocolate bar (1½ oz)	25g	6¼ tsp
5 oz flavored yogurt or squeezie yogurt	22g	5⅓ tsp
Energy drink (1 bottle)	37g	9¼ tsp
Canned peaches in light syrup, 1 small serving cup	12g	3 tsp
Nutri-Grain Cereal Bars (all flavors): 1 bar	12g	3 tsp
Jarred pasta sauce (e.g., tomato, basil, or marinara): ½ cup	8g	2 tsp
V8 Fusion Vegetable Fruit 100% juice: 250ml 1 cup	26g	6½ tsp
Glaceau Vitamin Water: 2⅔ cup bottle	32g	8 tsp
One pop tart (1.76 oz)	16g	4 tsp
½ cup raisin bran cereal	10g	2½ tsp

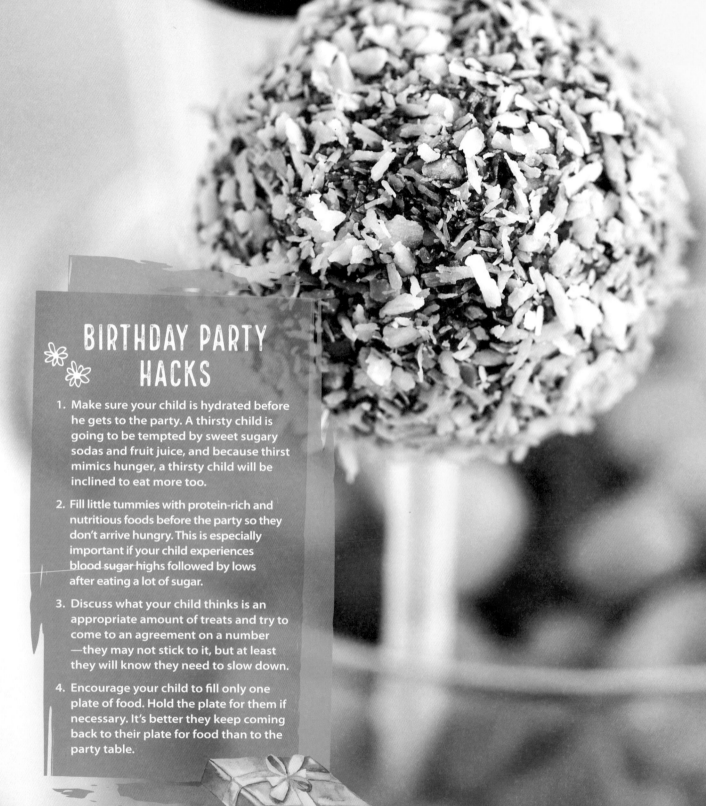

BIRTHDAY PARTY HACKS

1. Make sure your child is hydrated before he gets to the party. A thirsty child is going to be tempted by sweet sugary sodas and fruit juice, and because thirst mimics hunger, a thirsty child will be inclined to eat more too.

2. Fill little tummies with protein-rich and nutritious foods before the party so they don't arrive hungry. This is especially important if your child experiences blood sugar highs followed by lows after eating a lot of sugar.

3. Discuss what your child thinks is an appropriate amount of treats and try to come to an agreement on a number —they may not stick to it, but at least they will know they need to slow down.

4. Encourage your child to fill only one plate of food. Hold the plate for them if necessary. It's better they keep coming back to their plate for food than to the party table.

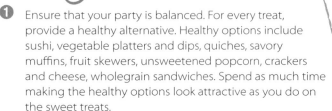

Top Tips for Party Hosts

① Ensure that your party is balanced. For every treat, provide a healthy alternative. Healthy options include sushi, vegetable platters and dips, quiches, savory muffins, fruit skewers, unsweetened popcorn, crackers and cheese, wholegrain sandwiches. Spend as much time making the healthy options look attractive as you do on the sweet treats.

② Serve a selection of treats, but don't go overboard with the sugar and food coloring. If you're going to have a bright red Elmo cake, a blue *Frozen* cake or a Ninja Turtle in green, it is best to avoid offering cupcakes with colored frosting and other frosted treats along with it. Instead use chocolate ganache or coconut cream frosting on the cupcakes (see recipes on page 91 and 281). Or better yet, try our Natural Rainbow Cake recipe made from natural food coloring (see page 281).

③ Don't follow the birthday cake with an offering of ice cream. Instead give your child a choice between a baked cake or an ice cream cake.

④ Younger children often only lick the frosting on cakes or cupcakes. Use cream cheese in the frosting to up the protein content and reduce the sugar amounts (see our recipe on page 92).

⑤ Instead of baking cupcakes, add frosting to nutrient-dense muffins, like the Chocolate Zucchini Muffins (see recipe on page 127).

⑥ Provide mini waters instead of individual cartons of juice for each child.

⑦ Offer only water or large jugs of pure fruit juice with no added sugar or preservatives, so parents can control how much they choose to give their children. The ideal balance would be 75 percent water and 25 percent fruit juice.

⑧ Choose unprocessed sweeteners for baked goods and avoid sprinkles and frostings that contain artificial colors or preservatives.

⑨ Leave packaged sweets or candies out altogether and offer squares of good, dark chocolate instead (start with 60%). You can even make your own healthier version of chocolate bears with homemade chocolate and fun molds (see our recipe on page 89).

⑩ Swap cake pops for delicious Choc Chia Pops (see recipe on page 89). They are a perfect healthy party treat and kids love them.

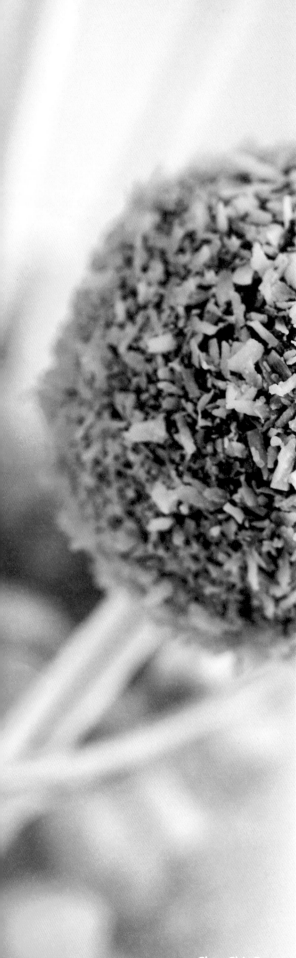

Choc Chia Pops
(see recipe on page 89)

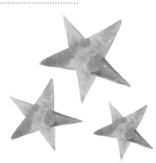

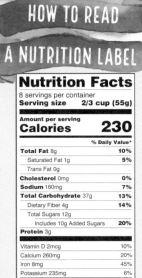

Nutrition Facts	
8 servings per container	
Serving size	**2/3 cup (55g)**

Amount per serving	
Calories	**230**

	% Daily Value*
Total Fat 8g	**10%**
Saturated Fat 1g	**5%**
Trans Fat 0g	
Cholesterol 0mg	**0%**
Sodium 160mg	**7%**
Total Carbohydrate 37g	**13%**
Dietary Fiber 4g	**14%**
Total Sugars 12g	
Includes 10g Added Sugars	**20%**
Protein 3g	
Vitamin D 2mcg	10%
Calcium 260mg	20%
Iron 8mg	45%
Potassium 235mg	6%

* The % Daily Value (DV) tells you how much a nutrient in a serving of food contributes to a daily diet. 2,000 calories a day is used for general nutrition advice.

To determine how much sugar a product contains, look at the column and then find the Total Sugar line (under Total Carbohydrate heading in the above example). A low-sugar product will contain less than 4.5 grams of sugar per 100 grams. A moderate sugar-containing product will have between 4.5 grams to 10 grams, and a high-sugar product will contain more than 10 grams per 100 grams. Sugar includes naturally occurring and added sugars. For example, if a squeezie yogurt listed 10 grams of sugar on the label, 4.5 grams would be naturally occurring (from lactose in milk) and the rest (around 5.5 grams) would be added in the form of fruit concentrate or cane sugar. To understand what forms of sugar have been added, always look at the ingredient list (found under or near the nutrition label). See a list of hidden names for sugar on page 67.

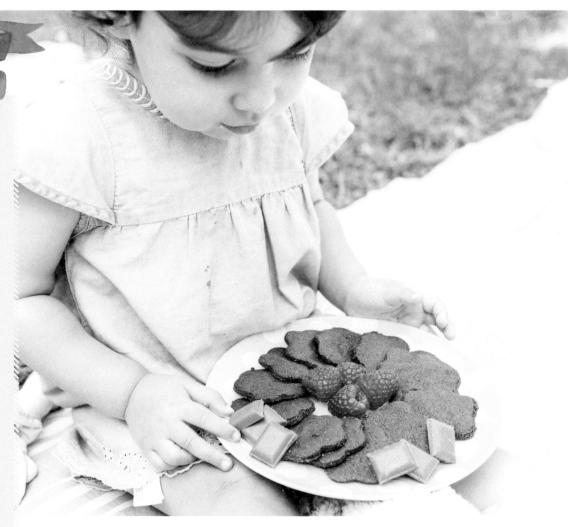

REFINED SUGAR 101

Refined sugar (sucrose) is extracted from sugar cane and sugar beets. Once harvested, the beets and sugar cane are pulverized and then boiled into a thick molasses-rich liquid. This liquid is then spun in a centrifuge to remove the molasses. In the final stages, the sugar goes through the refining process, which involves washing, filtration, and other purification methods to produce pure, white sugar crystals (sucrose).

Refined sugar, stripped of almost all fiber, vitamins and minerals, offers "empty" calories.

Sucrose (which is made up of equal molecules of the monosaccharides fructose and glucose) is digested quickly and has a high glycemic index, leading to rapid spikes in blood sugar and insulin levels (a hormone needed to reduce the concentration of blood sugar) after consumption.

Another worrying fact is that strong herbicides, fungicides and pesticides are used to grow sugar beets and sugarcane. Our challenge, when it comes to sweeteners, is to go back to using them in small amounts and

in their natural, unprocessed form, like pure maple syrup or raw honey, for example, which haven't been heated and stripped of vitamins and minerals.

I am definitely opposed to children having sweet snacks every day, but there is no harm in offering the occasional sweet treat if it's made with unprocessed sugars (see page 76). Depending on how much sugar they have been exposed to, each child will register sweetness at a different level. When you use or choose foods made with natural sweeteners, you have better control of what your child is eating and in what quantity.

According to Dr. Robert Lustig, Professor of pediatric Endocrinology at the University of California and author of *Fat Chance: The Bitter Truth About Sugar*, analysis of 175 countries over the past decade showed that when looking for the causes behind type 2 diabetes, the total number of calories consumed was irrelevant.

Rather, it was the specific type of calories that mattered. When people ate 150 calories more every day, the rate of diabetes went up 0.1 percent. But if those 150 calories came from a can of fizzy drink, the rate went up 1.1 percent, proving that added sugar is eleven times more potent in causing diabetes than general calories.

SUGAR AND FUSSY EATING

One of the leading nutritional causes of fussy eating is the introduction of sugary foods too early. When babies and toddlers are exposed to sugar, it alters their sweet taste receptors. For example, a child who has never eaten refined sugar will automatically rate a carrot as being sweet. If babies and young children with developing tastebuds are exposed to too many sweet foods too often, they develop a huge preference for those foods and fail to experience the natural sweetness of vegetables, and in some extreme cases fruit.

For fussy eaters, it's really important to start to balance their blood sugar levels and curb their cravings early on. For children who are already addicted to sweetened foods, it's important to go slowly and start to reduce the amount of sugar in their diets by finding healthier sugar substitutes and using transitional foods such as homemade sauces that are preservative free but may contain natural, non-processed sugars. The same goes for sweetened yogurts. Start by mixing a little plain yogurt into the sweetened yogurt and slowly up the ratio of plain versus sweetened.

MAKE SUGAR A "SOMETIMES" FOOD

Until my son was two-and-a-half years old, he was happy with my homemade snacks. Then one day we went to a party and he discovered Oreos and I found him holding one chocolate-covered cookie in each hand. From that moment on it has been a challenge for me to find the balance between knowing why he should not be eating refined sugar, to the reality that most of my friends and family do not adhere to a strict non-refined sugar way of life, so temptation is always there.

When my son turned five he began to ask me constantly for packaged treats. I could see that he was getting angry with me, as I stood firm. My intention was to try to keep him healthy. Knowing that banning sugar would only make it more appealing, I took a step backwards and worked out a way to appease his desire for packaged treats, while still maintaining a healthy home. I explained to him that as his mother, my job is to look after him and make sure he stays safe and healthy, but I realized that we needed to find a new system that worked for us both.

So the deal we came up with was that he could have a couple of sweet snacks of

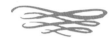

DID YOU KNOW?

Whether sugar is white, powdered, brown, or raw, it's all sucrose. In large amounts (more than 1/6 oz), it produces an immediate rise in blood-sugar levels.

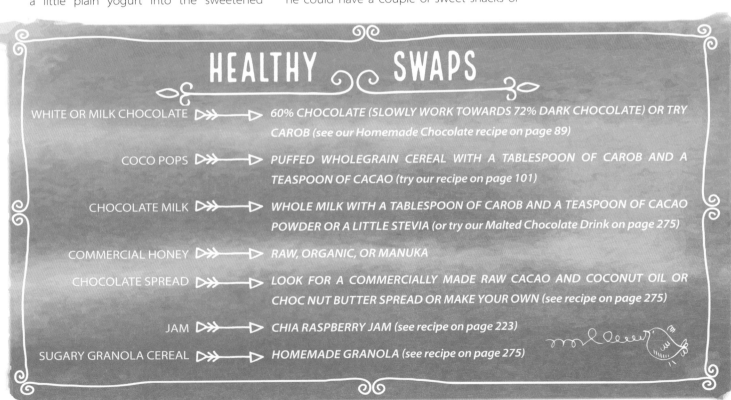

HEALTHY SWAPS

WHITE OR MILK CHOCOLATE ⟶ *60% CHOCOLATE (SLOWLY WORK TOWARDS 72% DARK CHOCOLATE) OR TRY CAROB (see our Homemade Chocolate recipe on page 89)*

COCO POPS ⟶ *PUFFED WHOLEGRAIN CEREAL WITH A TABLESPOON OF CAROB AND A TEASPOON OF CACAO (try our recipe on page 101)*

CHOCOLATE MILK ⟶ *WHOLE MILK WITH A TABLESPOON OF CAROB AND A TEASPOON OF CACAO POWDER OR A LITTLE STEVIA (or try our Malted Chocolate Drink on page 275)*

COMMERCIAL HONEY ⟶ *RAW, ORGANIC, OR MANUKA*

CHOCOLATE SPREAD ⟶ *LOOK FOR A COMMERCIALLY MADE RAW CACAO AND COCONUT OIL OR CHOC NUT BUTTER SPREAD OR MAKE YOUR OWN (see recipe on page 275)*

JAM ⟶ *CHIA RASPBERRY JAM (see recipe on page 223)*

SUGARY GRANOLA CEREAL ⟶ *HOMEMADE GRANOLA (see recipe on page 275)*

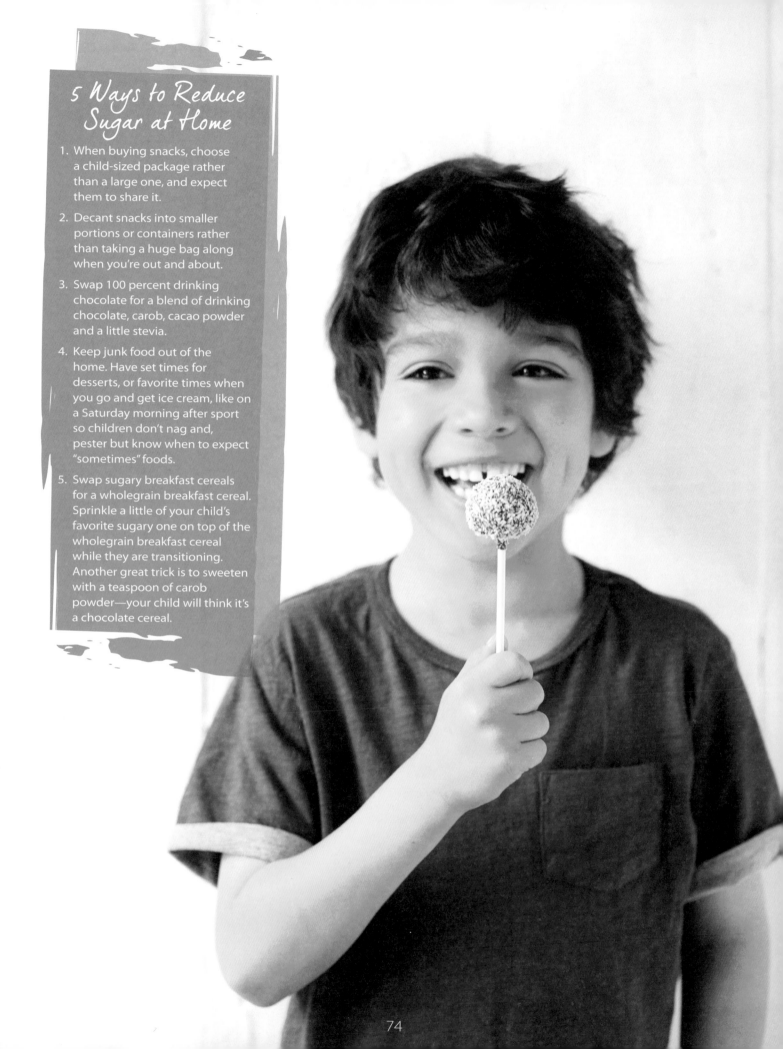

5 Ways to Reduce Sugar at Home

1. When buying snacks, choose a child-sized package rather than a large one, and expect them to share it.

2. Decant snacks into smaller portions or containers rather than taking a huge bag along when you're out and about.

3. Swap 100 percent drinking chocolate for a blend of drinking chocolate, carob, cacao powder and a little stevia.

4. Keep junk food out of the home. Have set times for desserts, or favorite times when you go and get ice cream, like on a Saturday morning after sport so children don't nag and, pester but know when to expect "sometimes" foods.

5. Swap sugary breakfast cereals for a wholegrain breakfast cereal. Sprinkle a little of your child's favorite sugary one on top of the wholegrain breakfast cereal while they are transitioning. Another great trick is to sweeten with a teaspoon of carob powder—your child will think it's a chocolate cereal.

his choice on the weekend, which were to be enjoyed outside of the home, with the focus on having a fun social time with his family and friends, but that when at home we stick to Mommy's choice of homemade goodies.

There are weeks when I don't adhere strictly to this, for example if he is going to a party or if I'm tired and the nag factor is strong! But at least we have some guidelines in place that we have agreed on together and that we can aim to stick to. This system works well for us, but you may need to experiment and work with your own child to see what suits you both best. If you come to an agreement together, it will be far easier to set boundaries than if you simply lay down the rules on your own. The key is to build an understanding and acceptance that these types of foods are to be enjoyed outside of the home and are not a typical part of everyday meals.

Consider this . . . Even if a food is labelled as having "no added cane sugar," check the ingredients list for fruit juice, fruit concentrate or honey.

MANAGE SWEET TEMPTATIONS

Up to eighteen months: There's no need to introduce refined sugar to babies or young toddlers. A muffin sweetened with pumpkin and banana will be enough to satisfy their sweet tooth and will appear to be the same as another child's cupcake.

Eighteen months and older: Be prepared with a homemade healthy snack for your child when you leave home, and learn to read nutrition labels when you're shopping so you can make the best choices when it comes to store-bought options (see page 72). When baking or preparing snacks, try to use use dates, raw honey, coconut sugar, or pure maple syrup, which are unrefined and contain trace minerals. Control portions by making mini muffins and smaller cookies.

Age three and older: Offer healthier versions of their favorite snacks, packed with whole fruits and vegetables. Explain that certain foods and drinks are "sometimes" foods. Keep these out of the home and enjoy them on occasion at the park, on a play date or at a sports event or party—this way your child will know when to expect these foods and will not nag for them daily. If you collect your child from school every day with a sweet snack it will become habitual and be expected.

Age four and older: Educate your child by talking to them and providing them with the facts about sugar. Let them help you bake and experiment with new foods. Use refined sugar alternatives such as coconut sugar, maple syrup, brown rice syrup (in moderation), and raw honey, as they are more nutritious than refined sugar, but remember they do have the same calorie content as sugar. You can also use stevia to reduce the sugar content in recipes, but remember it still creates the desire for sugar (see page 76 for more info).

Consider this . . . Most of the honey in supermarkets is pasteurized (which means it's been heated briefly at 140°F and then cooled rapidly), then filtered so it looks clearer and more appealing on the shelf. This reduces beneficial enzymes and possibly heat-sensitive antioxidants. Unlike processed honey, raw honey does not get robbed of its nutritional value and is a better choice for children. Active Manuka honey is a raw honey with the strongest antibacterial properties and is the best choice for adding to smoothies, layered bars, and truffles.

WHAT'S ALL THE FUSS ABOUT FRUCTOSE?

Fructose, the naturally occurring sugar in fruit, honey, and maple syrup, is the sweetest non-refined sweetener and has the lowest GI of all naturally occurring sugars. This means fructose produces a slightly slower increase in blood-sugar levels than sucrose. In whole fruit, it is loaded with vitamins, minerals, fiber, and antioxidants. And while a small amount of fructose (like that in a piece of fruit) isn't going to cause harm, if we eat too much of it, it cannot be converted into energy by the mitochondria inside our cells (which perform this function). Instead, the liver starts converting the excess fructose into fat in the form of triglycerides, putting us at risk of heart disease and diabetes. Fructose is overused in commercial food products and is often "hidden" in processed foods like salad dressing, bread, yogurt, and breakfast cereal, in the form high fructose corn syrup, agave nectar, fruit juice or fruit concentrate.

DID YOU KNOW?

Research now shows that 85% of children's taste preferences is due to the foods they are exposed to early on in life despite their genetic make-up.

Consider this...

One tablespoon of sugar is equal to 4 teaspoons. Keep this in mind when you're baking so you can track how much sugar is in the recipe and choose to lower the overall amount if necessary.

Healthy Sweeteners: The Lowdown

MAPLE SYRUP (GI 54)	HONEY (GI 35–64)	AGAVE SYRUP (GI 30)	MOLASSES (GI 55–60)	STEVIA (GI 0)

What is it?

An amber-colored liquid made from the sap of maple trees. Seventy percent sucrose and 30 percent fructose.

PROS

Lower glycemic index and lower in fructose than table sugar. It also contains 1/3 less sugar than table sugar. Pure maple syrup contains more antioxidants and minerals such as zinc and manganese than many other natural sweeteners, including honey. It's our number one replacement for syrup and liquid sweeteners in recipes.

CONS

Contains fructose, which is hard for the liver to metabolize. Many supermarket varieties are "maple-flavored" syrup and contain artificial ingredients such as GM corn syrup and caramel color. They have a higher GI, and are lower in nutrients. Although it will cost more, check that the product is 100 percent pure and labeled as "Grade A."

How to use it

Can be used in place of sugar in most baked goods, raw treats, and sauces—as it's a liquid you'll need to reduce other liquids in the recipe. Best practice: Use maple syrup in place of liquid sweeteners such as golden syrup.

What is it?

Flower nectar collected by bees, naturally broken down into simple sugars.

PROS

While sugar is 100 percent sucrose, honey is made up of around 35–40 percent glucose and 35–40 percent fructose (these proportions may vary depending on the source of the nectar). The remaining 20–25 percent is water with a trace of protein, a trace of fat and a trace of fiber. Some floral honeys have a lower GI (around 35) compared with commercial brands that usually have a GI of around 64. Raw or Manuka honey is packed with vitamins and also has antimicrobial properties.

CONS

Contains glucose which can cause a quick rise in blood sugar levels and fructose which is hard to metabolise. Most honey found in commercial food products has no benefits. Avoid in babies under the age of twelve months due to the risk of botulism.

How to use it

Add to smoothies, stir into plain unsweetened yogurt or drizzle on porridge, and use as a syrup replacement for cookies and biscuits. To preserve the benefits of Manuka or raw honey, avoid heating.

What is it?

Agave nectar is an amber-colored liquid extracted from the leaves of the blue agave plant.

PROS

It's intensely sweet, so you don't need as much as sugar.

CONS

It has an extremely high fructose content—75–90 percent, which is even more than that of high fructose corn syrup—meaning the liver cannot metabolise it well.

How to use it

It can replace sugar or honey in hot drinks, baking or other cooking, or be used as a topping for pancakes and French toast, but it's my least favorite natural sweetener because of the high fructose content.

What is it?

A byproduct of the sugar-cane refining process.

PROS

It's rich in all the nutrients extracted from sugar during the refining process—iron, copper, magnesium, zinc, calcium, and potassium. Thick and gooey blackstrap molasses, from the last press in the process, is particularly rich in minerals and often recommended as a great vegan source of iron.

CONS

High fructose levels.

How to use it

It's quite thick and viscous and is best used in baking. It is also sweeter than sugar and so should be used in smaller amounts.

What is it?

A powder or liquid crushed or extracted from the leaves of the *Stevia Rebandiana* plant.

PROS

It's three hundred times sweeter than sugar, natural, has no carbs or calories, and doesn't raise blood sugar (low GI), making it suitable for diabetics.

CONS

It can taste bitter and is often found mixed with erythritol (a sugar alcohol), which I do not recommend for young children.

How to use it

Available as both dried leaves (good for smoothies), powders or liquids. I like the dried leaves best, but if you can't find them look for brands that contain 100 percent stevia. Due to its slightly bitter after taste, it is best to use 1/2 tsp of pure stevia in baking to replace 1/2 cup of sugar. This is the best way to reduce overall sugar content, while transitioning children toward enjoying homemade treats.

Be aware that any added sweetener—natural or otherwise—will encourage our desire for sweetness. Moderation is always key when it comes to sweet foods, so although homemade versions made with the following sweeteners are more nutritionally dense, I still don't advise feeding children too much of them as they can displace other types of food in the diet and can ultimately have the same effect on their long-term health as refined sugar.

SUGAR ALCOHOLS (GI AVG 10)	MONK FRUIT (GI 0)	BROWN RICE SYRUP (GI 98)	COCONUT SUGAR (GI 35)	DATE SUGAR (GI 44–68)
What is it? The common sugar alcohols—sorbitol, mannitol, maltitol, erythritol, and hydrogenated starch hydrolysates—do not contain alcohol. They are manufactured from cornstarch. Xylitol is manufactured from such sources as cornhusks, sugar cane bagasse (stalk residue remaining after sugar extraction), or birch wood waste. **PROS** Very few calories, don't raise blood-sugar levels (meaning they're good for diabetics). Xylitol, unlike sugar, can actually fight tooth decay if used properly. It's often added to chewing gum. **CONS** Sugar alcohols can cause headaches, stomach upsets, and have a laxative effect, especially in young children. Because they're derived from cornstarch or cornhusks, they could contain inherent GMOs.	**What is it?** Extracted from China's Lo Han fruit (monk fruit). **PROS** Rich in antioxidants and with zero calories, the Chinese have used it for centuries to treat obesity and diabetes. **CONS** Creates a desire for sweets.	**What is it?** Brown rice, which is cooked and then exposed to enzymes which breaks it down into syrup. **PROS** It contains no fructose. **CONS** High GI and not recommended for use with anyone susceptible to insulin resistance or diabetes. It's also heavily processed and contains no nutrients and, like brown rice itself, could contain arsenic. Safe levels of arsenic are calculated per kg and children with lower weights are more susceptible to having too much arsenic in their body. For that reason I don't recommend it for children under five.	**What is it?** The extracted sap of the coconut palm flower. **PROS** One of the most nutritious and sustainable natural sugars available. Low GI, unrefined, contains vitamins and minerals such as potassium, phosphorous, calcium and magnesium, as well as inulin, antioxidants and amino acids such as glutamic acid, which is an important component in metabolism. **CONS** Contains only slightly less fructose, plus the same carbs and calories as table sugar.	**What is it?** Dehydrated, ground dates. **PROS** No additives. Contains fiber and is high in antioxidants and potassium. **CONS** High fructose content.
How to use it Avoid using for children and check ingredients lists to ensure there are no sugar alcohols present.	**How to use it** Look for monk fruit extract, monk fruit sweetener or dried monk fruit which can be found at many Chinese markets. This sweetener can be substituted for sugar, however, when it comes to baked foods it's recommended to substitute monk fruit extract for only half the sugar to ensure consistency and texture remains. You can use the dried fruit in soups.	**How to use it** Best used in baked goods, sauces, and salad dressings.	**How to use it** A perfect substitute for brown sugar in baking, but it won't work as a replacement for confectioners' sugar.	**How to use it** Its rich, sweet flavor makes it an ideal alternative to brown sugar. Unfortunately it doesn't melt and is difficult to dissolve. Best practice: use date sugar in baking nut breads, fruit breads, muffins, fruit crumbles, or sprinkling on cinnamon scrolls before baking. Avoid using in thin cookies as it burns easily.

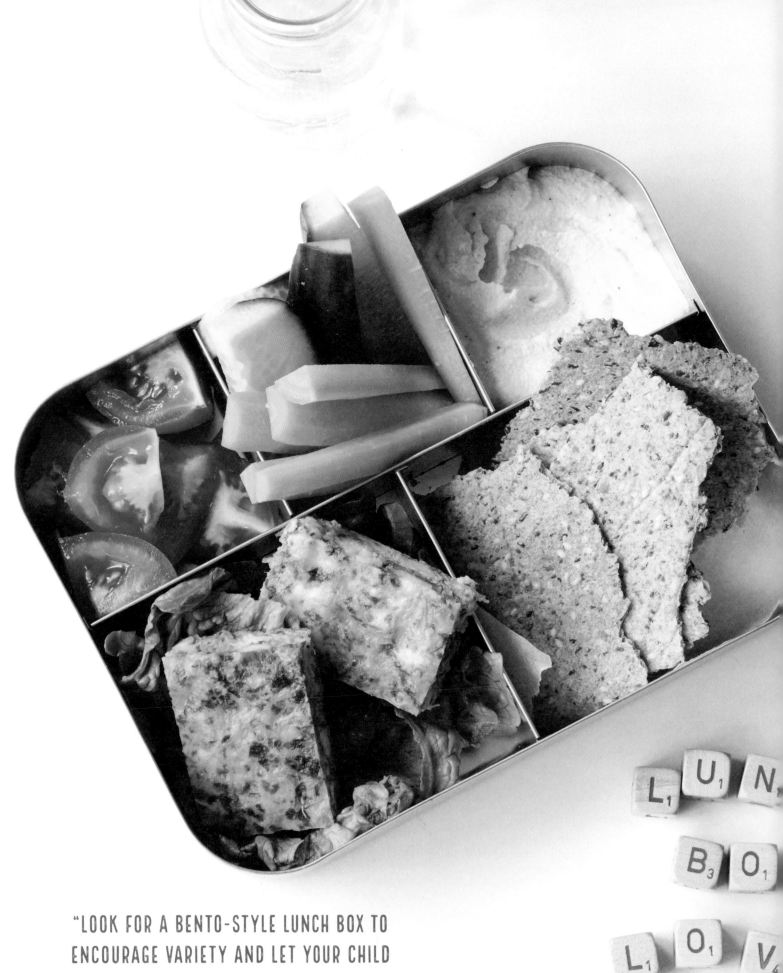

"LOOK FOR A BENTO-STYLE LUNCH BOX TO
ENCOURAGE VARIETY AND LET YOUR CHILD
CHOOSE WHAT TO EAT FIRST."

SIMPLE LUNCH BOX SWAPS

As filmmaker Damon Gameau demonstrated in *That Sugar Film*, some kids' lunch boxes can contain up to forty teaspoons of sugar in the form of '"healthy" foods, such as organic apple and blackcurrant juice, sesame snaps, fruit bars, organic golden raisins, a muffin bar, fruity bites, a fruit jelly pack, and a jelly sandwich.

Here are ten simple and easy swaps that will help you slash your child's daily sugar intake. The benefits are HUGE: your child will have better concentration at school, more stable moods after school (less whining, tantrums and tears!), and will go to sleep more easily at night as a result.

Golden raisins Grapes. A small pack of golden raisins contains five teaspoons of added sugar. Five to six (cut) grapes contain only one teaspoon of naturally occurring sugars by comparison.

Sweet popcorn Plain or lightly salted popcorn.

Squeezie yogurt Reusable pouches or other small, reusable containers filled with natural yogurt sweetened with a teaspoon of maple syrup or honey. Most squeezie yogurts contain around three teaspoons of sugar.

Chocolate milk Half chocolate milk, half plain milk.

Fruit Juice Diluted fruit juice: One quarter fruit juice and three quarters water.

Sports drinks Flavored coconut water. Gatorade has nine teaspoons of sugar while flavored coconut water contains just one to two teaspoons (you ultimately want your child to drink water instead of milk, fruit juice or sports drinks).

Jelly or honey sandwich Raw honey mixed with school-friendly sunflower butter or tahini which has a higher protein content than most nut butters.

Granola bars, muesli bars Low-sugar homemade versions (see recipe on page 193).

Are artificial sweeteners safe for kids?

I'm going to let the famous US pediatrician and author Dr. William Sears answer this one for me. He recently wrote in his column on Parenting.com: "Even though the US Food and Drug Administration (FDA) has granted artificial sweeteners like aspartame or sucralose (Splenda) the status of "generally regarded as safe (GRAS)," there have been several controversial findings, especially where kids are concerned. In his book *Excitotoxins*, board-certified neurosurgeon Dr. Russell Blaylock reviews the studies on aspartame and concludes that it is not safe, especially for the growing brains of children. In regards to Splenda, the manufacturer states that, because the body doesn't digest or metabolize Splenda, it is a 'no calorie' sweetener. According to the research reports in the Federal Register (the official publication of the US Food and Drug Administration), however, 20 to 30% of ingested Splenda is indeed metabolised by humans. And animal studies have resulted in wide individual variations concerning the amount of Splenda absorbed. Consider, also, that there are no studies on the long-term effects of the sweetener on humans, either adults or children. Even if most of the Splenda is not absorbed, as the manufacturer claims, it still hangs around in the gut for many hours—and I'm not convinced that this contributes to intestinal health!"

DID YOU KNOW?

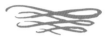

A recent landmark study in the US of more than 3000 infants and toddlers found that close to half of seven- to eight-month-olds are already consuming sugar-sweetened snacks, sodas and fruit drinks, a percentage that increases dramatically with age.

SUGAR AND HYPERACTIVITY: IS THERE A LINK?

Eating too much sugar can create a "sugar low" following a situation, like a birthday party, where blood sugar levels rise too high. It is commonly acknowledged that as blood sugar levels fall, the body responds by producing a large amount of insulin and there is a compensatory release of adrenaline. When blood sugar levels drop too quickly, some children may feel shaky and this might alter their thinking and behavior.

Contrary to popular belief, sugar may not be the only culprit behind sudden bursts of hyperactivity in children, a.k.a. the sugar rush (or the post-birthday party meltdowns that invariably follow). Scientists started looking into this in earnest in the 1970s after an American allergist, Benjamin Feingold, advocated the removal of food additives to treat hyperactivity in children. More recent research would suggest that Feingold was onto something. It seems that artificial colors, flavors, and preservatives packed into the sugary foods are a contributing factor to hyperactivity. One famous study into groups of three-year-olds found that artificial food coloring (particularly red, yellow, and orange), and the preservative sodium benzoate, made children more likely to lack concentration, lose their temper, interrupt others, and struggle to get to sleep. Foods to avoid include—no surprises here—many popular children's foods, like baked goods, soft drinks, cordials, flavored milk, colorful sprinkles, and frosting on cakes and cookies.

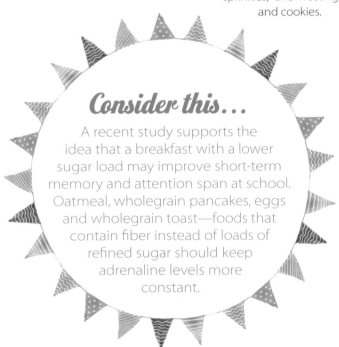

Consider this...

A recent study supports the idea that a breakfast with a lower sugar load may improve short-term memory and attention span at school. Oatmeal, wholegrain pancakes, eggs and wholegrain toast—foods that contain fiber instead of loads of refined sugar should keep adrenaline levels more constant.

The bottom line is to treat sugar as a "sometimes" food and make it a normal part of festive occasions, but use healthy sweeteners like those suggested in this book and avoid food colorings and other additives (learn more about this on page 258). Make your own cakes and cookies without using artificial food coloring whenever possible (see our recipe for Natural Rainbow Cake on page 281). If you're buying packaged food, choose foods containing "natural colors" made from fruit, vegetables, and spices like beetroot, carrot, paprika, and turmeric.

SUGAR'S EFFECT ON CHILDREN'S GUTS

More and more research is emerging to point to a healthy gut, one with flourishing beneficial bacteria, being the cornerstone of our children's health. Many conditions such as ADHD, autism, allergies and even obesity are being attributed to a disturbance in the microbiome-gut-brain axis (the biochemical signaling that takes place between the gastrointestinal tract and the central nervous system). Proper development of this critical relationship during infancy and childhood is vital for long-term health.

As our children's systems are still developing, they are extremely vulnerable to toxins in their environment. Their gastrointestinal tract provides vital functions for immunity and by protecting and maintaining healthy gut flora you ensure the integrity of your child's immune system. When there are changes to the microflora in your child's gut through antibiotic use or an overgrowth of yeast or bacteria, this can change the balance of the flora and deplete the beneficial bacteria. Sugary foods create the perfect environment for harmful bacteria to flourish as well as for yeast overgrowth. When sugar causes dysbiosis (microbial imbalance) it can lead to leaky gut syndrome where toxins enter into the bloodstream and can cause a range of inflammatory conditions

When we think about sugar, it's important to understand the overall impact it has on our children's health. Even if there is no immediate impact, we can be certain that overconsumption is detrimental to their long-term health.

GOAL 2: INTRODUCE STRUCTURE

I was inspired to specialize in early childhood nutrition after I joined a mothers' group with my then six-month-old son and saw other unsuspecting mothers introducing their six-month-old babies to squeezie yogurts, which contained added sugar. I realized then that a child's journey to junk food begins with the first teething biscuit, yogurt or sweetened porridge. Babies have a natural predisposition for sweet foods and if we introduce them to these from the get-go, we inhibit their ability to build up and enjoy a taste for other flavors.

Often, this desire for sweet food grows and leads to constant snacking and cravings. Consequently, when children get used to eating outside of mealtimes, their intake of nutritious food decreases at meals. Snacking is important so that kids can keep their energy up, but the ideal eating structure is three meals and two snacks per day with an extra snack added in on days when a child does sport. Often, however, snacking involves convenience foods that are high in sugar, salt, and fat. Like adults, children experience these snacks as palatable and ultimately addictive.

A recent study found that high-calorie snacking is a major cause of childhood obesity. Chips, candy, and other snack foods account for up to 27 percent of the daily caloric intake for children, age two to eighteen, according to findings by researchers at the University of North Carolina. Once we begin to reduce the amount of sugar in our children's diets, we need to ensure that we replace it with delicious, blood stabilizing foods offered at a consistent time each day to help ensure they do not crave more sugar.

There's no need to quit sugar outright. Instead transition from processed, refined sugar snacks to healthier homemade ones. Serving a healthy snack to a child is a great way to fill in the nutritional 'gaps' that may occur at mealtimes. To do this, it's important to create a structure for them as this helps their bodies know when to expect food. Structure also assists parents or caregivers to plan ahead.

One of the main contributing factors to the overconsumption of sugary foods is a reliance on convenience food. If you're rushing to pick up your child from school and have forgotten to bring a healthy snack, once they're in the car and nagging for food it's only human to reach for something convenient like an ice cream while you're filling up at the gas station. The problem is that the resulting blood sugar dip once they get home will lead to more nagging for sugary food. Create structure and ensure that your child knows to expect a nutritious snack when they get home from school that will keep them satisfied until dinner.

If you're on the run after school to sports or other lessons, with a structure in place, you will be able to prepare ahead of time by batch cooking so you always have nutritious after school snacks. If dinner is delayed and your child is genuinely hungry, offer a part of the dinner meal early if ready. Otherwise, a raw veggie platter with dips is a good idea.

👍 DO...	👎 DON'T...
make your own food as often as you can, beginning with the first purees or finger foods.	offer too many commercially prepared foods. It's impossible to compete with processed foods that contain sugar and salt (two of the most highly addictive tastes that can interfere with children getting used to natural foods).
choose foods in their natural state that have been minimally processed.	go for low-fat processed foods. They're usually loaded with added sugars to round out the taste.
teach children that sweet treats are "sometimes" foods and limit when they can expect to eat them and in what portions.	make sugar the "bad guy." The more we villainize sugar or deny our children foods which they see their friends eating, the more they will want it.
aim to remove sugar from staples like bread and crackers by making sure they contain no hidden sugars.	buy products that are marketed as being healthy without first checking the ingredients list.
keep baked goods and sweet treats out of the home. Instead prepare healthy versions of muffins and snacks for times when your child wants something sweet at home or for the school lunch box and after sports.	deny sweet treats when your child is with other children who are indulging, such as at birthday parties or on other special occasions. See our birthday party hacks to minimize the damage on page 70.
replace refined sugar with unrefined alternatives.	use more of these healthy sweeteners than the recipe calls for. While they offer more nutrition, they still have the same calories as refined sugar.

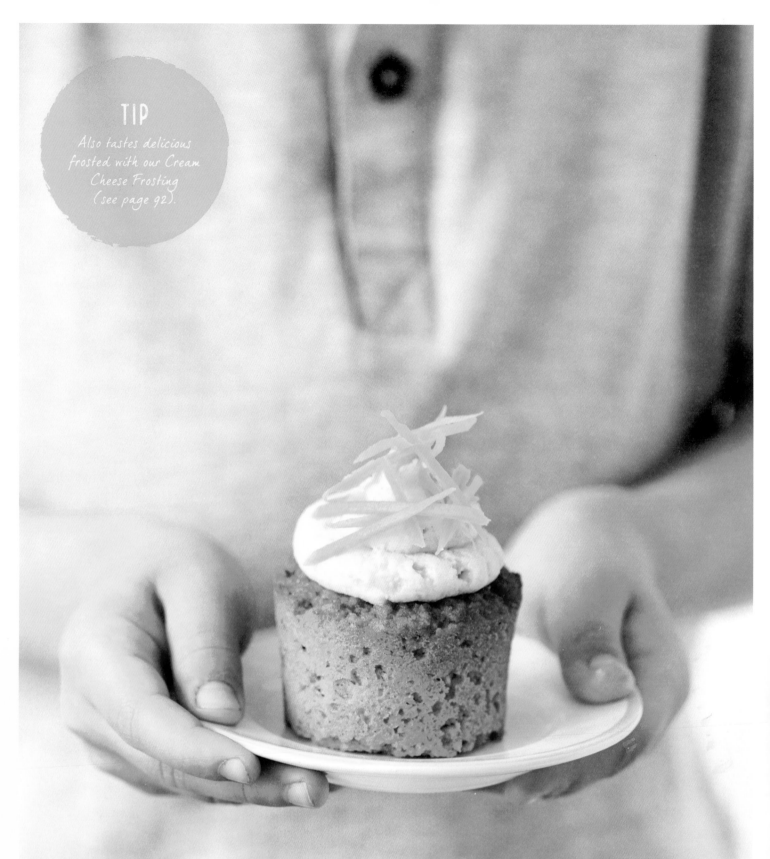

TIP

Also tastes delicious frosted with our Cream Cheese Frosting (see page 92).

"MADE FROM ALMOND MEAL AND EGGS, THIS CARROT MUFFIN WILL NOT SPIKE BLOOD-SUGAR LEVELS PLUS CARROTS ARE HIGH IN BETA-CAROTENE AND FIBER."

VEG Vegetarian | **Gluten Free** | **Dairy Free**

Prep time: 20 mins
Cooking time: 30–35 mins
Makes: 10 regular muffins or
24 mini muffins

Carrot & Cinnamon Muffins

My mom always served carrot cake at family celebrations when I was a child. Now my kids love this healthier version topped with macadamia cashew nut frosting when we have friends over for afternoon tea.

INGREDIENTS

1¼ cups (5¼ oz) almond meal

½ cup (2⅘ oz) pumpkin or sunflower seeds, processed into a fine meal

⅓ cup (1¾ oz) coconut sugar

1 tsp baking powder

pinch Himalayan rock salt

½ tsp ground cinnamon

⅛ tsp nutmeg

⅛ tsp ground ginger

2 large eggs

⅓ cup coconut oil, melted

½ tsp pure vanilla extract

1½ cups (4¾ oz) carrot, peeled and finely grated

EQUIPMENT

electric hand mixer

INSTRUCTIONS

Preheat oven to 355°F and line a muffin tray with muffin liners.

In a large bowl, place all dry ingredients and whisk until well combined.

In a small bowl, beat the eggs with an electric mixer.

Add coconut oil and vanilla extract and beat with an electric mixer until well combined. Pour this mixture into the bowl with the dry ingredients and whisk to combine.

Gently fold in the grated carrot.

Pour batter into the muffin liners and bake for around 30 to 35 mins, or until a cake tester comes out clean.

Remove from oven and allow to cool.

Serving and storing leftovers: Serve immediately, store in the fridge for up to 4 days or freeze for up to 4 months.

V Vegan | **Gluten Free**

Prep time: 10 mins
(+7 hours soaking and 30 mins refrigeration time)
Makes: 2½ cups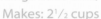

Macadamia Cashew Frosting

INGREDIENTS

1½ cups (8½ oz) cashews, soaked for 2–4 hrs, rinsed and drained

½ cup (2½ oz) macadamia nuts, soaked overnight or for at least 7 hours, rinsed, drained

½ cup coconut cream

2 tsp lemon juice

2 tsp pure vanilla extract

½ cup maple syrup

4 tbs coconut oil, melted

½ tsp sea salt

EQUIPMENT

high-speed food processor or blender

INSTRUCTIONS

Place all ingredients in a high-speed food processor or blender and blend, scraping down the sides occasionally, until smooth and creamy.

Chill in the fridge for about half an hour to firm up before spreading on your cake.

Serving and storing leftovers: Serve immediately, store in the fridge for up to 4 days or freeze for up to 4 months.

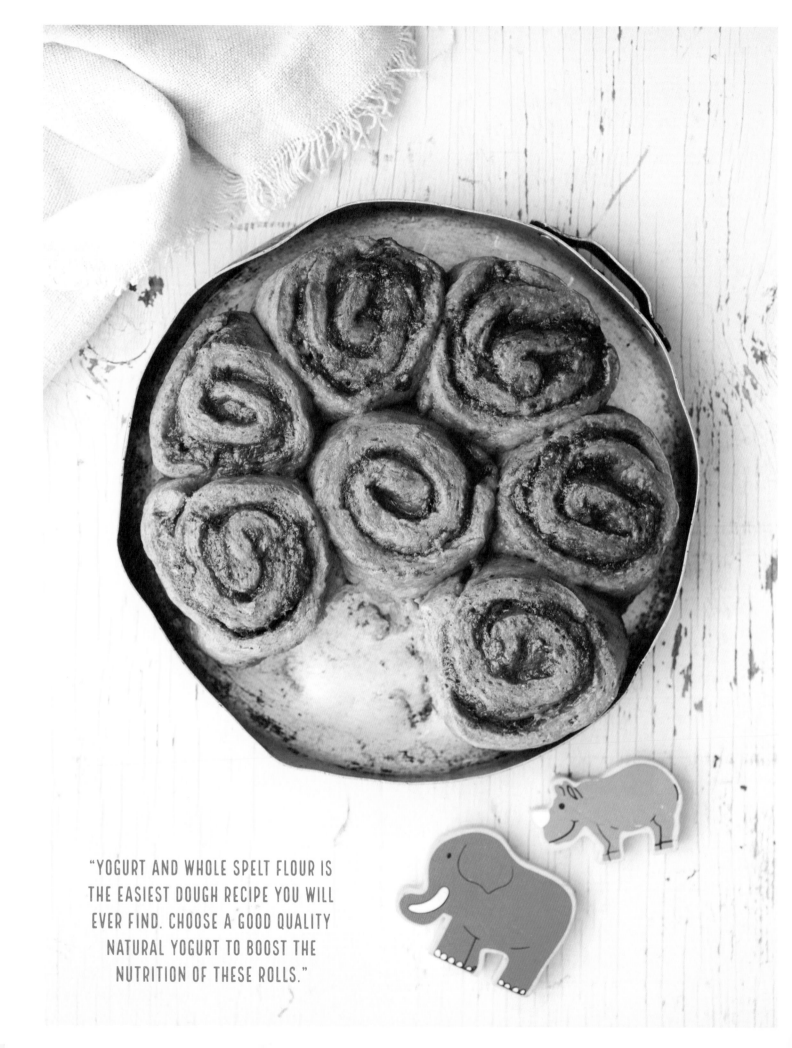

"YOGURT AND WHOLE SPELT FLOUR IS THE EASIEST DOUGH RECIPE YOU WILL EVER FIND. CHOOSE A GOOD QUALITY NATURAL YOGURT TO BOOST THE NUTRITION OF THESE ROLLS."

VEG
Vegetarian

Egg Free

Nut Free

Prep time: 20 mins
Cooking time: 20–25 mins
Makes: 8 scrolls

Banana Cinnamon Rolls

Growing up, my best friend used to order a cinnamon bun from the cafeteria every day. I love eating these scrolls with my kids and knowing that they are free from refined sugar and flour.

TIP

For a gluten-free version use 1 1/2 cups buckwheat flour, 1 cup almond meal and 1 tsp psyllium husk powder instead of the 2 cups of spelt flour.

Choose from any of our delicious fillings to use in this recipe. My kids love our Healthy Chocolate Spread (see page 275) or Chia Raspberry Jam (see page 223). Or for a savory version see recipe on page 251.

INGREDIENTS

DOUGH
2 cups (11¹⁄₈ oz) whole spelt flour

1 cup (9¹⁄₆ oz) natural Greek yogurt or coconut yogurt

1 tsp baking powder

¼ tsp baking soda

1–2 tbs coconut sugar (optional)

pinch of sea salt

FILLING
1 ripe banana 4¹⁄₄ oz, mashed

2 tsp ground cinnamon

1 tsp pure vanilla extract

1–2 tbs coconut sugar (optional)

EQUIPMENT
high-speed food processor

INSTRUCTIONS

Preheat oven to 355°F and line a baking tray with baking paper.

Place all dough ingredients into a food processor and process until smooth.

Remove the dough, shape it into a ball, and place between two sheets of baking paper and roll it into a rectangle shape about ¹⁄₆"–¹⁄₃" thick. If dough seems too sticky, lightly flour the baking paper and sprinkle some flour on top of the dough before rolling out. Remove the top sheet.

Mix the filling ingredients together in a small bowl.

Top dough with the banana mixture. Be careful to leave ³⁄₄" free of filling on the longer sides of the dough.

Roll dough into a log shape and cut into even slices to make scrolls.

Brush or drizzle scrolls with olive oil or coconut oil.

Place on the lined baking tray and bake for 20–25 mins.

Leave to cool on a wire rack before serving.

To ensure this recipe works best, use a thick yogurt.

Serving and storing leftovers: Serve immediately, store in an airtight container in the fridge for up to 4 days or freeze for up to 4 months. Warm before serving.

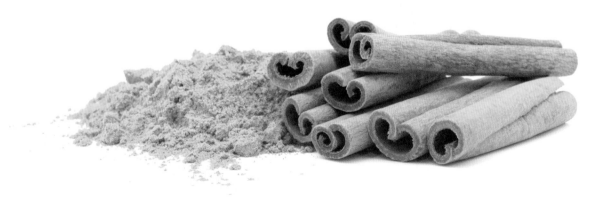

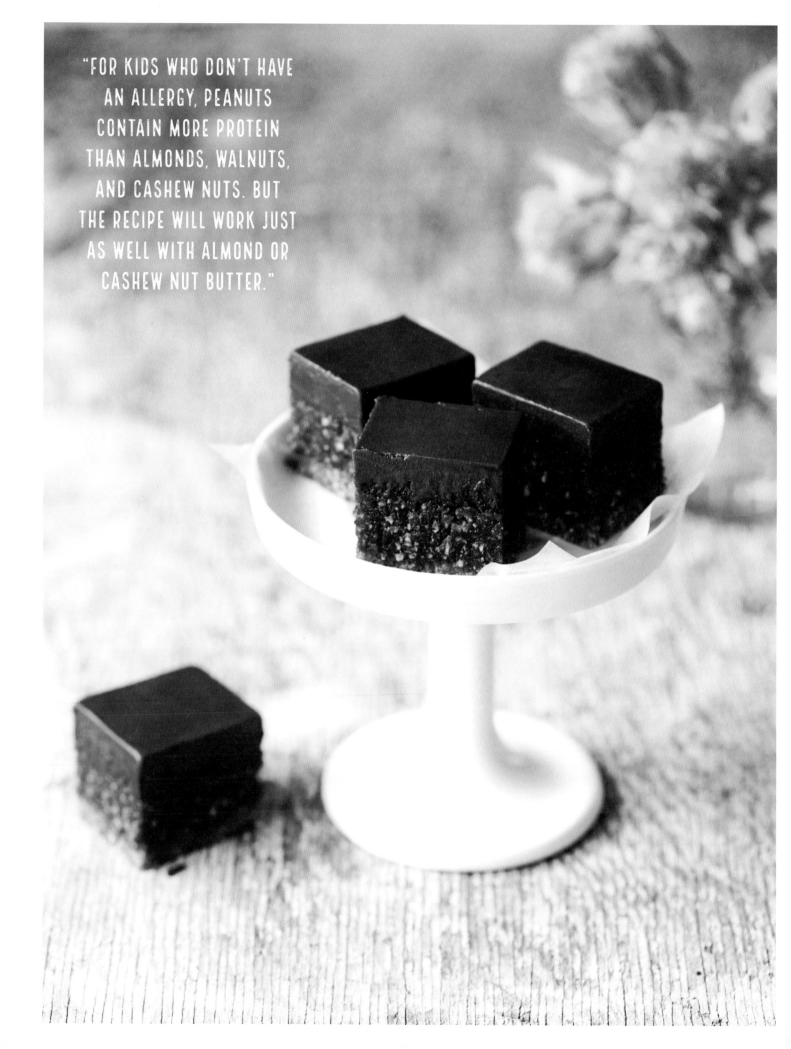

"FOR KIDS WHO DON'T HAVE AN ALLERGY, PEANUTS CONTAIN MORE PROTEIN THAN ALMONDS, WALNUTS, AND CASHEW NUTS. BUT THE RECIPE WILL WORK JUST AS WELL WITH ALMOND OR CASHEW NUT BUTTER."

Vegan　　Gluten Free

Prep time: 25 mins (+ 1 hour freezing time)
Makes: 36 squares

Raw Caramel Chocolate Squares

I created these raw squares sweetened with dates and maple sugar for the whole family to enjoy. It's a great replacement for refined sugar and preservative-filled chocolate squares.

INGREDIENTS

BASE:
½ cup (1½ oz) coconut flakes

1 cup (8½ oz) Medjool dates, pitted

½ cup (2⅕ oz) almond meal

1 tbs chia seeds

CARAMEL:
1 cup (9⅘ oz) organic crunchy peanut butter (no added sugar or vegetable oil)

1⅓ cups (11¼ oz) soft Medjool dates, pitted

3 tbs maple syrup

1 cup (2⅗ oz) shredded coconut (optional)

2 tbs cacao powder

2 tbs carob powder

pinch Himalayan rock salt

1 tsp vanilla extract, or 1 vanilla pod

2 tbs coconut oil, melted

2–4 tbs almond milk (4 tbs if not using maple syrup)

CHOCOLATE:
1 cup coconut oil, melted

½ cup cacao powder

½ cup maple syrup

EQUIPMENT
high-speed food processor

INSTRUCTIONS

FOR THE BASE:
Line a 8" x 8" square cake pan with baking paper.

Place all ingredients in a food processor and process until it reaches a fine but still crumbly consistency. Firmly press mixture into the cake pan and place in the freezer.

FOR THE CARAMEL:
Place all caramel ingredients in a food processor and process until smooth and creamy. Pour mixture evenly on top of the base and put back in the freezer.

FOR THE CHOCOLATE:
Whisk all chocolate ingredients in a small bowl until well combined. Pour chocolate on top of the caramel layer and put back in the freezer for at least an hour before cutting into squares, and serving.

Serving and storing leftovers: Serve immediately or store in an airtight container in the freezer for up to 4 months.

TIP

If your dates are not soft, soak them in hot water for 5-10 mins before using. Swap almond milk with coconut milk or milk of choice.

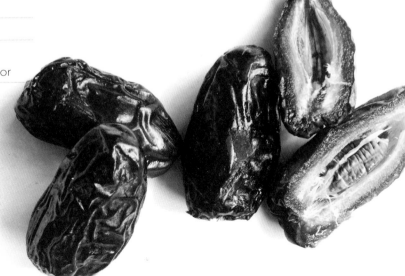

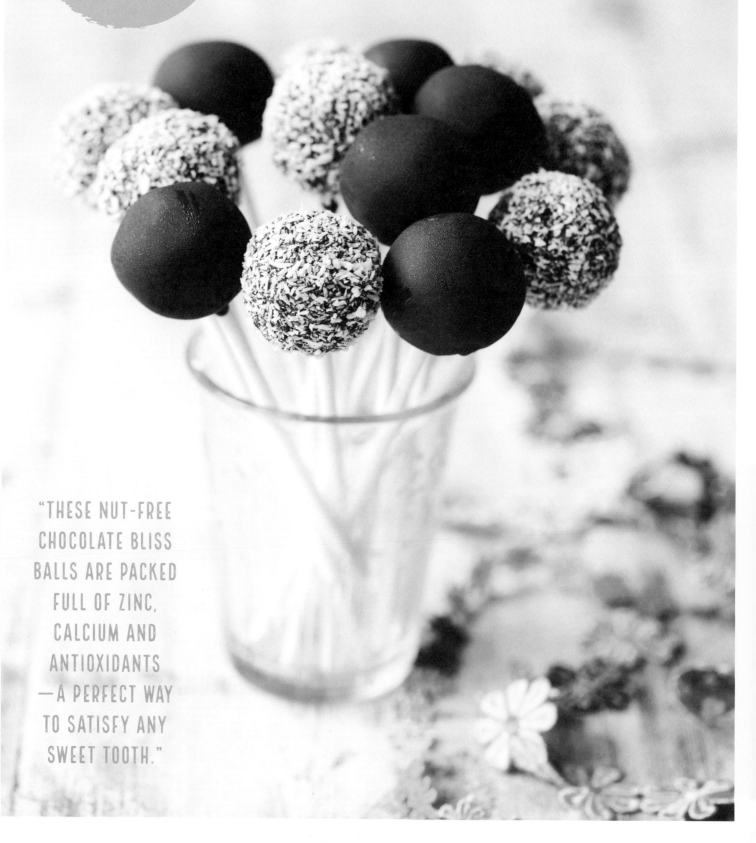

TIP

Leave out the chocolate and roll in coconut flakes instead for a yummy truffle treat (sticks optional).

"THESE NUT-FREE CHOCOLATE BLISS BALLS ARE PACKED FULL OF ZINC, CALCIUM AND ANTIOXIDANTS —A PERFECT WAY TO SATISFY ANY SWEET TOOTH."

V — Vegan · Gluten Free · Nut Free

Prep time: 20 mins (+1 hour freezing time)
Makes: 30

Choc Chia Pops

This healthy take on cake pops have become my go-to for school birthday treats instead of cupcakes. The kids love them and the teachers do too!

INGREDIENTS

1 cup (5³⁄₅ oz) mixed seeds (pumpkin, sunflower, sesame). If you don't require this to be school-friendly, use 1 cup (5³⁄₅ oz) of mixed nuts instead of seeds.

¼ cup (1³⁄₄ oz) chia seeds

1 cup (8¹⁄₂ oz) soft Medjool dates, pitted

¼ cup coconut oil, melted

1 tbs cacao powder

1 tbs carob powder

1 tsp ground cinnamon

pinch Himalayan rock salt

1 tbs coconut sugar (optional)

30 lollipop sticks

TOPPING:
Homemade Chocolate (see below), in liquid form OR 8³⁄₄ oz dark chocolate, melted

¹⁄₂ cup (1¹⁄₂ oz) coconut flakes (optional)

EQUIPMENT

high-speed food processor

INSTRUCTIONS

Place all seeds including chia seeds into high-speed processor and process until smooth.

Add half the dates and the coconut oil and process again until smooth.

Add remaining dates and process again.

Add the remaining ingredients and process until smooth consistency is reached.

Roll into little balls and place into freezer for an hour on a lined baking tray.

To make topping, place chocolate in small pot and melt over low heat. Once melted, remove from heat.

Remove bliss balls from freezer and place each one on top of a lollipop stick. Dip in melted chocolate then roll in coconut flakes (if using). Place choc pop in glass cup with chocolate end sticking up to let chocolate set before placing on a lined baking tray to go into the freezer. Leave to set in freezer for at least an hour before serving.

Serving and storing leftovers: Remove from freezer at least 10 minutes before serving. Store in the freezer for up to 4 months.

VEG — Vegetarian · Gluten Free · Dairy Free · Nut Free · Egg Free

Prep time: 8 mins (+1–2 hours to set)
Makes: 20 pieces

Quick & Simple Homemade Chocolate

INGREDIENTS

¹⁄₂ cup (2¹⁄₅ oz) organic cocoa butter

¹⁄₂ cup (1³⁄₄ oz) cacao powder

4 tbs raw honey or Manuka honey

¼ tsp pure vanilla extract

Himalayan rock salt

Toppings: coconut flakes, chopped nuts, raisins, goji berries, freeze-dried fruits (optional)

INGREDIENTS

tray of 20 small chocolate molds

INSTRUCTIONS

Pour some water into a small cooking pot and place over medium heat. Place the cacao butter in a small bowl and put it on top of the pot.

Once cacao butter is completely melted stir in all other ingredients until well combined and smooth.

Pour chocolate into small molds and sprinkle with toppings if desired.

Leave to harden in the fridge for 1–2 hours and remove from molds.

Serving and storing leftovers: Serve immediately after it has set, store in an airtight container for up to 1 month in the fridge, or freeze for 4–6 months.

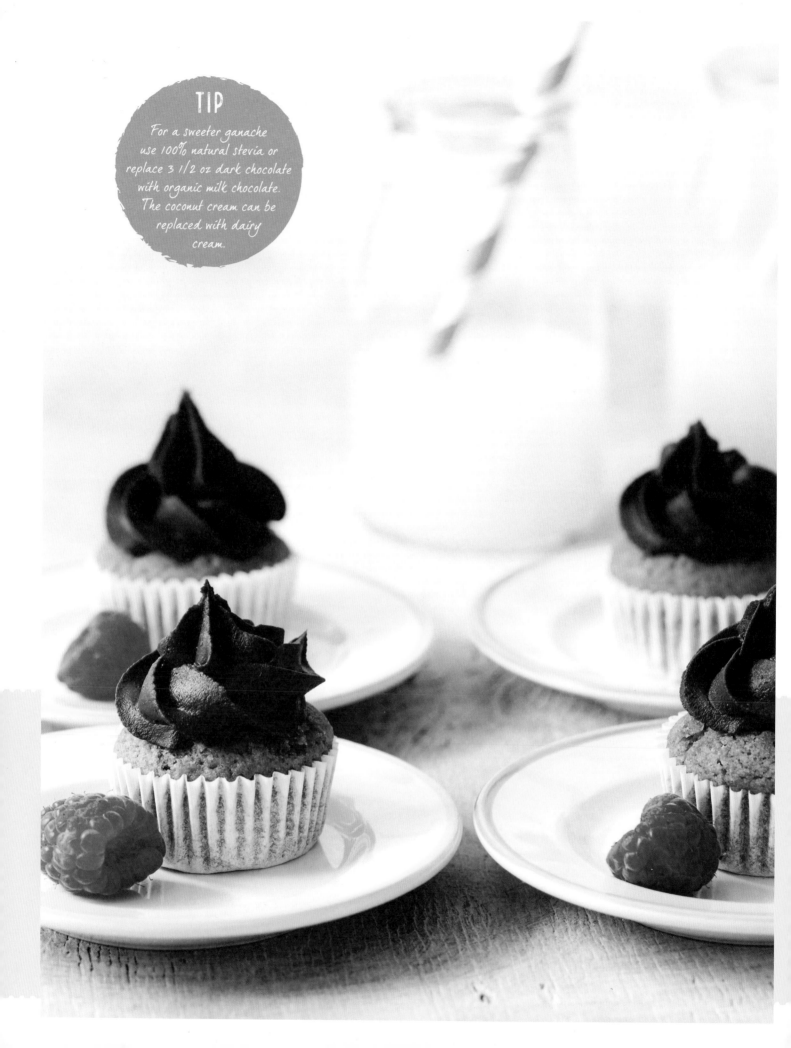

TIP

For a sweeter ganache
use 100% natural stevia or
replace 3 1/2 oz dark chocolate
with organic milk chocolate.
The coconut cream can be
replaced with dairy
cream.

VEG			
Vegetarian	Gluten Free	Dairy Free	Nut Free

Prep time: 15 mins
Cooking time: 15 mins
Makes: 24 mini cupcakes

Mini Vanilla Cupcakes

These gluten-free mini cupcakes are easy to make and I love the fact that they are free from refined wheat flour and sweetened with maple syrup.

INGREDIENTS

1½ cups (6⁴/₅ oz) Wholesome Child gluten-free flour mix (see page 32)

1 tsp xanthum gum or psyllium husk powder

1 tsp baking powder

¼ tsp baking soda

pinch Himalayan rock salt

1 egg

½ cup coconut milk or milk of choice

½ cup maple syrup

2 tbs coconut oil, melted

2 tsp pure vanilla extract

EQUIPMENT

electric hand mixer

INSTRUCTIONS

Preheat oven to 355°F and line a mini muffin tray with 24 mini muffin liners.

Combine all the dry ingredients in a medium-sized bowl.

Place all wet ingredients in a bowl and beat until smooth.

Slowly add dry ingredients to the wet mixture until well combined. Be careful not to overmix the batter as it can get too dense.

Pour batter into prepared mini muffin liners and bake for 15 mins or until a cake tester comes out clean. Allow to cool completely before frosting.

Serving and storing leftovers: Serve immediately, store in the fridge for up to 4 days or freeze for up to 4 months.

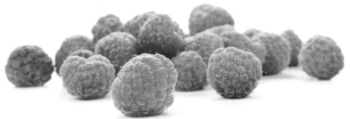

V		
Vegan	Nut Free	Gluten Free

Prep time: 10 mins
Cooking time: 5 mins
Makes: 2 cups

Decadent Chocolate Ganache

INGREDIENTS

1 cup coconut cream

8¾ oz organic dark chocolate (>70%), chopped

½ tsp pure vanilla extract

a generous 3–5 tbs maple syrup or pinch stevia (optional)

pinch sea salt

INSTRUCTIONS

In a medium-sized saucepan heat coconut cream until just before boiling. Remove from heat and add chocolate, vanilla extract, maple syrup and salt and let sit for 3–4 mins without stirring through.

Stir through until well combined. Allow to cool for 5 mins before using.

Serving and storing leftovers: Use immediately to frost your cake or, if you want to pipe it onto cupcakes, put in the fridge for an hour to set. Store in the fridge for up to a week or freeze for up to 6 months.

VEG
Vegetarian

Gluten Free

Dairy Free

Prep time: 25 mins
Cooking time: 15–20 mins
Makes: 50 small/25 large cookies

Gingerbread Cookies

INGREDIENTS

2 cups (8½ oz) almond meal

½ cup (2 oz) coconut flour

¼ cup (³/₅ oz) coconut flakes

½ tsp baking powder

¼ tsp baking soda

2¾ tsp ground ginger

1 tsp ground cinnamon

1 tsp pure vanilla extract

½ cup (2²/₃ oz) coconut sugar (to reduce sugar, substitute ¼ cup sugar with pinch of stevia)

1 egg

2 tbs maple syrup or raw honey

2 tbs apple sauce

⅓ cup coconut oil, melted

EQUIPMENT
High-speed food processor

INSTRUCTIONS

Preheat oven to 325°F and line two baking trays with baking paper.

Place all dry ingredients in a high speed food processor and process until well combined.

Add the wet ingredients and process until a smooth dough is formed (you can also mix by hand).

Roll the mixture out on a well-floured surface, using a rolling pin. If sticky, add flour onto rolling pin or cover dough with cling wrap and roll over plastic.

Using a cookie cutter, cut out gingerbread men shapes.

Bake for approximately 15–20 mins.

Remove cookies from oven and allow to cool.

Serving and storing leftovers: Serve immediately or store in an airtight container in the fridge for up to 2 weeks. Freeze for up to 4 months.

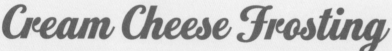

VEG
Vegetarian

Gluten Free

Nut Free

Egg Free

Prep time: 5–10 mins
Makes: 1½ cups

Cream Cheese Frosting

INGREDIENTS

⅓ cup (2⁴/₅ oz) unsalted butter, softened

1 cup (8¾ oz) cream cheese, softened

2 tbs maple syrup

1 tsp pure vanilla extract

1 tsp lemon juice

¼ tsp lemon zest

EQUIPMENT
electric hand mixer

INSTRUCTIONS

Using an electric mixer whip butter and cream cheese together on medium-high speed until smooth and fluffy.

Add in maple syrup, vanilla extract, lemon juice and zest and whip until well combined and creamy. Refrigerate frosting for half an hour to firm up if it seems a bit runny.

Use to ice cupcakes, muffins or carrot cake.

Serving and storing leftovers: Serve immediately on cupcakes, muffins or cake or store in an airtight container in the fridge for up to 4 days.

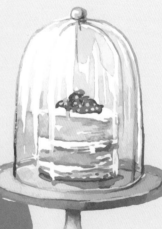

TIP

You can also use 100% natural stevia instead of the maple syrup. Double the recipe if you want to frost a cake.

Prep time: 10 mins
Cooking time: 15 mins
Makes: 20 cookies

Wholesome Almond Cookies

INGREDIENTS

1 cup (4¼ oz) almond meal

1 cup (¾ oz) puffed quinoa

1 cup (2⅘ oz) coconut flakes

1 tsp ground cinnamon

¼ cup coconut oil or butter

¼ cup maple syrup

½ tsp baking powder

2 tbs boiling water

INSTRUCTIONS

Preheat oven to 340°F and line two baking trays with baking paper.

In a medium-sized bowl, combine almond meal, puffed quinoa, coconut flakes and cinnamon.

In a small saucepan over low heat, melt the coconut oil and maple syrup, stirring until the mixture starts to bubble. Remove from the heat.

Combine the baking soda with boiling water together in a small bowl, then add to coconut oil mixture, stirring until foamy.

Pour coconut oil mixture into dry ingredients and combine well.

Roll 1 tbs of mixture into a ball and place on tray, flattening into a disc. Repeat with remaining mixture, allowing room for spreading.

Place in the middle of the oven and bake for 15 mins or until golden brown.

Allow to cool on trays before transferring to a wire rack. Store in an airtight container.

Serving and storing leftovers: Serve immediately or store in an airtight container outside the fridge for up to 3 days or in the fridge for up to 2 weeks. Freeze for up to 4 months.

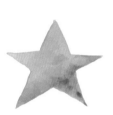
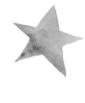

Vegan Gluten Free Nut Free

Prep time: 5 mins (+30 mins refrigeration time)
Makes: 1½ cups

Chocolate Avo Frosting

INGREDIENTS

2 large ripe avocados
14 oz, peeled and pitted

⅓ cup (1 oz) cacao powder

¼ cup (⅞ oz) carob powder

¼ cup coconut cream

½ cup maple syrup

¼ tsp pure vanilla extract

pinch of 100% pure stevia (optional)

EQUIPMENT

Hand-held blender

INSTRUCTIONS

Place all ingredients in a bowl and blend until smooth.

Refrigerate for at least half an hour before icing your cake or cupcakes with it.

Serving and storing leftovers:
Serve immediately, store in an airtight container in the fridge for up to 3 days or freeze for up to 4 months.

So often kids lick the frosting off a cupcake and leave the rest. I wanted to make sure they got a healthy boost in the process!

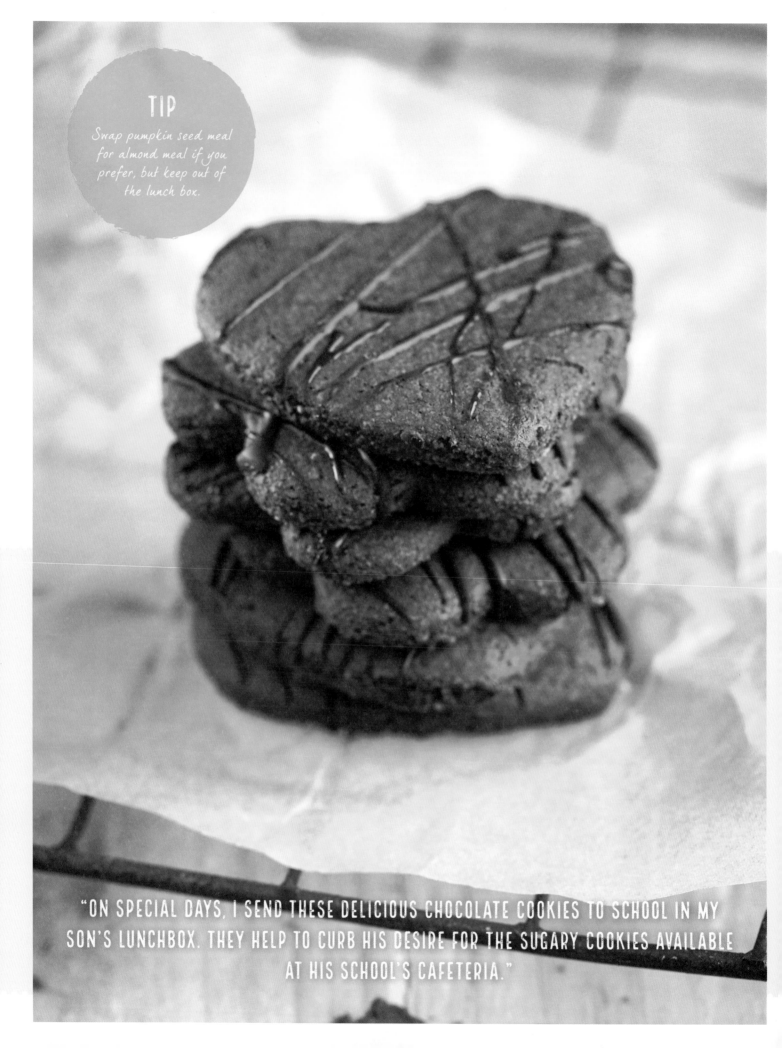

"ON SPECIAL DAYS, I SEND THESE DELICIOUS CHOCOLATE COOKIES TO SCHOOL IN MY SON'S LUNCHBOX. THEY HELP TO CURB HIS DESIRE FOR THE SUGARY COOKIES AVAILABLE AT HIS SCHOOL'S CAFETERIA."

Vegan   Gluten Free   Nut Free

Prep time: 30 mins
Cooking time: 10 mins
Makes: 30 cookies

Gluten-free Chocolate Cookies

These choc cookies are a great alternative to store-bought options. My kids love making them with me and sharing them with friends when they come over for lunch.

INGREDIENTS

¾ cup (3¾ oz) Wholesome Child gluten-free flour mix (see page 32)

¼ cup (1 oz) pumpkin seed meal

½ tsp psyllium husk powder or xanthum gum

¼ cup (⅞ oz) coconut flour

½ cup (2⅗ oz) coconut sugar

2 tbs maple syrup (optional)

2 tbs carob powder

¼ cup (⅞ oz) cacao powder

pinch of Himalayan salt

¼ tsp baking soda

1 tsp pure vanilla extract

¼ cup coconut oil, melted

3 tbs coconut milk or milk of choice

EQUIPMENT

high-speed food processor

INSTRUCTIONS

Preheat oven to 325°F. Line two baking trays with baking paper.

Place all the ingredients in a high-speed food processor and process until you reach a doughy consistency.

Press mixture together and use your hands to form an oval shape.

Place dough in between two sheets of baking paper and roll out to ⅙" using a rolling pin.

Remove the top baking sheet and cut out shapes using a cookie cutter. Repeat with remaining dough. Place baking paper with cut out shapes on a baking tray and bake for 10 mins.

Remove cookies from oven and allow to cool.

Serving and storing leftovers: Serve immediately, store in an airtight container in the fridge for 2 weeks or freeze for up to 4 months.

Vegan   Nut Free

Prep time: 30 mins
Cooking time: 10 mins
Makes: 30 cookies

Chocolate Spelt Cookies

INGREDIENTS

¾ cup (3¾ oz) whole spelt flour

¼ cup (1 oz) pumpkin seed meal

¼ cup (⅞ oz) coconut flour

½ cup (⅞ oz) coconut sugar

2 tbs maple syrup (optional)

¼ cup (⅞ oz) cacao powder

pinch of Himalayan rock salt

2 tbs carob powder

¼ tsp baking soda

1 tsp pure vanilla extract

¼ cup coconut oil, melted

3 tbs coconut milk

EQUIPMENT

high-speed food processor

INSTRUCTIONS

Preheat oven to 325°F and line two baking trays with baking paper.

Place all the ingredients in a high-speed food processor and process until you reach a crumbly consistency.

Press dough together and using your hands form an oval shape.

Roll dough out on a well-floured surface, using a rolling pin. If sticky, add flour to rolling pin or place dough in between 2 sheets of baking paper and roll out to ⅙". Remove top baking sheet.

Using a cookie cutter, cut shapes and place on lined baking trays. Bake for 10 mins.

Remove from oven. The cookies will be soft to touch so allow to cool before eating so they can harden up.

Serving and storing leftovers: Serve immediately. Store in an airtight container for up to 2 weeks or freeze for up to 4 months.

TIP

For a special treat, drizzle the cookies with some melted good-quality organic dark chocolate.

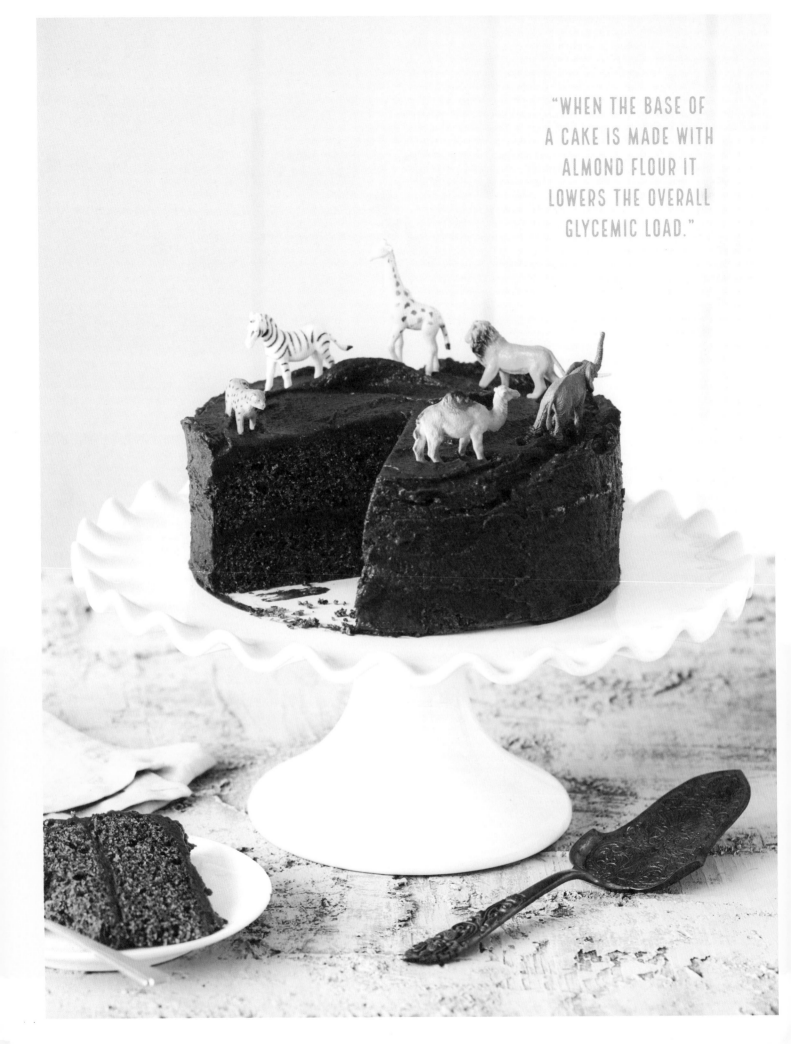

"WHEN THE BASE OF A CAKE IS MADE WITH ALMOND FLOUR IT LOWERS THE OVERALL GLYCEMIC LOAD."

VEG Vegetarian

Gluten Free

Dairy Free

Prep time: 25 mins
Cooking time: 35 mins
Serves: 12

Chocolate Almond Cake

For special celebrations I double the ingredients to make two layers and ice with Choc Date Frosting (see below).

TIP

If your child is used to more sweetness, use 3 1/2 oz dark chocolate and 3 1/2 oz good quality milk chocolate (visit www.wholesomechild.com.au for a list of store-bought chocolates we love).

INGREDIENTS

4 large eggs

½ cup (2³/₅ oz) coconut sugar

1 tsp lemon juice

½ tsp pure vanilla extract

1½ cups (6⅓ oz) almond meal or flour

1 tsp baking powder

pinch sea salt

7 oz organic dark chocolate (70%), finely grated

EQUIPMENT

electric hand mixer

INSTRUCTIONS

Preheat oven to 350°F and grease and line one 8¼" round cake pan with baking paper.

In a large bowl, lightly beat the eggs together with coconut sugar, lemon juice and vanilla.

In another bowl, mix the almond flour, baking powder, sea salt and chocolate.

Add the almond mixture to the egg mixture and stir to combine.

Scoop the batter into the prepared pan and bake for 35 mins. Leave to cool in the pan for 10 mins before carefully placing on a wire rack.

Leave to cool completely, then ice the cake with chocolate date frosting or your favorite frosting.

Serving and storing leftovers: Serve immediately, store in an airtight container in the fridge for up to 4 days or freeze for up to 4 months.

V Vegan

Gluten Free

Nut Free

Prep time: 15 mins (+1 hour to set)
Makes: 1 cup

Choc Date Frosting

INGREDIENTS

1 cup (8½ oz) soft Medjool dates, pitted

½ cup boiling water

1 tbs coconut oil

1 tbs coconut cream

2 tbs cacao powder

1 tbs carob powder

1 tbs maple syrup

1 tsp pure vanilla extract

pinch of Himalayan rock salt (optional)

EQUIPMENT

hand-held blender and blender bowl

INSTRUCTIONS

Place dates in a small bowl. Cover with boiling water. Add coconut oil. Allow to sit for at least 10 mins. Once the dates are soft, place the mixture in the blender bowl and add remaining ingredients. Process until it reaches a smooth consistency.

Refrigerate for at least an hour before using on cupcakes.

Serving and storing leftovers: Use immediately, or store in the fridge in an airtight container for up to 4 days or in the freezer for up to 4 months.

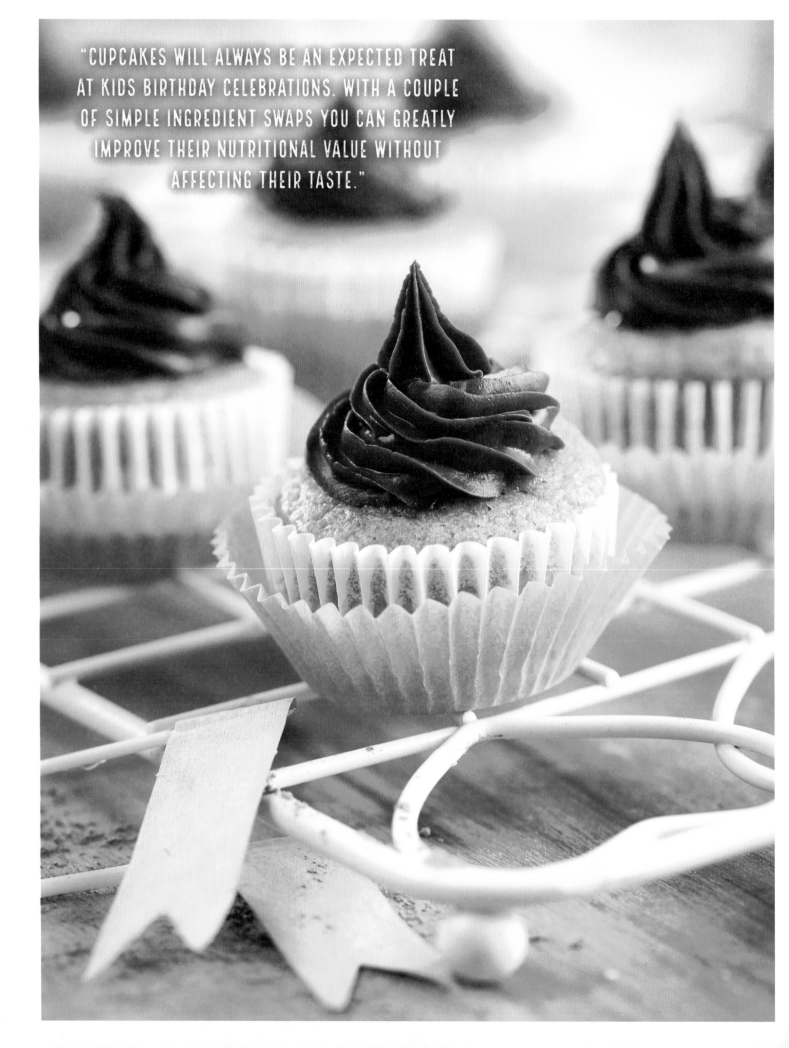

"CUPCAKES WILL ALWAYS BE AN EXPECTED TREAT AT KIDS BIRTHDAY CELEBRATIONS. WITH A COUPLE OF SIMPLE INGREDIENT SWAPS YOU CAN GREATLY IMPROVE THEIR NUTRITIONAL VALUE WITHOUT AFFECTING THEIR TASTE."

VEG
Vegetarian

Dairy Free

Nut Free

Prep time: 10 mins
Cooking time: 15 mins
Makes: 24 mini cupcakes

Easy Vanilla Cupcakes

Cupcakes are always a favorite of kids big and small. Substituting cupcake recipes with wholesome ingredients creates a delicious, healthier version that is free from processed sugars and additives.

INGREDIENTS

1 cup (5 oz) whole spelt flour

¼ cup (1 oz) arrowroot

1 tsp baking powder

¼ tsp baking soda

pinch Himalayan rock salt

1 egg

½ cup coconut milk (or milk of choice)

½ cup maple syrup

2 tsp pure vanilla extract

2 tbs coconut oil, melted

EQUIPMENT
electric hand mixer

INSTRUCTIONS

Preheat oven to 355°F and line a mini muffin tray with 24 mini muffin liners.

Combine all the dry ingredients in a medium-sized bowl.

Place all wet ingredients in a bowl and beat until smooth.

Slowly add dry ingredients to the wet mixture until well combined. Be careful not to overmix the batter as it can get too dense.

Pour batter into prepared mini muffin liners and bake for 15 mins or until a cake tester comes out clean.

Allow to cool completely before frosting.

Serving and storing leftovers: Serve immediately or store in the fridge for up to 4 days or freeze for up to 4 months.

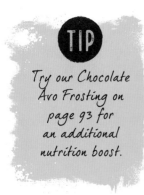

TIP

Try our Chocolate Avo Frosting on page 93 for an additional nutrition boost.

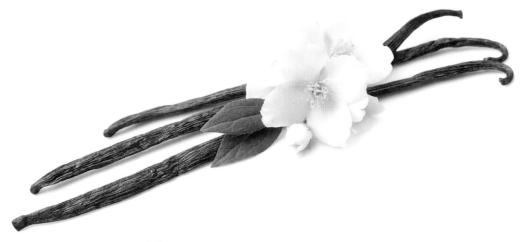

Vegan — Dairy Free — Gluten Free

Chocolate Quinoa Treats

INGREDIENTS

5 tbs (3¼ fl oz) coconut oil

¼ cup (⅞ oz) cacao powder

¼ cup (⅞ oz) carob powder

1 tsp pure vanilla extract

2 tbs of almond butter, peanut butter, cashew nut butter or sunflower seed butter

¼ cup–⅓ cup maple syrup

pinch of Himalayan rock salt (optional)

1½ cups (1 oz) puffed quinoa

INSTRUCTIONS

Place the coconut oil, cacao powder, carob powder, vanilla, almond butter, maple syrup and Himalayan rock salt in a small pot and gently heat over low heat.

Continue to stir until it's totally smooth and melted. Turn off heat and set aside.

Place quinoa puffs in a medium-sized bowl and cover with the chocolate sauce. Mix together, ensuring that all the quinoa puffs are completely covered with chocolate.

Spoon the chocolate puffs into mini muffin cupcake holders.

Place in freezer to set (approximately 1 hour).

Remove from freezer at least 10 mins before serving.

Serving and storing leftovers: Store in the fridge for up to 4 days or in freezer for up to 4 months.

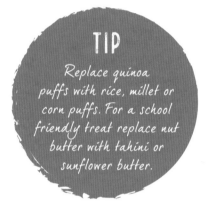

TIP

Replace quinoa puffs with rice, millet or corn puffs. For a school friendly treat replace nut butter with tahini or sunflower butter.

Vegan — Wheat Free

Prep time: 12 mins
Cooking time: 20–23 mins
Serves: 8

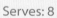

Crunchy Chocolate Coconut Granola

INGREDIENTS

2 cups (8½ oz) whole rolled oats

½ cup (1¼ oz) shredded coconut

½ cup (2⅘ oz) mixed nuts, chopped

¼ cup (1½ oz) pumpkin seeds

¼ cup (1¾ oz) chia seeds

pinch sea salt

¼ cup (⅞ oz) cacao powder

3 tbs coconut oil, melted

¼ tsp pure vanilla extract

2–4 tbs maple syrup or raw honey

INSTRUCTIONS

Preheat oven to 325°F and line a baking tray with baking paper.

In a large bowl, combine oats, shredded coconut, nuts, seeds and salt.

In a smaller bowl, add cacao powder, coconut oil, vanilla extract and honey and whisk to combine.

Pour chocolate mixture over dry ingredients, stirring until well combined and the granola is coated in chocolate.

Transfer mixture onto the baking tray and spread out evenly. Bake for 15 mins, stir through and bake for another 5–8 mins.

Remove from oven and allow to cool before transferring into a jar.

Serving and storing leftovers: Serve immediately with some almond milk and fresh raspberries or store in a glass jar for up to two weeks.

V — Vegan Gluten Free Nut Free

Prep time: 10 mins
Cooking time: 15 mins
Makes: 6

Apple & Cinnamon Doughnuts

INGREDIENTS

¾ cup (3¾ oz) Wholesome Child gluten-free flour mix (see page 32)

½ tsp psyllium husk powder

1 tsp baking powder

¼ tsp ground cinnamon

pinch sea salt

¼ cup maple syrup

⅓ cup coconut milk

½ tsp apple cider vinegar

½ tsp pure vanilla extract

2 tbs apple sauce

2 tbs coconut oil, melted

TOPPING:

1 tbs coconut oil, melted

½–1 tbs coconut sugar (optional)

1 tsp ground cinnamon

EQUIPMENT

doughnut tray

INSTRUCTIONS

Preheat oven to 355°F and lightly coat a doughnut tray with coconut oil.

In a medium-sized bowl, combine flour mix, psyllium husk, baking powder, cinnamon and sea salt.

In a small bowl, combine maple syrup, coconut milk, vinegar, vanilla extract, apple sauce, and coconut oil.

Add wet mixture to dry mixture and whisk until well combined.

Pour batter into prepared doughnut tray and bake in oven for 15 mins.

Leave to cool on a wire rack.

For the topping, add coconut sugar and cinnamon to a small bowl and stir to combine. Brush doughnuts with a little coconut oil and dip into the coconut-cinnamon mixture to coat.

Serving and storing leftovers: Serve immediately, store in an airtight container in the fridge for up to 4 days or freeze for up to 4 months.

You can replace the gluten-free flour mix with whole spelt flour or whole wheat flour.

V — Vegan Gluten Free Nut Free

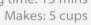

Prep time: 5 mins
Cooking time: 15 mins
Makes: 5 cups

Chocolate Rice Puffs

INGREDIENTS

5 cups (3½ oz) rice puffs

2 tbs cacao powder

2 tbs carob powder

3 tbs maple syrup or raw honey

3 tbs coconut oil, melted

¼ tsp pure vanilla extract

INSTRUCTIONS

Preheat oven to 200°F and line a baking tray with baking paper.

Place rice puffs in a large bowl. Combine cacao, carob, maple syrup, coconut oil, and vanilla extract in a small bowl and pour over rice puffs. Stir through until all puffs are coated in the chocolate mixture.

Spread over the baking tray and bake for 12–15 mins, stirring halfway through.

Leave to cool before transferring to a glass jar.

Serving and storing leftovers: Serve immediately with a splash of milk or store in a glass jar for up to 4 weeks.

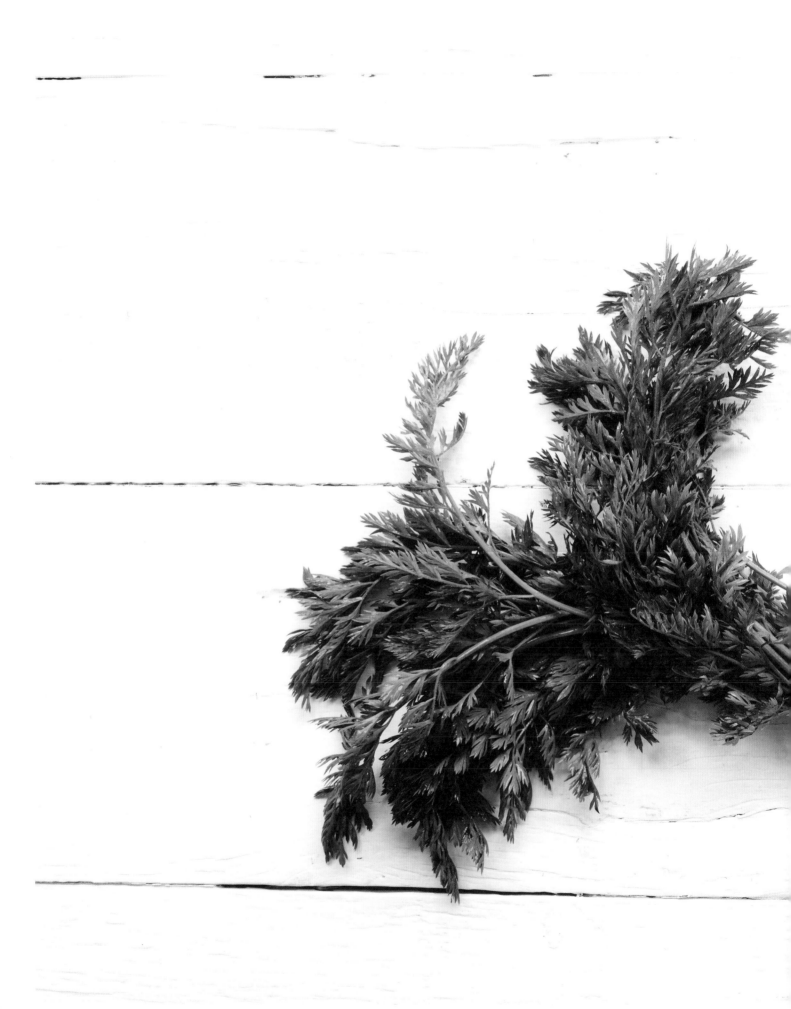

Increase Vegetables

GET CREATIVE AND PERSEVERE

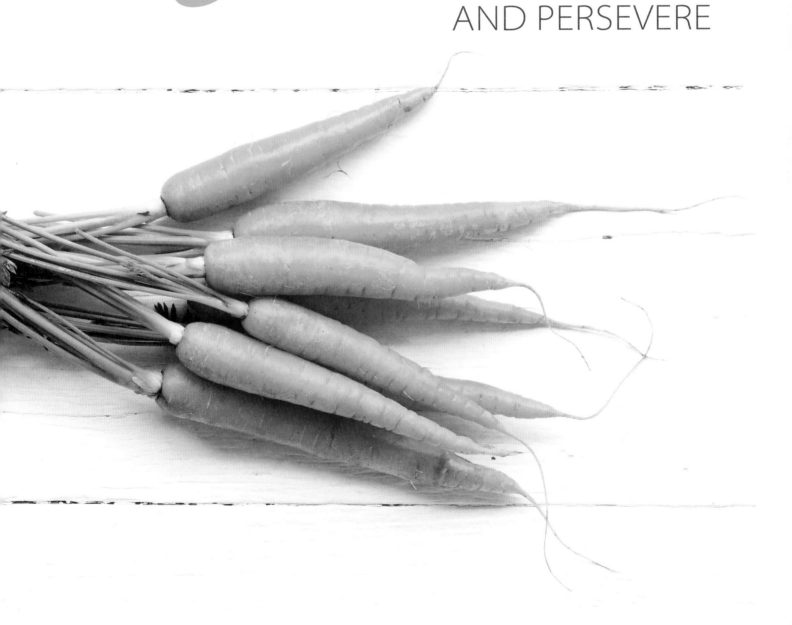

Getting children to eat their greens (and reds, oranges, blues, purples, and browns) on a daily basis is a constant battle for the majority of parents I see in my practice.

So why is there so much focus on the amount of veggies children consume? We all know that vegetables contain essential vitamins and minerals, but they're also nature's greatest insurance policy against disease, thanks to their awe-inspiring phytonutrients.

Scientists have found that the combination of vitamins and these unique plant compounds play an important role in everything from maintaining a healthy immune system to skin health, bone health, eye health, and heart health as well as helping to prevent and manage many illnesses, such as recurrent childhood infections and asthma. Along with the powerful disease-fighting potential that vegetables offer, their high fiber and low calorie content help children feel fuller for longer and maintain a healthy weight.

GETTING STARTED

For many children, eating the recommended servings will take time to achieve. Patience is always key!

1. Use positive reinforcement. Focus on vegetables that your child *is* willing to eat and make sure to praise him each time.

2. Provide opportunity by offering vegetables at snack times, in the lunch box and with main meals.
3. Work on slowly building up the amount of vegetables in each portion.
4. Once your child is eating more servings, focus on broadening variety.

Vegetables contain:

✓ essential vitamins and minerals that ensure proper growth and development, including calcium, folate, iron, magnesium, potassium and vitamin C.

✓ different phytonutrients, each with a unique set of disease-fighting chemicals (hence the need to eat a wide variety).

✓ life-preserving antioxidant and anti-inflammatory properties that protect young bodies against diseases.

✓ high levels of fiber which helps prevent illness and promote healthy digestive function.

PHYTONUTRIENTS AND ANTIOXIDANTS

Along with fruits, vegetables are nature's greatest source of antioxidants and phytochemicals.

Antioxidants, such as vitamins E and C, selenium and zinc, can help stabilize the effects of free radicals (harmful atoms with the ability to cause cellular damage that can lead to disease).

Phytochemicals, such as lycopene in tomatoes and anthocyanins in cranberries, are believed to have even greater antioxidant effects than vitamins and minerals, offering further protection from disease. The damage caused by an overload of free radicals can, over time, lead to illnesses such as heart disease and some cancers. By including a wide range of vegetables in your child's diet, you ensure they receive a daily antioxidant and phytonutrient boost.

Phytonutrients and antioxidants:

✓ provide plants with their colors, flavors, and smells.

✓ remove toxins from our bodies.

✓ boost the immune system.

✓ help regulate hormones.

WHAT DOES ONE SERVING LOOK LIKE?

¼ cup vegetables including broccoli, spinach, cauliflower, pumpkin, beetroot, sweet corn, sweet potato		¼-cup
¼ cup cooked beans, peas or lentils		¼-cup
½ cup salad vegetables (lettuce, cucumber, carrot, and pepper).		½ cup

✓ are anti-inflammatory (fight off inflammation that may lead to diseases like cancer).

✓ fight off free radicals.

As they age, kids who eat vegetables on a daily basis, or even every other day, may have a lower risk of:

✓ developing high blood pressure

✓ developing high cholesterol

✓ developing heart disease

✓ developing diabetes

✓ having a stroke

✓ developing bowel cancer

7 WAYS TO INCREASE VEGGIE VARIETY

Getting most kids to eat a range of vegetables once they are past the baby food stage (at around age one) can leave parents pulling their hair out. While it's necessary to stay calm if your child refuses to eat vegetables, continue to work on increasing their veggie consumption as long-term studies prove the vegetables your child eats now make an enormous difference to their health for the rest of their lives.

How many servings of veggies should my child be eating?

For optimal nutrition, children aged one through four should aim to eat five child-size servings of veggies per day. From ages four to eight the recommendation jumps to 4½ adult-sized servings per day (a child-sized serving doubled). From age nine onwards the goal is five or more servings of veggies daily.

1   CREATE A RAINBOW PLATE

Most children I see in my practice eat the same veggies each day. And while all vegetables are beneficial, the ultimate goal is to eat veggies from all the color groups to get the maximum benefit from their phytonutrients. We eat with our eyes first, so it makes sense to engage your child visually when encouraging them to eat more of a variety. Keep fresh and frozen produce on hand, and get your child to create his own rainbow plate, filled with veggies from all the color groups. It's a great way to teach young kids their colors too. See recipe for Rainbow Salad on page 129.

DID YOU KNOW?

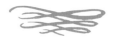

Most children eat 2–3 preferred vegetables day in and day out. Some studies have shown that among 4–8 year olds these are usually tomatoes and potatoes.

Aim to include

GREEN	Broccoli, spinach, cucumber, green beans, zucchini, asparagus, lettuce, kale, celery, Brussels sprouts, cabbage, snow peas, okra, spinach, peas, edamame (soy beans)	Iron, folate, zinc calcium, vitamin B6, potassium, lutein, chlorophyll
WHITE/BROWN	Cauliflower, potato, garlic, onion, leek, artichoke, parsnip, bamboo shoots, mushrooms, tofu, navy beans, lima beans, chickpeas, turnip, Jerusalem artichokes	Magnesium, beta-glucans, lignans, potassium, calcium
RED	Red pepper, radish (skin on), rhubarb, radicchio, beetroot	Folate, vitamin C, vitamin A, lycopene, quercetin, hesperidin
ORANGE/YELLOW	Carrot, pumpkin, sweet potato, corn, butternut or yellow squash, yellow or orange pepper	Beta-carotene, vitamin A, vitamin C, vitamin B6, vitamin B1, flavonoids, lycopene
BLUE/PURPLE	Eggplant, kohlrabi, Spanish onion, purple cabbage, Kalamata olives, purple carrots, purple sweet potato (skin on)	Vitamin K, potassium, phosphorous, zeaxanthin, resveratrol, vitamin C, fiber, flavonoids, quercetin

Phytonutrients like capsaicin (found in Pepper) protect us from harmful carcinogens, while saponins (found in beans) prevent the spread of cancer cells and allicin, (found in garlic) has antibacterial properties.

(Continued on page 110 after Vegetables table)

❷ TRY ONE NEW VEGGIE A WEEK

I usually find a strong connection between children who eat the same vegetables over and over and their parents who do the same. If this sounds like your family, start by looking at your own diet. I often see clients who say they eat a lot of veggies but when I ask them to keep a food diary, I see they eat only carrots, cucumber, peas, and potatoes, for example, even though they eat them every day. By expanding your own repertoire of vegetables, you give your child the opportunity to see a variety of veggies being eaten and to try some of them too. You can also expand their range by including different vegetable groups. Try salad veggies, cruciferous vegetables like cauliflower and brussels sprouts, and starchy vegetables like taro or sweet potato. While there's nothing wrong with focusing on accepted vegetables, sometimes we forget there is a huge selection out there which, given the opportunity, children may actually enjoy. See the table on pages 108–109 for some of my favorite 'non-typical' veggies to try.

❸ INCLUDE BEANS AND LEGUMES

These are our most nutritious plant foods, high in protein, B-vitamins, iron, potassium, fiber, minerals and phytochemicals like saponins, isoflavones, and phytosterols. Beans are an excellent way to ensure optimum protein intake in vegetarians, prevent constipation, and keep away other nasty illnesses such as colon cancer, heart disease, and high cholesterol. To prevent bloating and "wind," soak dried beans overnight in water with a tablespoon of apple cider vinegar and then rinse before cooking. (See page 30 for more info on preparing beans.) For canned varieties, look for BPA-free cans wherever possible and rinse well. Try kidney beans, navy beans, black beans, adzuki beans, chickpeas and lentils. (See recipe for Lentil & Vegetable Soup on page 121.)

❹ ADD SEA VEGETABLES

Seaweed, thanks to its high calcium content, strengthens bones and teeth. It's also high in iron, has antimicrobial properties, and is a good source of essential vitamins, minerals, and dietary fiber which helps prevent constipation. Nori, rich in vitamins A, B1, B2 and C as well as iodine, also contains protein. Use it for sushi, shred it over salad or create veggie-filled seaweed wraps, filled with julienned carrots, cucumber, shredded chicken (or protein of choice) and avocado. Despite the nutritious benefits of seaweed, it is possible for it to contain heavy metals. Hijiki, for example, contains high levels of arsenic and should be avoided. If your child likes the seaweed snack packs that have become common at supermarkets, seek out certified organic varieties, as they are less likely to contain heavy metals and other contaminants, and always check the ingredients to make sure there is no MSG or added sugar. Moderation is key, so don't offer your child seaweed on a daily basis.

❺ DON'T FORGET HERBS AND SPICES

Basil is packed with essential oils such as eugenol, citronellol, linalool, citral, limonene and terpineol, which are known to have anti-inflammatory and anti-bacterial properties. Use in tomato-based pasta sauces, sprinkle on pizza, and mix into rissoles.

Mint soothes upset stomachs and improves digestion. Chill mint tea or add fresh mint leaves and orange slices to water and serve in place of juice. Use in our Rainbow Salad (see recipe 129).

Oregano is often used to treat respiratory tract disorders, gastrointestinal (GI) disorders, and urinary tract disorders. Add to chicken, lamb, or beef dishes.

Parsley, rich in many vital vitamins, including Vitamin A, C, B12 and K, keeps your immune system strong, tones your bones, and heals the nervous system. It helps flush out excess fluid from the body, thus supporting kidney function. Add to smoothies, chicken soup, and pasta sauces.

Spices: As well as adding flavor, spices such as turmeric (anti-inflammatory), ginger (great for digestion), and cinnamon (balances blood sugar levels) are packed with nutrients too. Add turmeric and ginger to chicken soup, sprinkle turmeric on cauliflower, and cinnamon onto pumpkin or butternut squash.

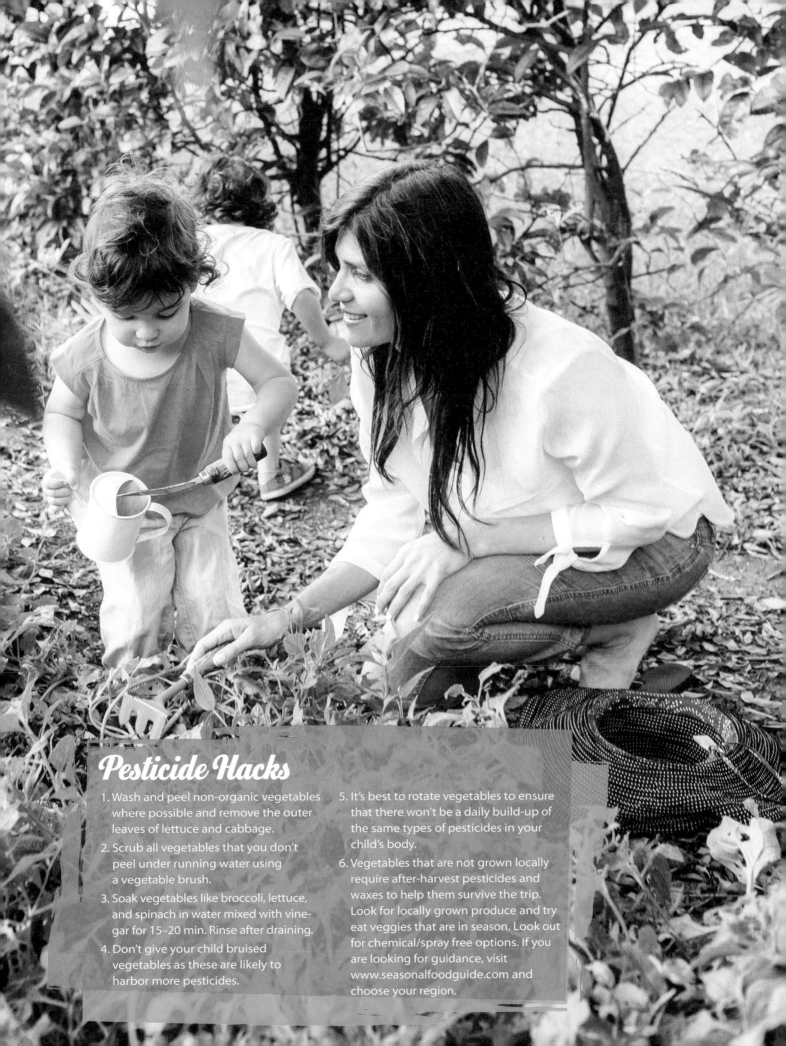

Pesticide Hacks

1. Wash and peel non-organic vegetables where possible and remove the outer leaves of lettuce and cabbage.

2. Scrub all vegetables that you don't peel under running water using a vegetable brush.

3. Soak vegetables like broccoli, lettuce, and spinach in water mixed with vinegar for 15–20 min. Rinse after draining.

4. Don't give your child bruised vegetables as these are likely to harbor more pesticides.

5. It's best to rotate vegetables to ensure that there won't be a daily build-up of the same types of pesticides in your child's body.

6. Vegetables that are not grown locally require after-harvest pesticides and waxes to help them survive the trip. Look for locally grown produce and try eat veggies that are in season. Look out for chemical/spray free options. If you are looking for guidance, visit www.seasonalfoodguide.com and choose your region.

Vegetables

ARTICHOKES	ASPARAGUS	BEETROOT	BRUSSELS SPROUTS	JERUSALEM ARTICHOKES	KALE

Benefits

ARTICHOKES: High in potassium, vitamin K, calcium, and folate and packed with health boosting antioxidant activity. They also contain a compound called cynarin which helps to reduce indigestion and bloating.

ASPARAGUS: A good source of fiber, folate, vitamins K, C and E, as well as chromium, a trace mineral that helps to keep blood sugar levels stable by enhancing the ability of insulin to transport glucose from the bloodstream into cells. It may cause your child's urine to have a pungent odor but this is harmless and caused by the sulphur compounds.

BEETROOT: A powerhouse of healthy nutrients such as folate, calcium, iron, fiber, potassium and vitamin C. They are also rich in phytochemicals such as anthocyanins and saponins. Don't discard the greens, which are rich in calcium, iron, and vitamins A and C. They can be sautéed and used in place of spinach or hidden in bolognaise sauce.

BRUSSELS SPROUTS: Aside from their vitamin C, folate, and beta-carotene content, it's their antioxidant content that really stands out. This small cabbage-like veggie helps clean up free radicals—scientists have proven these close cousins of broccoli are packed with molecules our bodies convert into diindolymethane (an immune-system booster) that helps protect new brain cells. They also have plenty of bitter sulforaphane, as well as compounds called isothiocyanates, which detoxify cancer-causing substances in the body.

JERUSALEM ARTICHOKES: Rich in iron—containing one of the highest levels among all the root vegetables. Also high in potassium, copper, and fiber.

KALE: Rich in cancer-fighting antioxidants and vitamins, kale is also an excellent source of vitamin C and beta-carotene and contains an impressive combination of phytonutrients lutein and zeaxanthin. It also contains more iron and calcium than almost any other vegetable.

How to use it

ARTICHOKES: Cut off the stem and remove any tough outer leaves. Cut off the top 3/4" and trim tips of remaining leaves. Cook whole by steaming. Cut in half, and remove the inedible, fuzzy center. Once cool show your child how to pull off the curved outer leaves and use his teeth to scrape off the tender part. You can also make the artichoke heart into a dip or slice it onto a pizza.

ASPARAGUS: Sauté in a pan, grill, bake or steam, then add a few shavings of Parmesan cheese and let your child squeeze lemon juice over the asparagus. Or use in our delicious Asparagus & Cheese Tart on page 255.

BEETROOT: Roast, steam or bake them. Alternatively, grate raw beetroot and mix with grated apple and carrot for a colorful summer salad. Thanks to their bright pink color, they are also a great addition to smoothies; try our Beetroot Berry Smoothie recipe on page 225—the berries help to disguise their slightly earthy taste. Or use in our delicious Beetroot Bliss Balls on page 115.

BRUSSELS SPROUTS: Steam or roast, sprinkle with olive oil and a touch of Himalayan rock salt. Kids love peeling the leaves off these teeny cabbage lookalikes.

JERUSALEM ARTICHOKES: Once peeled, Jerusalem artichokes can be eaten raw in salads, steamed and mashed like potato, roasted, or deep-fried in a healthy oil to prepare as chips. Steamed Jerusalem artichoke can also be puréed and used as a dip or in pasta sauce or added to stews and soups.

KALE: Put a handful of kale leaves into a berry-packed smoothie and it'll virtually disappear. Toss roughly chopped kale leaves in olive oil, sprinkle with sesame seeds, and roast to make kale chips. Slice very finely and add to stir-fries or rissoles, or add to soups and simmer until soft. For a great kale packed smoothie, see our Avocado Chocolate Smoothie on page 225.

To increase variety, here are some of Wholesome Child's favorite nutrient packed, non-typical veggie choices

KOHLRABI	PARSNIPS	PURPLE CARROTS	RED CABBAGE	SPAGHETTI SQUASH
Benefits	**Benefits**	**Benefits**	**Benefits**	**Benefits**
Mildly sweet, knobby purple or green, kohlrabi is a rich source of phytonutrients as well as vitamin C, B-complex groups of vitamins such as niacin, vitamin B-6 (pyridoxine), thiamin, pantothenic acid and minerals such as manganese, iron, and calcium.	Parsnips, a cousin of the humble carrot, contain a wide variety of minerals and nutrients, including dietary fiber, folate, potassium, and vitamin C. An added bonus for children is they are slightly sweet.	Not only do they have the vitamin A and beta-carotene of ordinary carrots, they're also rich in anthocyanins, the antioxidant compounds that give blueberries their color and health benefits. The pigments in purple carrots are thought to improve memory, enhance vision, protect against heart attacks and act as anti-inflammatories.	Red cabbage is unique among the cruciferous vegetables, as it provides about 30 milligrams of the antioxidant anthocyanin per half cup. Anthocyanins have anti-inflammatory benefits and are partly responsible for red cabbage's cancer prevention powers too.	High in vitamins A and C as well as beta-carotene, lutein, and zeaxanthin, which are all linked to healthy vision and optimal eye health.
How to use it	**How to use it**	**How to use it**	**How to use it**	**How to use it**
Always peel the tough outermost layer of the bulb. Then steam, roast, add to soups and stews, grate raw into salad or fritters. Kohlrabi leaves can be sautéed or steamed too. Or try our Rainbow Salad on page 129.	Prepare and bake parsnips as you would French fries. It's often easier to introduce to children if they are mixed in with sweet potato or regular homemade chips. Remember, parsnips need approx ten min longer to cook than regular potatoes. Or try our delicious Shepherd's Pie with parsnip mash (see recipe on page 169).	Serve and enjoy in the same manner as regular carrots: raw, baked, steamed, or roasted. Perfect for a fun lunch box alternative.	Grate raw to create a more colorful coleslaw and serve with a homemade mayonnaise. Add to stir-fries or cut in half and separate the large leaves and place in steamer. Use the cooked leaves as wraps or roll-ups, and fill with our bolognaise sauce, black bean mix, or shredded chicken and cheese.	Bake or steam. Add olive oil or butter, and sprinkle with a favorite cheese, or serve with a tomato-basil sauce. Allow to cool and then using a fork separate the long strands and serve as spaghetti.

⑥ SHOP FOR VEGETABLES TOGETHER

Encourage your little ones to touch, smell and engage with their food. Let them help with grocery shopping. Encourage them to pick up a carrot, an apple, or a zucchini from the shelf and place it in the basket or shopping cart themselves—this begins the engagement with the new food. Can they put the dish or new veggie onto the table for the family? Don't be disappointed if they don't eat the new food the first time it's offered—stay positive and freeze what is not eaten and offer it again—repetition is key here.

⑦ COOK VEGETABLES TOGETHER

Children love to eat what they have helped to prepare, and it is important for them to be exposed to vegetables in their raw state and understand how the texture and look of a vegetable changes when it's cooked. Let them help by peeling carrots and potatoes (look for kid-friendly graters), cutting lettuce with a plastic lettuce knife, pouring beans into soups, adding grated zucchini into the muffin batter or grated carrot into the bolognaise.

HOW TO BUY ORGANIC WITHOUT BREAKING THE BANK

I would recommend buying organic vegetables whenever you can. Increase variety by looking for organic flash-frozen vegetables in the freezer section. Studies have frequently shown that organic vegetables have higher antioxidant activity (between 19 percent and 69 percent). Babies and young children have lower levels of the enzymes needed to detoxify pesticide chemicals from their bodies, compared to adults. Their developing brains and nervous systems are also more vulnerable to chemicals than adults. The consumption of pesticides and other chemicals at an early age therefore may have a detrimental impact to their long-term health.

A visit to your local farmer's market is a better option than the supermarket as locally grown seasonal vegetables often contain fewer pesticides. Often, while they might not carry the "certified organic" label, some vegetables sold at farmer's markets are organically grown.

Farmer's markets are also usually more affordable than supermarkets, and make a fun outing with the kids.

We all know that buying organic produce can be costly. So to understand when it's worth the extra dollars, it pays to be informed which produce contain the highest pesticide residue levels and make your organic choices accordingly. Look at the Environmental Working Group's Dirty Dozen and Clean List of fruit and vegetables: www.ewg.org/foodnews/list.php.

This website contains a list of the most popular fresh produce items, and ranks these by "cleanest" to "dirtiest." The produce listed as "dirty" are hard to clean, and even when washed and scrubbed, still contain significant amounts of pesticide residue. Note: although the data on the EWG website is compiled by the US Department of Agriculture and Food and Drug Administration, there is a considerable overlap with Australian produce, as Australian commercial farming practices closely correlate to those in the USA.

BEST TO CHOOSE ORGANIC:

Celery (64 different pesticides applied)
Pepper (49 different pesticides applied)
Spinach (48 different pesticides applied)
Potatoes (37 different pesticides applied)
Kale
Lettuce
Cucumber

OKAY TO CHOOSE NON-ORGANIC:

Onions
Avocado
Asparagus
Peas
Cabbage
Eggplant
Broccoli
Mushrooms
Sweet potato
Corn (as long as it is labelled non-GMO)

Consider this . . . If your child is still a baby or a young toddler, you may be able to use repetition to your advantage when it comes to adding new vegetables to the menu. Don't give up if your child protests. In one study, researchers identified mothers who had given up after their babies rejected a particularly protested vegetable on two or three occasions. The mothers were then asked to offer this same disliked vegetable, every second day for two weeks, at first the baby's intake of the disliked vegetable was low. However, by the time they had sampled it seven or eight times, surprisingly over 70 percent of these children not only accepted the previously spurned vegetable, but really liked it, readily eating as much of it as their other favorite veggies.

RAW VS COOKED: IS THERE A NUTRITIONAL DIFFERENCE?

A veggie in its raw state is the most nutritious choice because the enzymes, vitamins, and phytonutrients are intact, right? Not always. Some vegetables are actually healthier when cooked, as applying heat increases the levels of some nutrients by breaking down the cell walls of the plant, releasing the nutrients contained within. Roasting can boost a carrot's levels of beta-carotene by over 30 percent. This key antioxidant supports our night vision, guards against heart disease, several cancers (bladder, cervix, prostate, colon, esophagus), and is a particularly potent lung protector.

Another great example is steamed spinach, which has higher levels of lutein, an antioxidant that helps prevent cataracts and macular degeneration. Heating Popeye's favorite veggie can also help your child absorb more calcium. Spinach is also more compact when cooked, so your child gets more nutrients per mouthful. Lightly cooking vegetables such as Pepper, broccoli, and cauliflower can also make them easier to digest for some children.

WHAT IS THE BEST WAY TO COOK VEGGIES?

The method you use can make a big difference in how many vitamins and minerals your child ultimately gets from his vegetables. High temperatures can diminish some of the vitamins and minerals by 15–30 percent, with boiling being the biggest culprit, so avoid boiling vegetables. Steaming until crisp-tender is the most nutritious way to prepare vegetables, as this methods retains most of the vegetable's natural liquids. Sautéing and grilling are also good options. And remember, roasting vegetables is a great way to get rid of their bitter taste.

WHAT ABOUT FERMENTING VEGETABLES?

The *lactobacilli* in fermented vegetables, such as pickled cucumbers, carrots or sauerkraut, enhances their digestibility and increases vitamin levels. Numerous helpful enzymes are produced as well as antibiotic and anti-carcinogenic substances. These bacteria promote the growth of healthy bacteria or flora throughout our intestines. Start slowly when offering to your child; one tablespoon per mealtime is adequate. See our recipe for a great child-friendly Fermented Carrot Sticks on my website, www.wholesomechild.com.au.

SO WHY WON'T KIDS EAT VEGGIES?

We are born with a natural predisposition to prefer sweet and salty flavors, and to reject bitter or sour tastes. Nature intended it to be this way to protect us when we were hunters and gatherers, helping us stay away from poisonous bitter plants. Although toddlers may start loathing any food, vegetables tend to take the biggest hit. Here are a few common reasons why:

1. No predictability

Of course there is no predictability when it comes to vegetables. A local seasonal carrot can be delicious and sweet. A carrot that has been imported or has been in cold storage for a few months may have an entirely different consistency and not be as sweet. An experience with a bitter carrot can easily turn a child off carrots for good. Visually, they do not appear the same either. My son is an avid veggie eater, but will turn his nose up at the sight of a brown spot in a favoured veggie. And if you are buying organic, you will know that nature does not always turn out the best looking produce.

2. Too many sweet foods too early on

One of the leading nutritional causes of fussy eating happens when children are exposed to sugar too early, as it alters their sweet taste receptors. If a young child's developing taste buds are exposed to too many sweet foods too often, they develop a preference for that kind of food and will fail to appreciate the natural sweetness of vegetables.

GOAL 3: INSPIRE AND MODEL

1. PERSEVERE

Because we know human beings are genetically predisposed to enjoy sweet foods and reject bitter ones from a young age, it's important to make the effort to offer our children vegetables in their natural state over and over again. Repeated exposure to veggies from as early on as possible is the best way to avoid fussy eating.

Always give your child a chance to experience the true flavor of foods, even in the face of

DID YOU KNOW?

Thanks to its thick skin, the cleanest produce with the least amount of pesticides is avocado.

TIP

If you're out of the baby phase and don't have time to make your own vegetable purees keep a few bottles of organic baby food handy to add into recipes.

initial rejection. Their little tastebuds are forever changing, so what is not eaten today might become a firm favorite in the future. With older children, learn to hide your exasperation.

Instead, play it cool and focus on being a role model during family dinners. When your child sees you snacking on baby carrots or having a salad day after day, it may not be too long before a little hand reaches in there to swipe some for themselves.

2. MAKE SALAD AND VEGETABLES READILY AVAILABLE

Put the bowl and serving dishes onto the dinner table and supply tongs so that children can easily serve themselves. Good habits start young, so even if your child refuses to touch a vegetable, it's important to train them to expect a salad and serving of cooked vegetables at each meal. Dressing salad with healthy options, such as olive oil and balsamic vinegar or one of our delicious salad dressings can entice children to try it.

3. USE YOUR IMAGINATION

When my kids were going through a particularly fussy stage with broccoli, one day I got up on a table and started doing a crazy dance each time they took a bite of their broccoli. It worked! They were both laughing so hard they forgot about the fact that they didn't like the taste. A green bean becomes a wriggly worm, a piece of cauliflower is a cloud and a carrot is a snowman's nose.

4. VISIT A COMMUNITY GARDEN OR START YOUR OWN VEGGIE PATCH

You don't have to have a huge plot of land to have a vegetable garden. You can grow veggies or herbs in pots on the kitchen windowsill, patio or on a balcony. Include your kids every step of the way, from choosing what to grow, to packing the soil, watering, weeding, and of course, picking. The more they're involved, the more they'll enjoy it and keep helping . . . and eating.

👍 DO . . .	👎 DON'T . . .
ensure that the emotional environment at mealtimes is pleasant. Simply give your child their vegetables and act as if you don't mind whether they eat them or not.	get into a power struggle over veggies (no commands, orders, threats, punishments, bribes). As soon as you let go of the power struggle, children may become more willing to try new veggies because they have nothing to gain by refusing it.
praise your child for trying small amounts of new veggies. Over time continuing to do this will lead to familiarity with the new vegetables and a greater desire to eat them.	introduce new foods in a coercive way, or use threats, and never force your child to eat large quantities of new foods.
try offering them vegetables cut into fun shapes, laid out in color patterns, steamed rather than raw. For older children, using star charts is a good way to get them to try a new vegetable.	use food, especially dessert or treats, as a reward.
discuss the health benefits of eating vegetables with older children in a fun and engaging way.	lecture your children about the healthy benefits of vegetables without speaking about the fact that they are delicious too.
let your child decide whether you'll have green beans or broccoli. Simple choices will help him feel a sense of control.	dictate the menu. Offer choices, for example: Would you like your sweet potato mashed, baked or cut into chips?
make eating veggies fun. Try making a veggie face (like cucumber eyes, tomato nose, green bean mouth, and shredded carrot hair). Toddlers also love dipping, so try serving veggies with yogurt.	take it personally when the vegetables you have lovingly prepared are picked at or passed over entirely.
keep veggies in plain view in the fridge or pantry. What the eyes see the tummy wants.	force a child to eat when they are genuinely not hungry. Look over the day . . . did they have a big afternoon tea? What did they eat at their grandmother's house? Was there a birthday party at school?

Eight Veggie Tricks

There is nothing wrong with bumping up recipes with hidden veggies, as long as you offer these same veggies to your child in their raw state too. The bottom line is you can never have too many veggies in a child's diet. Going over the recommended five veggie servings a day is nothing but beneficial. And disguising vegetables becomes appropriate if a child is going through a fussy eating stage that is making it impossible for them to reach even half of their recommended daily veggie intake. However, it's always best to involve your child in the process of adding veggies to their food. Prepare a choc muffin with added zucchini, and see the surprise on their face when they realize it tastes really good! Work within the framework of your child's favorite foods. If he loves pancakes, make them with pumpkin and sweet potato puree; if he loves pasta make your own pasta sauce and puree peas, onions, garlic and zucchini into it. Veggies can be added into muffins (see recipe for Chocolate Zucchini Muffins on page 127) or cookies too.

1 If your child only likes one vegetable such as carrots or potatoes, you can try pureeing similar colored veggies and add them in as small quantities. For example, sweet potato and carrot, cauliflower and potato, broccoli and zucchini, mashed potato and parsnip, or parsnip chips added to homemade French fries.

2 If your child will only eat sweet foods, bake vegetables in a honey sauce. Sweet potato, pumpkin, carrot, parsnip, or zucchini drizzled with raw honey and extra virgin olive oil and a pinch of cinnamon may be more palatable. Or put a drizzle of maple syrup into the water if you're boiling vegetables.

3 Use the nutrient-packed water from steamed or boiled vegetables to water down fruit juice, or add to other dishes.

4 If your child loves burgers it's easy to add vegetables to beef or chicken patties, or try lentil burgers. The same goes for bolognaise sauce, pasta sauce, or meatballs (see our recipe on page 155).

5 Veggie stocks are an absolute powerhouse of nutrients (see recipe on page 277). Cook up an assortment of veggies, including leek, carrots, onion, parsley, and bay leaves and add to any food you're cooking. You can even boil pasta or rice in the veggie stock. Avoid stock cubes where possible, as they contain preservatives, sugar and excess salt. Instead, freeze homemade vegetable stock into cubes to use at a later stage.

6 Homemade sauces like hummus, tzatziki, babaghanoush (made with eggplant), sweet pepper relish, ketchup, broccoli cheese sauce, and pesto sauce are all a great way to boost your child's veggie intake. The list is endless. If your child is used to processed sauces, use a 1:3 ratio and slowly reduce the amount of processed sauce. See our delicious dips in Steps 5 and 8.

7 Experiment with thinly sliced sweet potato, parsnip, beetroot, and butternut tossed in extra virgin olive oil and roasted to make homemade oven chips.

8 Add vegetables to smoothies too. Use yogurt as the base and add one banana, the juice of half an orange, frozen blueberries, raw spinach or kale, pepper or carrot, and any of the following cooked and cooled vegetables: baked pumpkin, baked zucchini, or beetroot. You will need to experiment with sweetness. To start, use sweeter veggies like pumpkin, carrot, and sweet potato, then experiment with green veggies like celery and spinach. Freeze leftovers in ice trays or popsicle molds. See our smoothie recipes on page 225.

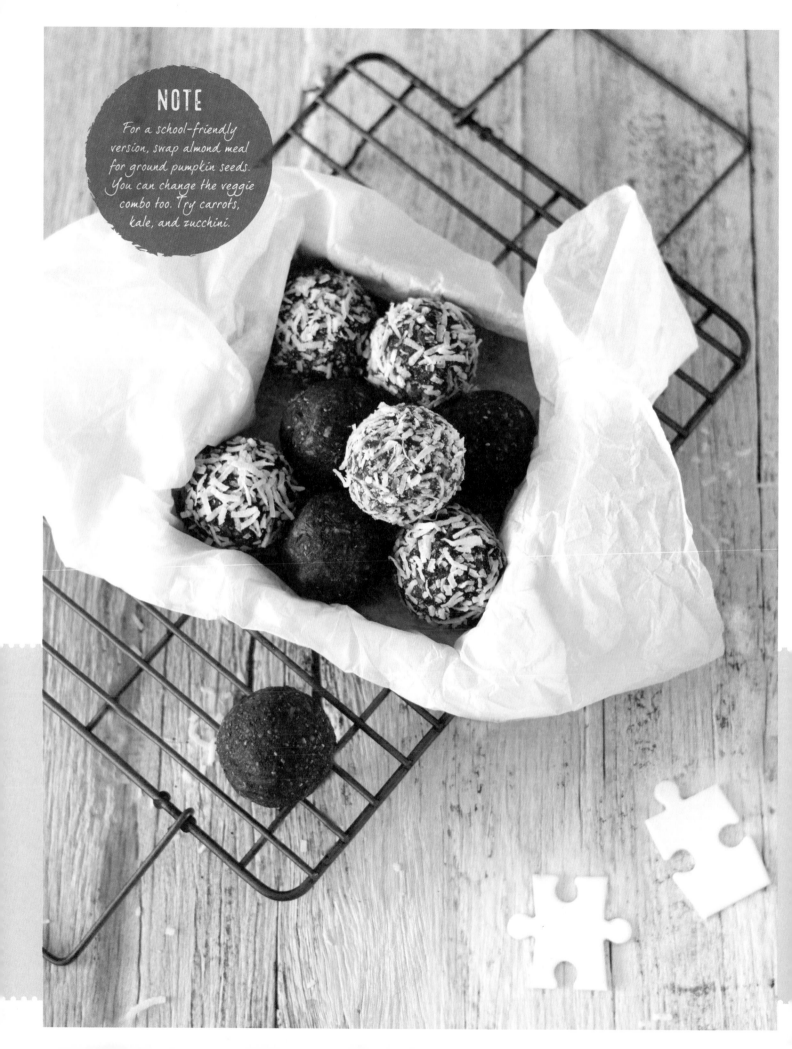

NOTE

For a school-friendly version, swap almond meal for ground pumpkin seeds. You can change the veggie combo too. Try carrots, kale, and zucchini.

Prep time: 25 mins (+ 1 hr refrigeration time)
Makes: 30 (approx.)

Beetroot Bliss Balls

This is a really clever way to disguise beetroot, a rich source of vitamin C, fiber, and cancer-fighting phytonutrients. Plus my three-year-old daughter had so much fun watching her hands turn red as she rolled them into balls.

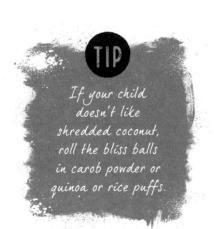

TIP

If your child doesn't like shredded coconut, roll the bliss balls in carob powder or quinoa or rice puffs.

INGREDIENTS

1 cup (8.46 oz) dates, pitted and chopped

½ cup (2⁴⁄₅ oz) beetroot, peeled and finely grated

½ cup (¹⁄₆ oz) baby spinach, finely sliced and chopped

1¼ cups (5¼ oz) almond meal

1 cup (2²⁄₃ oz) shredded coconut

1–2 tbs chia seeds

¼ cup (1¼ oz) coconut sugar

½ cup (1¼ oz) extra shredded coconut to roll balls in

EQUIPMENT

high-speed food processor

INSTRUCTIONS

Place all ingredients into a high-speed food processor and process until smooth.

Roll into little balls and then roll the balls in the shredded coconut.

Place bliss balls in freezer and leave to set for 1 hour.

Serving and storing leftovers: Keep bliss balls in the freezer for up to 6 months. Best eaten within 15 mins of removing from freezer.

Vegetarian Gluten Free Dairy Free Nut Free

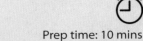

Prep time: 10 mins
Cooking time: 10 mins (1–2 mins each side)
Serves: 4

Sweet Potato Pancakes

INGREDIENTS

4 eggs

½ ripe banana

1½ cups (13¼ oz) sweet potato, peeled and steamed or roasted

1 tbs chia seeds

½–1 tsp ground cinnamon

pinch Himalayan rock salt

coconut oil, for frying

EQUIPMENT

high-speed food processor

INSTRUCTIONS

Place all ingredients into a high-speed food processor and process until smooth.

Brush a large frying pan with some coconut oil and heat over medium heat.

Spoon around ⅛ cup to ¼ cup of batter into the pan.

Cook pancakes for approximately 1–2 mins on each side. Continue with rest of the batter.

Serving and storing leftovers: Serve immediately, store in the fridge for up to 4 days or freeze for up to 4 months.

TIP

Replace the sweet potato with pumpkin and serve with ricotta cheese, coconut cream or natural yogurt.

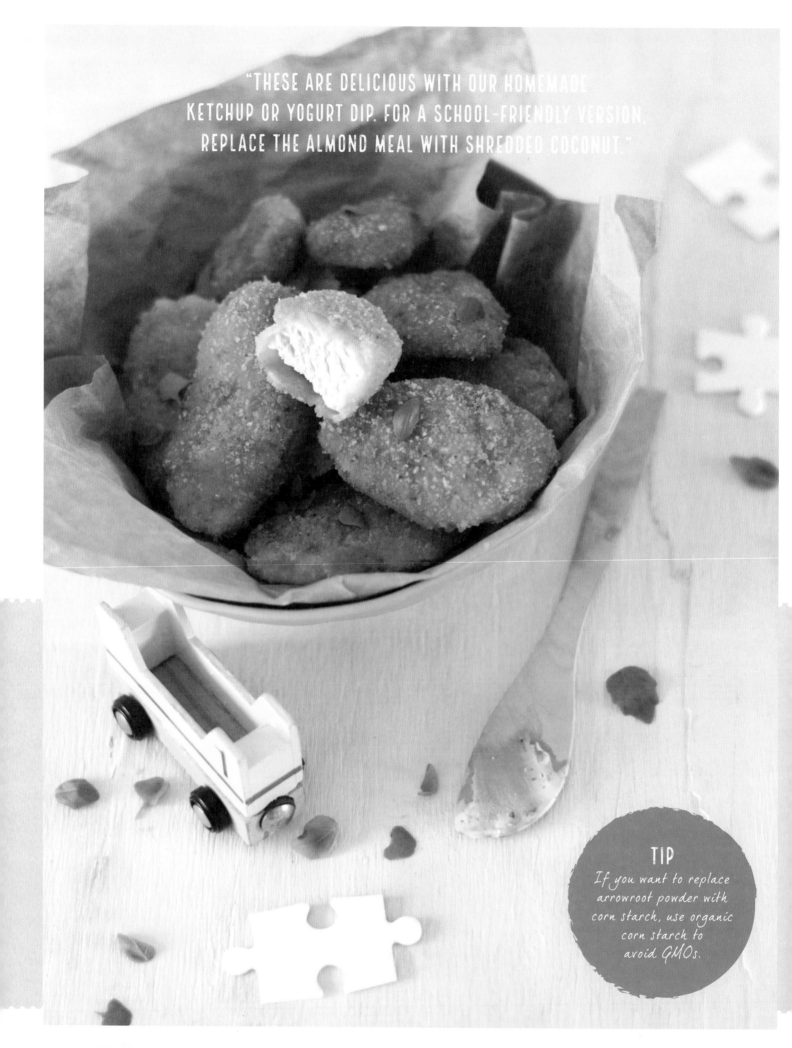

"THESE ARE DELICIOUS WITH OUR HOMEMADE
KETCHUP OR YOGURT DIP. FOR A SCHOOL-FRIENDLY VERSION,
REPLACE THE ALMOND MEAL WITH SHREDDED COCONUT."

TIP
If you want to replace arrowroot powder with corn starch, use organic corn starch to avoid GMOs.

Gluten Free   Dairy Free

Prep time: 30 mins
Cooking time: 10 mins
Serves: 5

Chicken Nuggets with Cauliflower

An excellent alternative to store-bought versions, with an added nutritional boost from the cauliflower. These are a firm favorite in my home and among the fussiest of my clients.

INGREDIENTS

1 cup (3¹/₅ oz) rice bread crumbs

¹/₂ cup (2 oz) almond meal

¹/₄ tsp sea salt

¹/₂ cup (2 oz) arrowroot

¹/₂ cup (4¹/₂ oz) cauliflower puree

3 large eggs, lightly beaten

1 lbs chicken tenderloins or breast, skinless cut into nugget-sized pieces

1–2 tbs olive oil for frying

INSTRUCTIONS

In a medium-sized bowl, combine the bread crumbs, almond meal, and ¹/₄ tsp sea salt and mix together.

In a separate bowl place the arrowroot powder.

In a shallow bowl, combine the cauliflower puree and egg and whisk together using a fork.

Place the chicken nuggets on a large plate and sprinkle with the remaining salt.

Dip each chunk separately into arrowroot powder then into the egg mix and finally into the bread crumbs. Press down firmly to ensure that each nugget has a thick coating of the breadcrumb mix.

Coat a large frying pan with 1–2 tbs olive oil and place over medium heat. Place the nuggets in the pan and make sure they are not touching each other and there is enough room to turn them over.

Cook for approx 3–4 mins on each side or until golden brown.

Serving and storing leftovers: Serve immediately, store in fridge for up to 3 days or freeze for up to 4 months.

Vegetarian   Gluten Free   Nut Free

Prep time: 10 mins (+30 mins refrigeration time)
Cooking time: 10 mins
Makes: 25 Patties

Cheesy Cauliflower Falafel Patties

INGREDIENTS

1¹/₂ cups (9¹/₂ oz) cooked chickpeas or 1 (14 oz) can chickpeas, rinsed, drained

1 cup (3¹/₂ oz) cauliflower florets

¹/₂ yellow onion, chopped

2 garlic cloves, crushed

1 egg

¹/₂ cup (1²/₅ oz) low-sodium cheese, grated

1 tsp tahini

1 tbs lemon juice

¹/₂ cup (2 oz) pumpkin seed meal

¹/₂ cup (1¹/₂ oz) rice bread crumbs

1 tbs chia seeds

¹/₄ tsp ground cumin

¹/₂ tbs fresh parsley, chopped

sea salt and pepper, to taste

coconut oil for frying

EQUIPMENT

high-speed food processor

INSTRUCTIONS

Place all ingredients except for the coconut oil in a food processor and process until it reaches a smooth consistency. Place mixture in the fridge for 30 mins.

Heat coconut oil in a large frying pan.

Wet your hands with a little water to prevent dough from sticking to your hands. Form small balls and place them in the frying pan, flattening down a bit with a spoon.

Cook for 2–3 mins on each side, or until crispy and brown on the outside.

Allow to cool before serving as consistency is best when cool.

Serve with a garden salad and dips.

Serving and storing leftovers: Serve immediately, store in an airtight container in the fridge for up to 4 days or freeze for up to 4 months.

For a dairy-free version simply leave out the cheese.

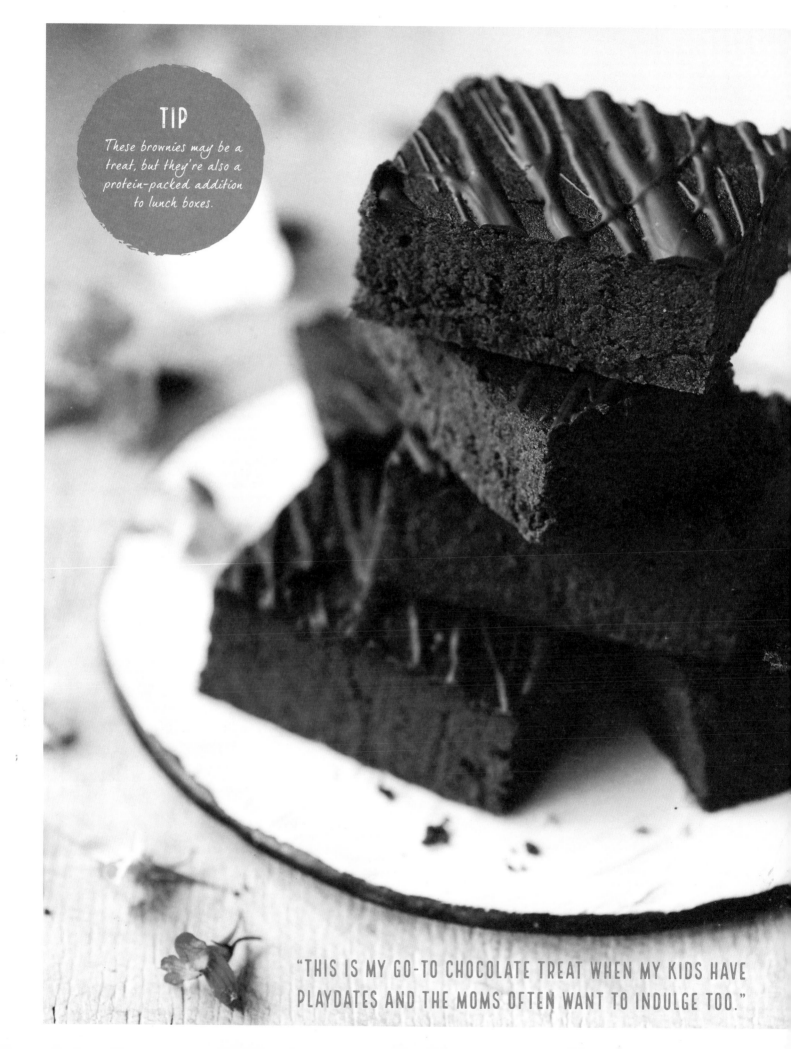

"THIS IS MY GO-TO CHOCOLATE TREAT WHEN MY KIDS HAVE PLAYDATES AND THE MOMS OFTEN WANT TO INDULGE TOO."

VEG Vegetarian

 Gluten Free

 Nut Free

 Dairy Free

Prep time: 10 mins
Cooking time: 25–30 mins
Makes: 16 mini brownies (approx)

Rich Chocolate Black Bean Brownies

It's hard to believe that the base of this chocolatey goodness is made from black beans, making them high in folate and a good source of iron and fiber.

INGREDIENTS

1½ cups (9½ oz) cooked black beans or (1 14 oz) can black beans, rinsed, drained

3 eggs

3 tbs coconut oil, plus a little more for coating the baking dish

⅓ cup (1 oz) cacao powder

2 tbs carob powder

pinch of sea salt

3 tsp pure vanilla extract

1 tsp baking powder

½ cup (2⅔ oz) coconut sugar (to sweeten further, add an extra ¼ cup (1¼ oz) coconut sugar or a pinch of stevia)

EQUIPMENT

high-speed food processor

INSTRUCTIONS

Preheat oven to 325°F.

Grease a small square 8" x 8" baking dish with coconut oil.

Place all the ingredients in a blender and process at a high speed until smooth.

Pour the mixture into the prepared baking dish.

Place in oven and bake for 25–30 mins. Check after 25 mins by sliding a knife into the brownie. If it comes away clean, the brownies are ready. Allow to cool before cutting into little squares.

Serving and storing leftovers: Serve immediately, store in fridge for 4 days or freeze for up to 4 months. Serve with coconut cream and fresh strawberries for a dessert treat.

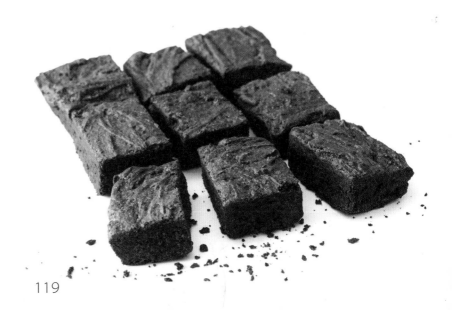

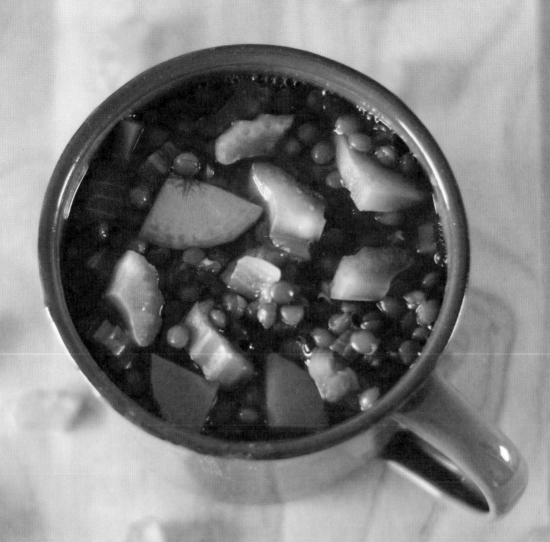

"A GREAT VEGETARIAN OPTION AND MEAL IN ONE. SERVE WITH BROWN RICE OR SOURDOUGH BREAD FOR A NUTRIENT-PACKED PROTEIN HIT."

TIP

Serve with brown rice for a complete protein-packed meal. Pairing plant-based proteins and whole grains enhances the benefits of plant-based proteins.

Vegan / Gluten Free / Nut Free

Prep time: 10 mins (+12 hours soaking time)
Cooking time: 50 mins
Serves: 8

Lentil & Vegetable Soup

High in fiber, vitamin B6 and iron, this hearty and warming soup is my son's favorite. It's perfect as an after school snack or as a main course for dinner.

INGREDIENTS

2 tbs extra virgin olive oil

1 yellow onion, finely chopped

1 garlic clove, finely chopped

2 medium-sized carrots, peeled and finely chopped

2 stalks celery, finely chopped

1 lb brown lentils, soaked for 12 hrs, rinsed, drained

1 cup (8¾ oz) diced tomatoes (if using store-bought buy tomatoes in a glass jar instead of a can to avoid the BPA that is often found in the lining of cans.)

2 quarts vegetable broth or bone broth (see recipe on page 277)

½ tsp ground cilantro

½ tsp ground cumin

sea salt to taste

EQUIPMENT

high-speed food processor (optional)

INSTRUCTIONS

Place a pot on a medium heat and add olive oil.

Sauté onion, garlic, spices, carrot, and celery for 5–7 mins.

Add the lentils, tomatoes, and broth and stir.

Increase the heat and bring to the boil.

Once boiling, reduce heat slightly and leave to simmer covered for approximately 40 mins or until the lentils are soft. Serve the soup as is, or puree for a smoother consistency.

Serving and storing leftovers: Serve immediately, store in the fridge for up to 4 days or freeze for up to 4 months.

Vegetarian / Gluten Free / Nut Free

Prep time: 10 mins
Cooking time: 25 mins
Makes: 1 quart

Veggie Pasta Sauce

INGREDIENTS

1 tbs extra virgin olive oil

1 leek, finely diced

2 garlic cloves, diced

1 cup (5 oz) butternut squash, peeled and finely diced

2 medium-sized zucchini, finely diced

1 medium-sized carrot, grated

½ cup (½ oz) baby spinach, chopped

4 medium-sized tomatoes, finely diced

14 oz tomato puree

1 tsp Italian herbs

sea salt and pepper, to taste

⅓ cup (1 oz) gouda or mozzarella, grated

INSTRUCTIONS

Heat oil in a large saucepan. Add leek and garlic and cook for 3 mins or until soft.

Add squash, zucchini, carrot, spinach, tomatoes, tomato puree, herbs, and salt and pepper and cook, covered on medium heat for 15–20 mins or until vegetables are soft.

Stir through cheese and serve on top of pasta or rice or with some meat.

Serving and storing leftovers: Serve immediately, store in the fridge for up to 4 days or freeze for up to 4 months.

If your child prefers a smooth texture blend the sauce. For a dairy-free version leave out the cheese.

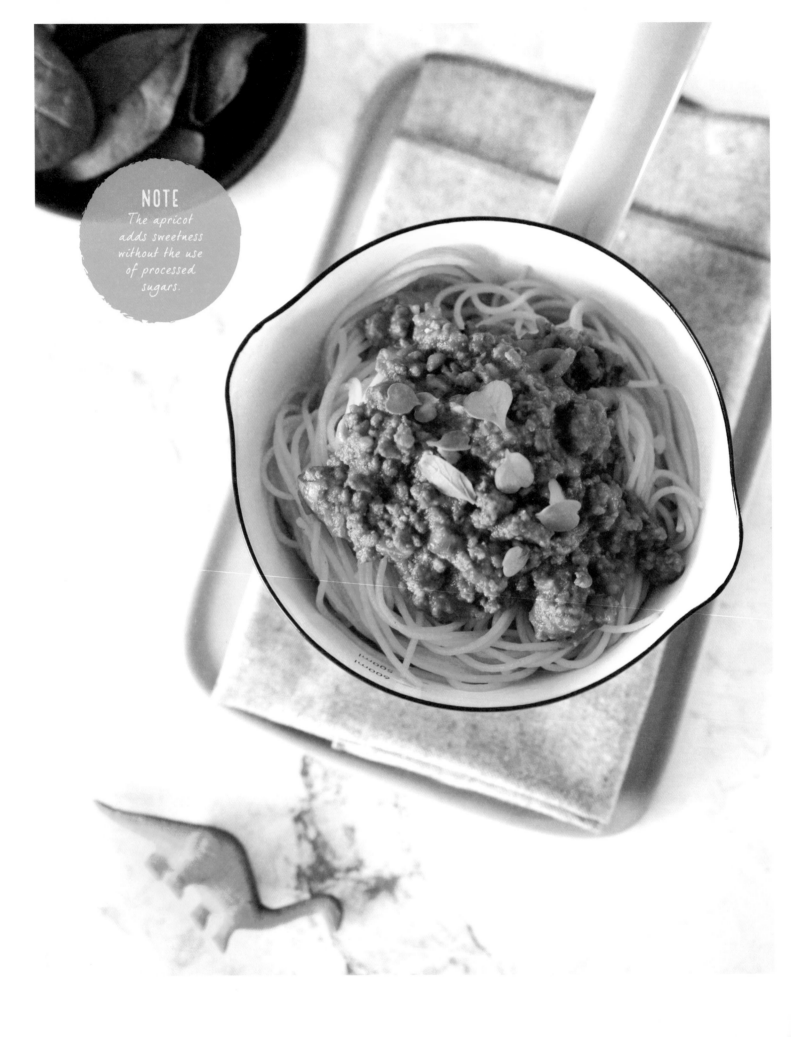

NOTE

The apricot adds sweetness without the use of processed sugars.

Dairy Free

Nut Free

Gluten Free

Egg Free

Prep time: 20 mins
Cooking time: 45 mins
Serves: 8

Supercharged Bolognaise

Even the fussiest of eaters won't be able to detect the veggies in this dish. It can be pureed into a smooth consistency for babies and picky eaters.

INGREDIENTS

1–2 tbs olive oil

1 large yellow onion, finely chopped

2–4 cloves garlic, finely crushed

2¼ lb beef or lamb mince

2 tbs mixed Italian herbs

2 tsp ground cinnamon

1½ lbs tomato puree in a glass bottle (not canned)

1 cup vegetable stock or bone broth (for bone broth recipe see page 277)

½ cup (4½ oz) butternut squash, steamed and pureed. (Do not throw away excess water)

½ cup (4½ oz) sweet potato, steamed and pureed

2 dried apricots, sulphur-free, finely sliced

1 cup (⅞ oz) spinach, finely chopped

sea salt and pepper, to taste

EQUIPMENT

hand-held blender or high-speed food processor

INSTRUCTIONS

In a medium to large pot, heat oil on medium heat and sauté onion and garlic until transparent.

Add mince, then turn up the heat and brown.

Add mixed herbs, cinnamon and salt. Keep stirring until mince is browned all the way through and no pink pieces can be seen.

Add tomato puree and vegetable stock and simmer covered on a low heat for 10 mins.

Add butternut, sweet potato, and apricot, cover and simmer for 15 mins.

Add spinach and check to make sure liquid level is not too low. If extra water is needed, add water from steamed vegetables to increase vitamin and mineral content. Simmer for 10 more mins.

Add salt and pepper to taste.

Turn off heat and leave to cool. Serve with wholegrain or gluten free pasta, or brown rice.

Serving and storing leftovers: Serve immediately, store in fridge for up to 3 days or freeze for up to 4 months.

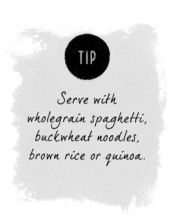

TIP

Serve with wholegrain spaghetti, buckwheat noodles, brown rice or quinoa.

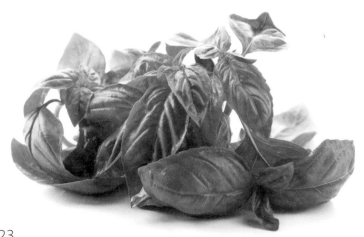

VEG Vegetarian **Gluten Free** **Nut Free**

Prep time: 5 mins
Cooking time: 20–25 mins
Serves: 4

Shakshuka With Quinoa & Greens

INGREDIENTS

1 tbs extra virgin olive oil

½ yellow onion, finely diced

½ red pepper, finely sliced

1–2 cloves of garlic, finely diced

1 large tomato, finely diced

1½ cups tomato puree

1 cup (5½ oz) cooked quinoa

sea salt and pepper, to taste

⅓ cup (⅓ oz) greens (kale, spinach, chard), finely sliced

4 eggs

⅓ cup (1¾ oz) feta or goat's cheese, crumbled

2 tbs fresh parsley, finely diced (optional, for garnish)

INSTRUCTIONS

Preheat oven to 350°F.

In a large frying pan or a skillet, heat oil and cook onions and pepper for about 3–5 mins or until soft.

Add garlic and tomato and cook for another 2 mins.

Add tomato puree and quinoa and simmer for 5 mins.

Season with salt and pepper and add ⅓ cup of greens.

Gently crack eggs into pan over tomato mixture. Season egg with a little salt.

Transfer pan or skillet to oven and bake for 10–15 mins.

Sprinkle with feta cheese and fresh parsley and serve with some homemade Pita Bread (see recipe on page 282).

Serving and storing leftovers: Serve immediately or store in an airtight container in the fridge for up to 3 days.

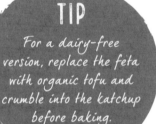

TIP

For a dairy-free version, replace the feta with organic tofu and crumble into the katchup before baking.

VEG Vegetarian **Gluten Free** **Nut Free**

Prep time: 15 mins
Cooking time: 15–20 mins
Makes: 20 mini muffins

Vegetable Muffins

INGREDIENTS

1 cup (8¾ oz) steamed vegetables (sweet potato/cauliflower/green beans)

2 eggs

½ cup (1⅖ oz) grated cheddar cheese, plus ⅛ cup extra to sprinkle on top

½ cup (2⅓ oz) Wholesome Child gluten-free flour mix (see page 32) or spelt flour

½ tsp baking powder

¼ tsp baking soda

pinch of sea salt (optional)

EQUIPMENT

High-speed food processor

INSTRUCTIONS

Preheat oven to 340°F and line a muffin tray with muffin liners.

Place all ingredients into a high-speed food processor and process until smooth.

Spoon batter into muffin liners, sprinkle extra cheese on top and bake for 20 mins or until a cake tester or knife comes out clean.

Place on a wire rack to cool before serving.

Serving and storing leftovers: Serve immediately, store in an airtight container in the fridge for up to 4 days or freeze for up to 4 months.

Use 1 cup of any leftover vegetables you have in the fridge. For a dairy-free version replace cheddar cheese with coconut cream.

VEG
Vegetarian

Nut
Free

Prep time: 40 mins (+ 1 hour chilling time)
Cooking time: 50–60 mins
Makes: 30 rolls

Vegetarian Sausage Rolls

INGREDIENTS

PASTRY

1¼ cups (6½ oz) cubed unsalted butter, chilled

2 cups (10 oz) whole spelt flour, plus more for work surface

¾ tsp sea salt

⅔ cup filtered ice-cold water

FILLING

1–2 tbs olive oil

1 (about 1 lb) large sweet potato, peeled and cubed

½ leek, finely sliced

½ yellow onion, finely sliced

2 garlic cloves, crushed

2–3 cups vegetable stock or filtered water

1 medium-sized zucchini, grated

1 cup (4¼ oz) frozen peas

½ cup (1½ oz) rice bread crumbs

¾ cup (2⅕ oz) cheddar, grated

2 tbs fresh parsley, chopped

1 tsp tamari

sea salt and pepper, to taste

1 egg yolk, beaten

sesame and black chia seeds (optional)

EQUIPMENT

high-speed food processor

INSTRUCTIONS

PASTRY

On a plate, place 1 cup (5¼ oz) of cubed butter in an even layer and transfer to freezer and allow to chill.

Place spelt flour and salt together in a high-speed food processor and pulse to combine.

Place remaining butter into the processor and pulse until no visible pieces of butter remain.

Add chilled butter cubes to the dough mixture and pulse twice for just about 3 seconds.

Add ⅓ cup water to the dough mixture and pulse twice for 3 seconds again. Repeat with remaining water, pulsing twice.

Scrape dough from bowl onto a well-floured work surface.

Lightly flour dough and, using your hands, squeeze and shape dough into a cylinder. Press down to flatten into a rectangle.

Roll dough out into a rectangle about ½" thick. You need to make sure to flour under and on top of the dough and roll dough away and back toward you in the length and once in the width.

Fold the two longer ends in toward the middle of the rectangle, leaving a ¾" space in the middle. Starting from the shorter end, roll dough into a snail, then press dough down and wrap in cling wrap. Refrigerate for at least an hour.

FILLING

Preheat oven to 390°F and line two baking trays with baking paper.

Heat olive oil in a large frying pan over medium heat. Add sweet potato, leek, onion, and garlic and cook for 5 mins, or until slightly browned.

Add 2 cups of stock or water, bring to a boil and simmer until sweet potatoes are soft and water is evaporated (about 15–20 mins; add ⅓ cup of water only if potatoes are still hard).

Once the sweet potatoes are soft and mushy, mash them with a fork.

Add zucchini and peas and cook for another 3–5 mins.

Turn off the heat, cool for 5 mins, and then add bread crumbs, cheese, parsley, tamari and salt and pepper. Set aside.

Take dough out of the fridge and halve it. On a floured surface, roll both halves into rectangles (about 6/32" thick).

Cut each pastry sheet in half. Divide the vegetable mixture into four equal portions and spoon mixture down along the long side of one pastry half, shaping veggie mix into a long sausage shape. Beat the egg in a separate bowl and brush opposite long edge with a little egg.

Roll to enclose, placing the pastry seam underneath. Cut into 1⅙" to 2" sausage rolls and place on the lined baking trays.

Brush with the egg yolk and sprinkle with sesame and/or black chia seeds. Bake for 20–25 mins or until golden and cooked through.

Serve warm with Homemade Ketchup (see page 283).

Serving and storing leftovers: Serve immediately. Store in the fridge for up to 3 days or freeze for up to 4 months.

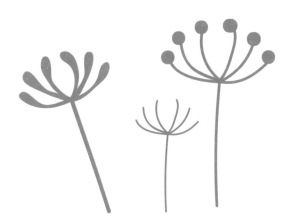

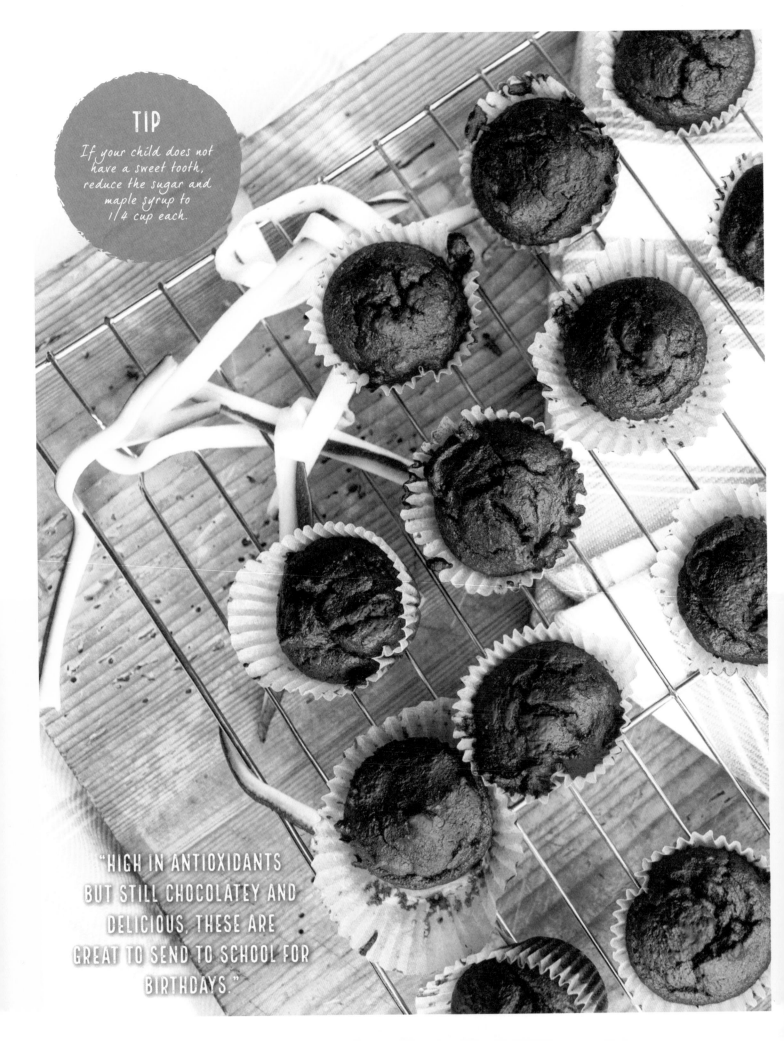

TIP

If your child does not have a sweet tooth, reduce the sugar and maple syrup to 1/4 cup each.

"HIGH IN ANTIOXIDANTS BUT STILL CHOCOLATEY AND DELICIOUS, THESE ARE GREAT TO SEND TO SCHOOL FOR BIRTHDAYS."

VEG — Vegetarian
Gluten Free
Nut Free
Dairy Free

Prep time: 25–30 mins
Cooking time: 35 mins
Makes: 30 mini muffins

Chocolate Zucchini Muffins

In my practice I had a nine-month-old client who would not eat anything other than chocolate. These muffins helped wean her off chocolate mudcakes while we worked towards improving her overall diet.

INGREDIENTS

1 cup (6¹⁄₃ oz) zucchini, grated

½ cup (4½ oz) sweet potato, steamed, pureed

1 egg

2 ripe bananas

¹⁄₃ cup (1¾ oz) coconut sugar

¹⁄₃ cup maple syrup

¹⁄₃ cup (2½ oz) coconut oil, melted

1 cup (5½ oz) brown rice flour

½ tsp baking powder

1 tsp baking soda

2 tbs cacao powder

1 tbs carob powder

1 tsp pure vanilla extract

pinch sea salt

¹⁄₃ cup (1¹⁄₅ oz) dark chocolate chips (optional)

EQUIPMENT

high-speed food processor

INSTRUCTIONS

Preheat the oven to 355°F.

Place the zucchini in a clean tea towel and squeeze to remove excess water.

Place the zucchini, sweet potato, egg, banana, coconut sugar, maple syrup and coconut oil in a processor and process at a high speed.

Add the rice flour, baking powder, baking soda, cacao powder, carob powder, vanilla and sea salt. Process at a high speed until smooth consistency is reached.

Gently fold in the chocolate chips by hand.

To make mini muffins, use mini paper inserts and add 1–2 tbs of batter per muffin and cook for 30–35 mins or until a cake tester comes out clean.

Serving and storing leftovers: Serve immediately, store in an airtight container in the fridge for up to 4 days or freeze for up to 4 months.

VEG — Vegetarian
Gluten Free
Nut Free
Dairy Free

Prep time: 15–20 mins
Cooking time: 15 mins
Makes: 24 mini muffins

Vanilla Muffins with Cauliflower

INGREDIENTS

5 Medjool dates, pitted

1 egg

1 tsp pure vanilla extract

¼ cup coconut oil, melted

¼ cup (2¼ oz) apple sauce (unsweetened)

½ cup (1¾ oz) cauliflower, steamed and drained

¼ cup maple syrup

1 cup (4³⁄₅ oz) Wholesome Child gluten-free flour mix (see page 32)

½ tsp baking powder

¼ tsp baking soda

pinch sea salt

EQUIPMENT

high-speed food processor

INSTRUCTIONS

Preheat oven to 355°F and line a mini muffin tray with muffin liners.

Place dates, egg, vanilla extract, coconut oil, apple sauce, cauliflower, and maple syrup into the processor and process until smooth.

Next, add all dry ingredients and process until well combined.

Place batter into mini muffin liners and bake for 15–20 mins or until a cake tester or knife comes out clean.

Allow to cool on a rack and enjoy them plain or topped with your favorite frosting.

Serving and storing leftovers: Serve immediately, store in an airtight container in the fridge for up to 4 days or freeze for up to 4 months.

Replace the gluten-free flour mix with spelt flour. If medjool dates are hard, soak for 3–5 min in hot water. Discard excess water.

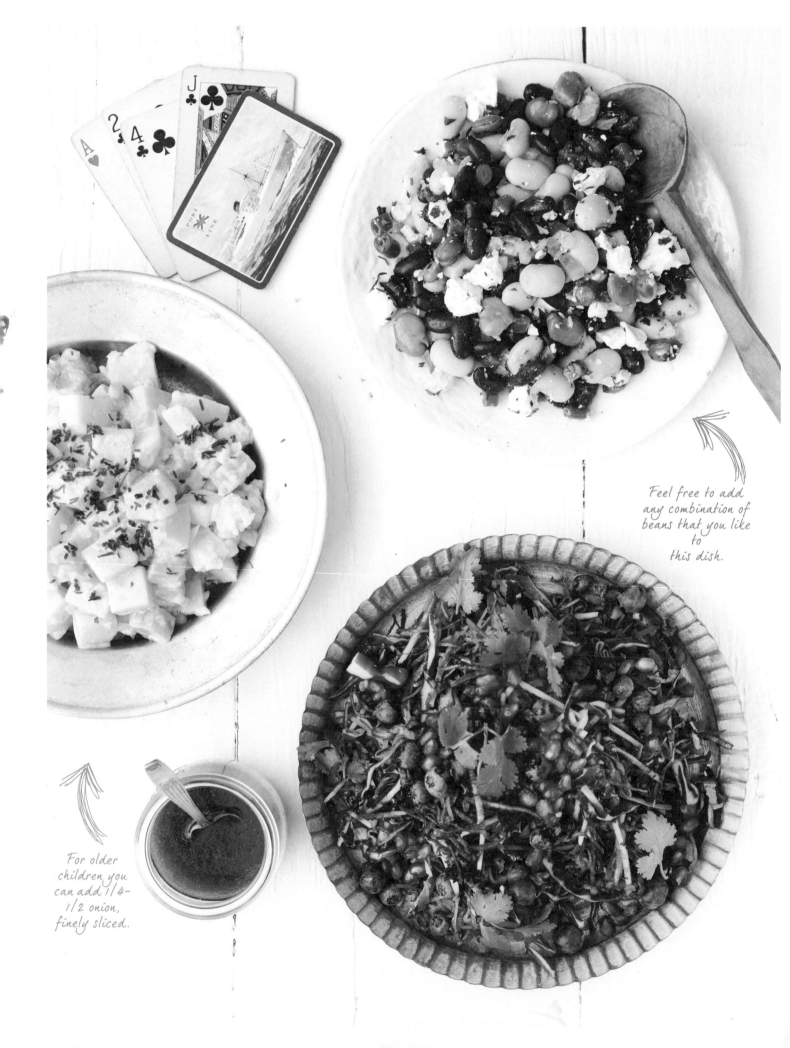

Feel free to add
any combination of
beans that you like
to
this dish.

For older
children you
can add 1/4–
1/2 onion,
finely sliced.

Vegetarian · Nut Free · Gluten Free

Prep time: 15 mins
Cooking time: 5–10 mins
Serves: 4–6
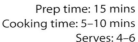

Mixed Bean Salad

INGREDIENTS

1½ cups (9½ oz) green beans, chopped

1 cup (5¼ oz) fava beans, peeled

1½ cups (9½ oz) cooked kidney beans or 1 (14 oz) can kidney beans, rinsed, drained

1½ cups (9½ oz) cooked lima beans or 1 (14 oz) can lima beans, rinsed, drained

1 garlic clove, crushed

1 cup (5¼ oz) feta, crumbled

¼ cup (⅙ oz) basil, chopped

¼ cup (⅙ oz) cilantro, chopped

2 tbs mint, finely sliced

DRESSING
2 tbs apple cider vinegar

1 tbs lemon juice

1–2 tbs avocado or olive oil

sea salt and pepper, to taste

INSTRUCTIONS

In a medium-sized pot, bring water to the boil and add green beans and fava beans. Cook for approximately 5 mins or until soft. Rinse, drain and allow to cool.

Combine all salad ingredients and the dressing in a large bowl and mix to combine.

Serving and storing leftovers: Serve immediately or store in an airtight container in the fridge for up to 4 days.

Vegan · Gluten Free

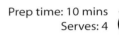

Rainbow Salad

INGREDIENTS

1 cup (2⅘ oz) purple cabbage, finely grated

½ cup (½ oz) kale, finely sliced

½ (1½ oz) medium kohlrabi, finely grated

2 large carrots, peeled and finely grated

1 large beetroot, grated

1 medium red apple, peeled and finely grated

½ cup (2⅘ oz) blueberries

¼ cup (1 oz) pomegranate seeds

¼ cup (⅙ oz) fresh mint, finely sliced (optional)

¼ cup (1.6 oz) fresh cilantro, finely sliced (optional)

DRESSING:
juice and zest of ½ an orange

2 tbs pomegranate molasses or maple syrup

½ tsp cold-pressed sesame oil

¼ cup macadamia nut oil, or olive oil

sea salt and pepper

INSTRUCTIONS

Place all salad ingredients in a large bowl.

For the dressing, add all ingredients to a small jar, put lid on top, shake and pour over salad.

Mix thoroughly to combine.

Serving and storing leftovers: Serve immediately or store in an airtight container in the fridge for up to 4 days.

Vegetarian · Nut Free · Gluten Free · Egg Free

Prep time: 10 mins
Cooking time: 15 mins
Serves: 2–4

Sweet Potato Salad

INGREDIENTS

1 medium-sized (8¾ oz) sweet potato, peeled

3 medium-sized (8¾ oz) potatoes

2 tbs chives, chopped

DRESSING:
2 tbs sour cream

2 tbs unsweetened Greek yogurt

1 tbs apple cider or white balsamic vinegar

2 tsp Dijon mustard

2 tbs filtered water

sea salt and pepper

INSTRUCTIONS

Steam sweet potato until just soft. Drain and let cool.

Peel potato and cook until soft but not mushy. Drain and let cool. Then cut into small cubes.

In a bowl, combine sweet potatoes, potatoes, and chives with dressing ingredients. Carefully stir through.

Serving and storing leftovers: Serve immediately or store in an airtight container in the fridge for up to 4 days.

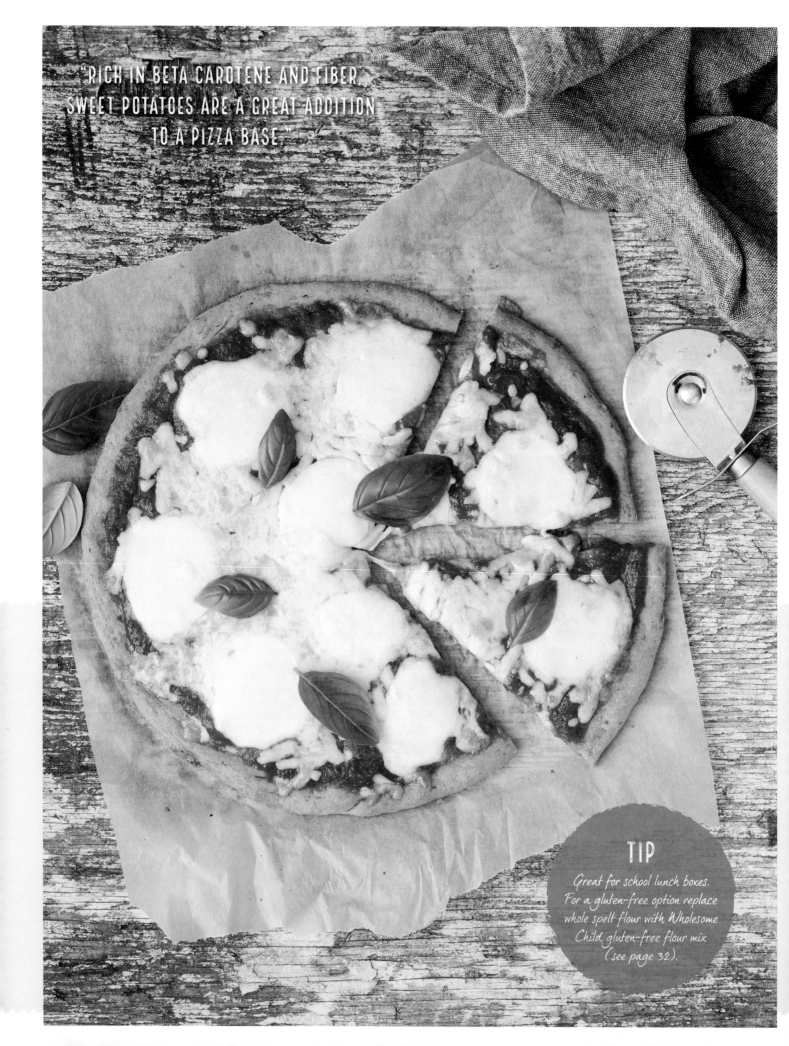

"RICH IN BETA CAROTENE AND FIBER,
SWEET POTATOES ARE A GREAT ADDITION
TO A PIZZA BASE."

TIP

Great for school lunch boxes.
For a gluten-free option replace
whole spelt flour with Wholesome
Child gluten-free flour mix
(see page 32).

VEG
Vegetarian

Nut Free

Egg Free

Prep time: 15 mins
Cooking time: 25–30 mins
Serves: 4

Sweet Potato Pizza

Kids love pizza but they don't always go for vegetable toppings. So I decided to create a pizza for my kids which had veggies in the base—and it worked best with sweet potato. This is one recipe that most fussy eaters will love.

INGREDIENTS

DOUGH:

1½ cups (13¼ oz) sweet potato, peeled, steamed and mashed

1½ cups (7²/₅ oz) whole spelt flour

2 tsp baking powder

½ tsp sea salt

1 tbs extra virgin olive oil

1 tsp oregano (dried)

TOPPING:

1 cup tomato paste or puree

2 cups (5½ oz) grated cheese (mozzarella, gouda, or swiss)

optional extras: basil, mushrooms, pepper, tomatoes, olives, grated carrot, grated zucchini, anchovies.

EQUIPMENT
high-speed food processor

INSTRUCTIONS

Preheat oven to 390°F and line a pizza pan or baking tray with baking paper.

To make the dough, place all ingredients into a high-speed food processor and process until well combined. Or you can add the ingredients to a large bowl and knead well together with your hands until the mixture resembles a ball of orange pizza dough.

Press out the dough into a large circle. If it's too sticky, oil your hands with olive oil. To achieve a crispy base, the dough should be about a ¹/₆" thick.

Bake in the oven for approximately 15–20 mins or until the edges of the dough are slightly browned. Twenty mins will ensure a crisp base.

Remove pizza base from oven, add the tomato paste, cheese, and preferred toppings, and grill for 5–8 mins until cheese is melted.

Allow to cool, then cut into slices.

Serving and storing leftovers: Serve immediately. Store in the fridge for up to 4 days or freeze the precooked base for up to 4 months.

VEG
Vegetarian

Gluten Free

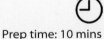

Prep time: 10 mins
Cooking time: 20–25 mins
Serves: 4

Cheesy Cauliflower Pizza Base

INGREDIENTS

2 cups (7 oz) cauliflower florets, roughly chopped

1 egg

½ cup (1½ oz) mozzarella/gouda/cheddar cheese, grated

1 cup (4¼ oz) almond meal

1 tsp dried oregano

½ tsp sea salt

1 tbs coconut oil, melted

EQUIPMENT
high-speed food processor

INSTRUCTIONS

Preheat oven to 355°F and line a baking tray with baking paper.

Place cauliflower florets into a food processor and process until finely crumbed.

Place processed cauliflower in a clean tea towel or cheese cloth and squeeze out excess water.

Add processed cauliflower and remaining ingredients into processor, except for coconut oil, and process until smooth.

Brush coconut oil over baking paper.

Add cauliflower dough and spread out until ¹/₆"–¹/₃" thick.

Bake in oven for 15–20 mins.

Remove from oven and layer with your toppings of choice.

Bake for another 5 mins or until cheese is melted and edges are golden and crisp.

Serving and storing leftovers: Serve immediately, store in fridge for up to 4 days or freeze pre-baked base for up to 1–2 months.

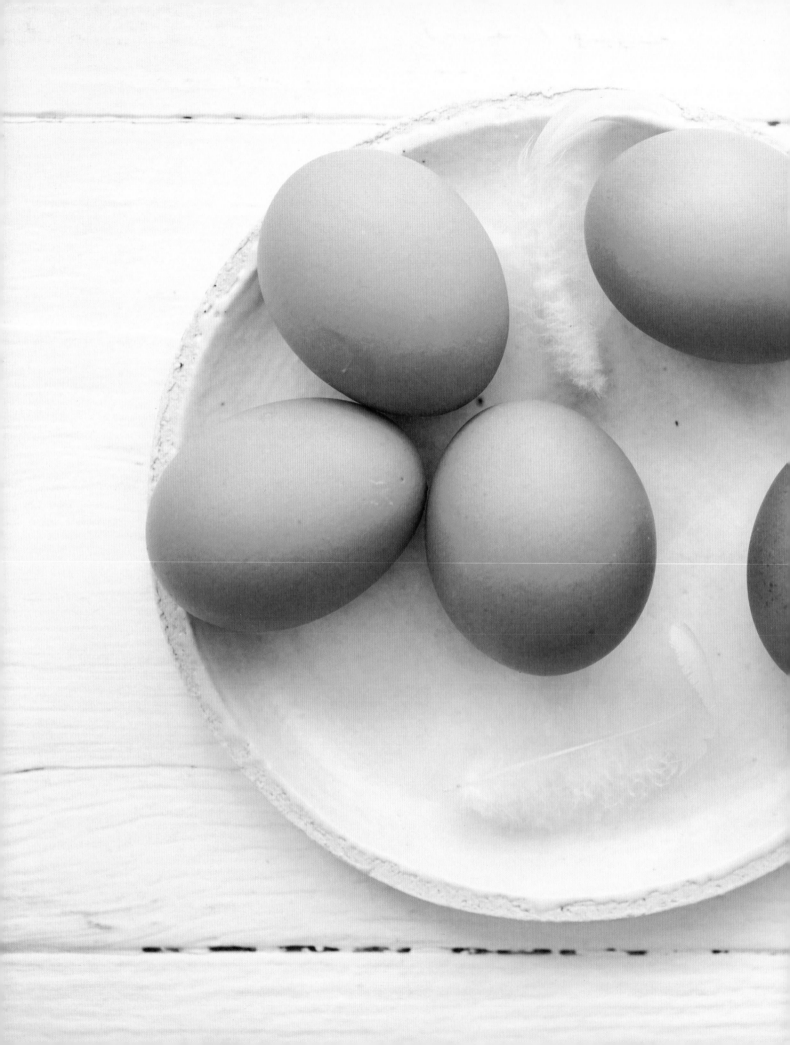

Boost
Protein

BALANCE HEALTHY ANIMAL PROTEINS WITH VEGETARIAN OPTIONS

In my practice I usually see kids avoiding two of the five food groups: vegetables and protein. While children will get some protein from the other food groups, studies show that it's usually the main nutrient lacking from their lunch boxes. A low-protein lunch can ultimately impact a child's ability to concentrate as well as their energy levels. The good news is that most kids (even vegetarians) can receive their daily quota and easily exceed their recommended protein requirements as long as they are eating a balanced diet that includes a variety of healthy protein choices.

WHY IS PROTEIN SO IMPORTANT?

Protein contains amino acids (the building blocks of our DNA) that the body uses to build and maintain muscle, bone, enzymes, and red blood cells. Proteins grow, maintain, and replace the tissues in our bodies. Therefore our muscles, organs, and immune systems are mostly made of protein. Protein-rich food also contains vitamins and minerals such as vitamin B12, zinc, and iron, all necessary for healthy appetite regulation as well as proper immune function.

According to the Franklin Institute, tyrosine, an essential amino acid found in cheese, beef, lamb, pork, beans, fish, chicken, nuts, seeds, and eggs is instrumental in producing the neurotransmitters, norepinephrine, and dopamine, that help kids stay alert and energised. Conversely when kids eat high-carbohydrate meals, often their brain's tryptophan levels increase and produce serotonin, which may make them feel tired.

EATING PROTEIN-RICH MEALS:

✓ helps kids stay fuller for longer.

✓ makes children less likely to snack between meals.

✓ keeps kids on their toes, mentally and physically.

✓ boosts the immune system.

WHAT ARE THE BEST SOURCES OF PROTEIN?

Animal sources of protein that tend to deliver all the amino acids a child's body needs are red meat, poultry, fish, eggs and dairy products. Two plant sources make the cut too: soy protein (such as soy beans, tofu, tempeh, and soy milk) and quinoa—the only legume and whole grain to be considered a complete protein (contains all essential amino acids). Other nuts, seeds, and whole grains can all help your child get an adequate amount of protein each day. However, it's important to be aware they all lack one or more of the essential amino acids.

ESSENTIAL VS NON-ESSENTIAL AMINO ACIDS: WHAT'S THE DIFFERENCE?

There are twenty amino acids found in proteins. Eleven of these amino acids are made by the body (non-essential) while the other nine must come from the diet (essential). To produce all twenty, kids need ample and varied sources of protein in their diets.

HOW MUCH PROTEIN SHOULD MY CHILD BE EATING?

Protein requirements differ at different ages based on the body's need for growth and repair. Babies and young children require more protein than adults per kg of body weight. This often equates to children eating one to two servings of good-quality protein on a daily basis.

The best sources of protein are lean meat, poultry, fish, eggs, and good-quality dairy products plus vegetable proteins such as legumes, beans, nuts and seeds.

Children aged one to three years require 1.1g/kg of body weight or 13g of protein daily. For children aged four to eight years the requirement is 0.95g/kg or 19g daily.

Consider this...

While eating raw egg has health benefits such as higher antioxidant activity, it can contain Salmonella, which is a potentially dangerous food-borne bacteria. When it comes to food safety, kids under four are extra vulnerable, so raw eggs are best avoided.

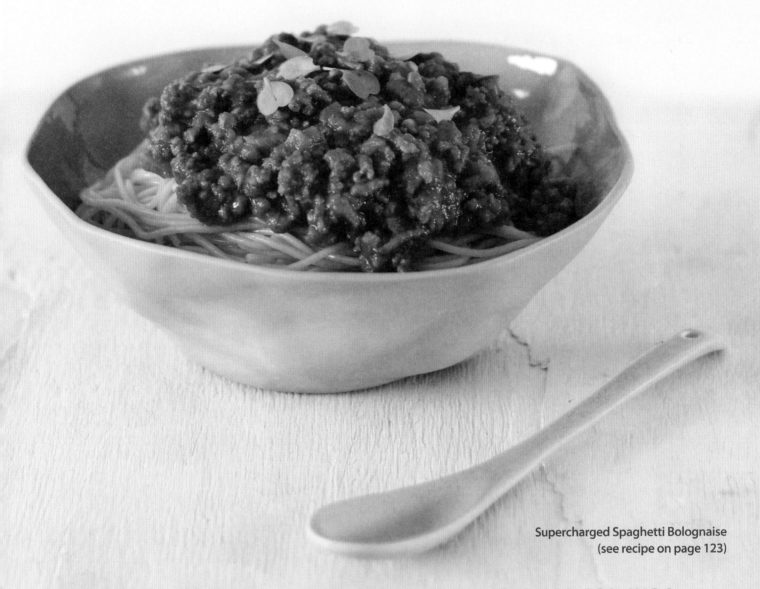

Supercharged Spaghetti Bolognaise
(see recipe on page 123)

AMOUNT OF PROTEIN IN TYPICAL SERVING SIZES FOR KIDS

PROTEIN	AMOUNT PER SERVING SIZE	PROTEIN	AMOUNT PER SERVING SIZE
COOKED LEAN BEEF, LAMB, VEAL OR PORK	17g of protein in a serving the size of your child's palm	SOAKED AND COOKED OR CANNED LENTILS, CHICKPEAS OR BEANS	5g of protein in 4 tbs
GROUND BEEF, LAMB OR PORK	4g of protein in 2 tbs	PEANUT, ALMOND, CASHEW OR SUNFLOWER BUTTER	7g of protein in 2 tbs
COOKED LEAN CHICKEN OR TURKEY	12g of protein in a serving the size of your child's palm	PEANUTS, ALMONDS OR SUNFLOWER SEEDS	3-6g of protein in 1 cupped handful or approx 10 nuts
FISH FILLET	13g of protein in a serving the size of your child's palm and fingers	COOKED QUINOA	4g of protein in ½ cup
TOFU	5g of protein in a serving the size of your child's palm	YELLOW CHEESE	7g of protein in 1 slice
1 EGG	6g of protein in 1 egg	YOGURT	6-7g in ½ cup

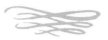
The protein contained in egg white is considered the highest quality protein of all foods.

IS IT OKAY TO EXCEED THE RDI OF PROTEIN?

A three-year-old who has eaten two medium eggs has already met their Recommended Daily Intake (RDI) of protein. However, there is no harm in your child eating more than the RDI as long as you're offering them high-quality protein, as no upper limits have been set for young children.

I recommend including protein with each meal, for example sourdough toast with peanut butter for breakfast, salmon for lunch, and spaghetti bolognaise for dinner. For vegetarians, try quinoa porridge with crushed almonds for breakfast, a spinach and feta slice for lunch, and adzuki bean stew for dinner. However, although no upper limit has been set, it's important to note that it is potentially dangerous for children to follow a very high-protein diet (like the popular Paleo or Atkins diets). Too much protein in a child's diet can put stress on the liver and kidneys. Eating too much red meat or processed meat has also been linked to certain cancers.

HOW MANY SERVINGS OF RED MEAT PER WEEK IS HEALTHY?

This is a topic of debate. According to the American Institute for Cancer Research (AICR), the consumption of red meat has been associated with a modest increased risk of colon cancer. It's safe to say a child who is eating a varied diet filled with protein and iron-rich foods from other sources such as chicken, lentils, and eggs needs only one to two servings of red meat per week. And vegetarian children, under the guidance of a health practitioner, may thrive without any red meat.

However, young children with limited diets will benefit from eating red meat two to three times weekly to ensure their vitamin B12, zinc, and iron levels remain sufficient. Aim to buy grass-fed over grain-fed meat and also look for organic grass-fed options. However when buying grass-fed meat, always ask if it is grass-finished as some farmers who call their meat "grass fed" raise animals in a pasture and then in the last eight weeks of their lives feed them growth-promoting grains.

RED MEAT: GRASS-FED, GRAIN-FED OR ORGANIC?

GRASS-FED MEAT	GRAIN-FED MEAT	ORGANIC MEAT
Animals do not consume genetically modified ingredients like corn, soy or canola oil, making meat naturally GMO free.	Corn feed can contain inherent GMOs.	Can be grass-fed or grain-fed or a combination of both.
Fewer antibiotics as cattle graze in more humane and sanitary conditions.	Overuse and misuse of antibiotics in farmed animals is a major source of antibiotic-resistant bacteria in humans.	No herbicides or pesticides have been used in the pasture.
Up to five times more CLA than grain fed-meat. CLA, or naturally occurring conjugated linoleic acid, is a fat also found in breast milk, that can help boost the immune system, improve bone mass, and control blood sugar levels.		If grain feed is used it is GMO-free.
A healthier ratio of omega-6 to omega-3 fatty acids.	Reduced CLA, vitamin A and E content.	No growth hormones or antibiotics have been used unnecessarily.
Higher levels of beta-carotene from grazing on natural pastures, which assists with immune health, visual health, and fat metabolism.	A higher ratio of omega-6s to omega-3s, meaning it can cause inflammation in the body.	Certified organic farm animals are allowed as much as possible to carry out their natural behaviors, form natural social groups, are not caged, and are allowed generous pasture access.
Higher levels of vitamin A, which is important for bone growth, sustaining healthy vision and protecting a child's body from infection. Vitamin A also promotes the health and growth of cells and tissues in the body.		
Up to four times higher in vitamin E, crucial for a child's health and development. Vitamin E helps boost a child's immune system, aid their body in fighting germs, and assist the cells of the body in working together.		

HOW TO CHOOSE THE BEST SAUSAGES

- If the nutrition panel reads "meat" or "sausage meat," it could be anything, including buffalo, camel, and rabbit. If you are purchasing a beef sausage and you want to be sure it contains only beef, then it needs to say "beef meat" as the first ingredient. The same applies for chicken, pork or lamb sausages.

- Look for a sausage that contains less than 5 percent saturated fat.

- Beware of sodium. Pick a sausage that contains less than 450mg of sodium per 3½ oz. There are no regulations limiting the level of sodium in sausages and this can be extremely harmful to young children.

- Choose a sausage with as high a percentage of meat as possible. Look for a sausage containing a minimum of 85–90 percent meat.

- Avoid sausages that contain cancer causing preservatives—nitrates and nitrites—these form nitrosamines in the body which increase risk of developing cancer.

- Other common preservatives to avoid include sulphur dioxide (220) and sodium and potassium sulphites (221–225 and 228). Sulphites can cause asthma attacks, hay fever, and hives in children who are sensitive to them.

- Empty fillers should also be avoided. These typically include soy, maize, maltodextrin (sugar), hydrolyzed vegetable protein (another name for MSG), potato and tapioca starch, and rusk (wheat). These fillers are commonly used to add bulk to mass-produced sausages that are sold by weight.

IS PROCESSED MEAT SAFE?

Processed meat differs from unprocessed meat in that it may be salted, cured, fermented, smoked, or contain added preservatives or other additives. It is far healthier for a child to eat grass-fed red meat rather than processed ham or sausages. The AICR advises limiting or avoiding processed meats such as sausages, frankfurters, salami, bacon, and ham to once every two weeks as there is strong evidence that processed meat increases the risk of stomach and colon cancer. Be aware that even with this recommendation, there is no real "safe limit" for children's consumption of processed meats.

However for many fussy eaters who are lacking zinc, iron and B12, processed meats such as sausages and roast ham are often the only way parents can get them to eat meat. In my practice, while trying to work on extending these children's meat choices to include healthier options, we have often needed to find processed meats that are the so-called "best of the worst." This is no easy feat as it is very hard to find a sausage, for example, that is free of fillers, preservatives and additives. So I was really pleased to find a gluten-free packaged sausage in my local supermarket that contains 92 percent beef, no fillers, no preservatives, no sugar, 5.5 percent saturated fat and 123mg of sodium—the options are there if you look for them.

Another good option is to choose a 100 percent grass-fed beef sausage from an organic butcher, or a butcher that you can trust. Ask the right questions: Do the sausages contain fillers, preservatives or nitrates? Is it gluten free? But again, I do not recommend processed meat unless a child is avoiding meat altogether. Ideally it is preferable to phase out all processed meat from a child's diet.

Consider this…

Often the main ingredient in a sausage—meat—accounts for less than 70% of the actual sausage. Up to 50% of this can be pure fat, depending on the type of sausage (pork versus beef versus breakfast, etc.). So the average sausage, which many parents think of as a great protein hit for their child, may only contain a third protein, not to mention fillers, preservatives, nitrates and other unwanted ingredients.

CAN KIDS EAT EGGS EVERY DAY?

Along with amino acids, eggs, provide vitamin A (important for healthy eyes, bones and teeth), vitamin D (also supports healthy bones and teeth), choline (important for brain function and heart health), and selenium (important for thyroid function).

While it's true that egg yolks contain cholesterol, studies have found that they have little significant impact on cholesterol levels. And since eggs also contain nutrients that may help lower the risk for heart disease, including protein, vitamins B12 and D, riboflavin and folate, it is safe to let your child eat an egg every day as long as they show no sensitivity to eggs (eggs are one of the top five allergens).

Eggs are an easy dinner or breakfast option, but if they are becoming an everyday fallback meal, aim for two to four times weekly to ensure variation in your child's diet. My rule of thumb for my own kids is to serve an omelette, scrambled, fried eggs, or frittata two to three times each week, not counting the eggs they may be consuming in other foods like pancakes, muffins, or cookies.

CHICKEN AND EGGS: ORGANIC VS FREE-RANGE

When I speak to parents, there is always great confusion as to the healthiest chicken and eggs to buy for their families. Many families have moved away from caged eggs due to the public awareness about the cruelty in which the chickens are raised. However, they still are unclear as to why one should pay extra for organic.

Organic chicken is much more expensive than free-range chicken (sometimes nearly double the price), and organic eggs often cost more too. So is it worth spending the extra money? Without a doubt, YES. Even though organic and free-range birds are both given fresh air, sunshine, and space to grow (although for some free-range chickens this can amount to a maximum of two hours outside per day) this is where the similarities end (see table below).

Consider this... Many chicken brands say they are free from unnatural additives or processes, however in the US, unless they are certified organic by a USDA-accredited certifying agent,

CHICKEN: FREE RANGE VS ORGANIC

FREE RANGE	ORGANIC
Free range is certainly more humane than caged, but it is often questionable as to how much time chickens spend outdoors during daylight hours. The latest USDA guidelines state that farmers can label their eggs "free range" as long as each bird has two square feet of space, have access to the outdoors, and must be outdoors at least six hours per day, weather permitting.	Organic chickens and their eggs contain higher omega-3 essential fatty acid levels, minerals, and vitamins such as beta-carotene because of greater access to forage for their natural diet and the organic feed they are supplemented with is more nutritionally balanced.
Chicken meal in non-organic chickens can vary from vegetarian to containing fishmeal, and many contain GM material from corn.	Organic chicken is more expensive because it costs more to ensure there's no exposure to "quick-fix" chemicals and to ensure higher Animal Welfare standards.
All chickens, unless certified organic, can be treated with antibiotics if they are unwell or, in some cases, if they are underweight.	Organic birds are raised without the use of antibiotics, hormones, or coccidiostats in their feed. Their food is also guaranteed free of chemicals, herbicides, and fertilizers.
Free-range chickens can be treated with therapeutic antibiotics under veterinary direction and sold with the use of coccidiostats (a chemical agent added to animal feed).	Organic chickens are slower to reach maturity with a recommended age of sixty days, which also adds to the heftier price tag.
Chickens are intensively raised to be ready for consumption in as little as thirty-two days.	

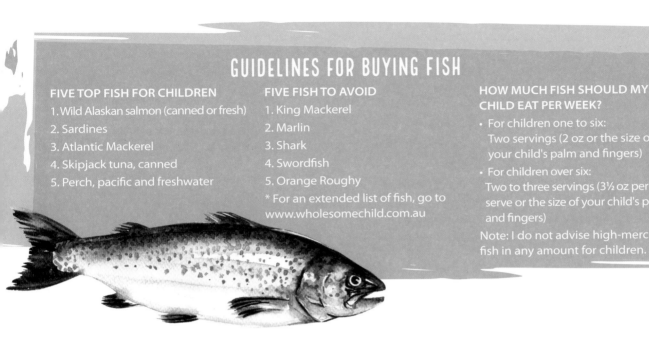

GUIDELINES FOR BUYING FISH

FIVE TOP FISH FOR CHILDREN

1. Wild Alaskan salmon (canned or fresh)
2. Sardines
3. Atlantic Mackerel
4. Skipjack tuna, canned
5. Perch, pacific and freshwater

FIVE FISH TO AVOID

1. King Mackerel
2. Marlin
3. Shark
4. Swordfish
5. Orange Roughy

* For an extended list of fish, go to www.wholesomechild.com.au

HOW MUCH FISH SHOULD MY CHILD EAT PER WEEK?

- For children one to six:
  Two servings (2 oz or the size of your child's palm and fingers)
- For children over six:
  Two to three servings (3½ oz per serve or the size of your child's palm and fingers)

Note: I do not advise high-mercury fish in any amount for children.

---

this cannot be guaranteed. Don't be fooled by labels that say "farm raised," "all natural," or "no added hormones or antibiotics." Look for the certifying body in your region to ensure best quality.

FISH

Fish is an essential part of a healthy and balanced diet. Aside from providing protein, it is the best source of omega-3s in the diet—real brain food and essential for heart health and eyesight too. (See Step 6 for more benefits of omega-3s). Fish is also rich in important vitamins and minerals such as vitamin D, iodine, and selenium. It has less overall fat than other animal proteins and is low in cholesterol. I recommend wasting no time in offering a wide variety of wild-caught, low-mercury fish to babies as soon as they are eating solids. However, in my practice I often see parents introducing canned tuna fish as the first fish.

In my Introducing Solids workshop, I highlight the fact that although canned tuna is a good source of protein, it does not contain the high amount of omega-3s that you'll find in canned salmon or sardines, and there is also the concern of mercury. Try to offer fresh or fatty fish over canned tuna, but if buying tuna, canned skipjack is the best option as it's lowest in mercury. (There is more information on introducing solids and fish recipes for babies at www.wholesomechild.com.au). There are so many wonderful ways to serve fish to children—grilled, steamed, homemade into fish fingers, rissoles, fish patties or fish cakes, mixed with pasta sauce or in a curry.

Consider this . . . I once created a menu planner for a daycare who were serving the children three servings of fish weekly—a selling point for parents until it turned out they were using basa (catfish), which is not recommended for consumption more than once a week due to its mercury content. The chef included it because it was so affordable. He was not aware of the mercury content—a good reminder to always ask what fish is being used.

FISH: WILD VS FARMED

The potential dangers of eating farmed fish are often raised by parents. So is wild-caught better than farmed? Yes, it is. The problem with farmed fish is in the way they are reared—not sustainable and also the feed often contains chicken feathers, GM ingredients, meat offcuts and in the case of salmon, astaxanthin, a synthetic coloring agent. Farmed fish may also contain higher amounts of contaminants like polychlorinated biphenyls (PCBs) due to their feed. Because of overcrowding and inhumane practices there is often a need for antibiotics use in farmed fish. Chemicals like copper may be added to the nets to prevent fish escaping. Pesticides are also used to treat sea lice. However, wild fish have their drawbacks too as the mercury, PCB, and dioxin levels remain unknown. So which fish are best for young children? Wherever possible purchase wild Alaskan canned or fresh organic-farmed fish, such as salmon, if available (these have been farmed in a sustainable manner and the feed is free from GMOs, chicken feathers, and meat offcuts). Researchers have found that both farmed and wild salmon are high in omega-3s compared to shrimp, tuna, and other fish, and they are generally very low in mercury.

FIVE TIPS FOR BUYING FISH

1. *Choose wild fish whenever possible as it's free from GMOs, antibiotics, and other chemicals.*

2. *Buy organic salmon if wild is not available and avoid conventional farmed salmon that is often fed processed high-fat feed in order to produce larger fish.*

3. *Choose canned fish in spring water or extra virgin olive oil. Start off with salmon or sardines as they contain higher levels of omega-3s.*

4. *Replace takeout fish and chips and store-bought fish fingers with homemade, low-mercury variations (see page 57).*

5. *Look for sustainably caught fish. According to Greenpeace, when shopping for canned tuna products, look for "pole and line" caught tuna and try to avoid buying yellowfin tuna. Make sure the tuna you buy has the species name (skipjack is best), where it was caught, and the fishing method used displayed clearly on the label.*

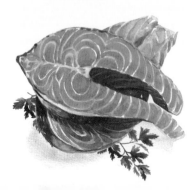

HEAVY METAL MERCURY: SHOULD I WORRY?

There is often discussion about the pros and cons of eating fish, as many parents are worried about the heavy metal mercury levels. Heavy metal mercury is a pollutant generated by coal plants and other industrial activity. It settles into oceans where bacteria convert it into methyl mercury, a form readily absorbed by the human body. This mercury builds up in fish, particularly large predators such as tuna, swordfish, and sharks.

Mercury is particularly dangerous for small children, because it can affect brain development. However, limiting or avoiding fish during early childhood can often mean missing out on important nutrients that can have a positive impact on growth and development as well as on general health.

It is recommended that children up to six years of age follow the same guidelines used in pregnancy, as an increased susceptibility to mercury may exist in the first few years of life when the brain is rapidly developing.

Choose fish wisely for children, focusing on low mercury fish that is either wild-caught or organically farmed. Some wild fish (usually predators) are higher in mercury, a particular concern for young children up until age six.

As a general rule, eating smaller species of fish is best. Avoid top predator fish like shark, swordfish, grouper, and marlin as they have more mercury, and instead choose seafood that is lower on the food chain, like sardines.

Whenever you buy fish, ask where it's from, whether it's wild or farmed and if it's sustainably fished. It is also wise to keep a smart phone handy when shopping for fish so that you can check the mercury content.

I suggest using the Fish4Health app, available for free through iTunes. If you do

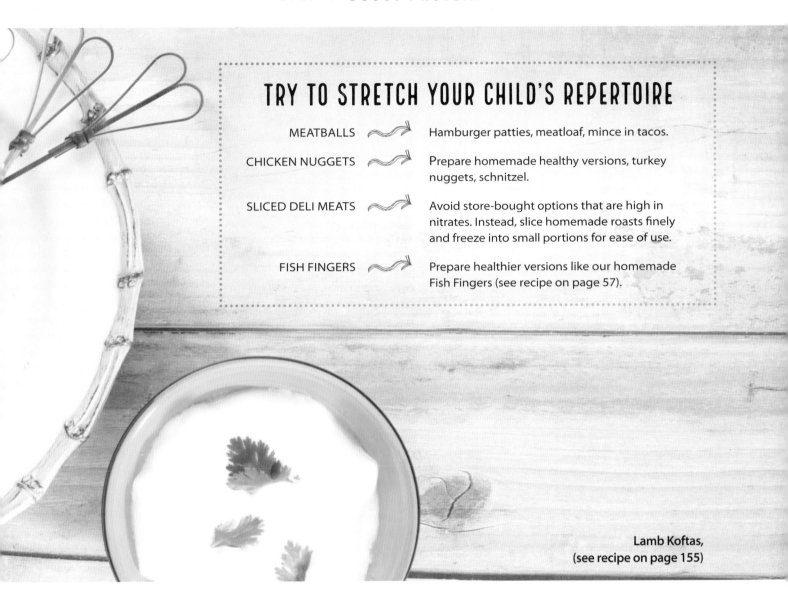

TRY TO STRETCH YOUR CHILD'S REPERTOIRE

MEATBALLS → Hamburger patties, meatloaf, mince in tacos.

CHICKEN NUGGETS → Prepare homemade healthy versions, turkey nuggets, schnitzel.

SLICED DELI MEATS → Avoid store-bought options that are high in nitrates. Instead, slice homemade roasts finely and freeze into small portions for ease of use.

FISH FINGERS → Prepare healthier versions like our homemade Fish Fingers (see recipe on page 57).

Lamb Koftas,
(see recipe on page 155)

feed your child a serving of fish that might be high in mercury, stay away from all other seafood for up to a fortnight.

FISH VS SHELLFISH

Shellfish are generally not as rich in omega-3s as most fish. Lobster, for example, contains very few omega-3s, and shrimp and clams are pretty modest contributors too. Shellfish allergies are also among the most common of food allergies.

Shrimp, crab, and lobster cause most shellfish allergies. While reactions vary, they do tend to be severe (such as anaphylaxis). To prevent a reaction, strict avoidance of shellfish and shellfish products is essential.

Always read ingredient labels to identify shellfish ingredients. If you are going to introduce shellfish to your child, start with one new type at a time at home rather than at a restaurant.

WHAT ABOUT SUSHI?

Raw seafood used in sushi or sashimi certainly has its health benefits, especially salmon which is high in omega-3s. However, raw fish or shellfish may contain common bacteria like Listeria or Salmonella and parasites, all of which can cause serious illnesses in young children. The FDA in the US recommends that children under five don't consume raw fish or shellfish. Raw shellfish is considered the most dangerous to eat because it's most likely to be contaminated. If you are going to eat sushi, buy it from a well-established restaurant and eat it as soon as possible. I do not recommend purchasing sushi and sending it to school.

HOW TO GET YOUR KIDS TO EAT MEAT (AND FISH)

Some children are born carnivores and will eat meat off the bone while others find it

DID YOU KNOW?

Plant-based omega-3 fats, such as flaxseed oil and walnuts, are important for good health. However less than 10 percent is converted into EPA and DHA. Fish oil, on the other hand, provides pre-formed EPA and DHA.

Eight ways to serve more protein

Do you have a fussy eater on your hands? Read on for ideas to up their protein intake. (See Fussy Eating section for more info).

1. Serve plain yogurt with crushed nuts and a fruit for a snack.

2. If your child is taking a jelly or honey sandwich to school every day, add a layer of tahini or sunflower butter. Sunflower butter has more protein than other nut butters and is school-friendly.

3. Mix canned red salmon with sweet potatoes and rice bread crumbs to make salmon cakes. Or try our Salmon & Millet Rissoles (see recipe on page 167).

4. Make your child a delicious egg wrap instead of a wheat wrap. Try our delicious Arrowroot Tortillas (see recipe on page 153).

5. Try a chicken sandwich. For younger children the dark meat from the chicken may be more palatable plus it's higher in iron. Instead of mixing it with mayonnaise try yogurt or our Miso & Tahini Dressing (see recipe on page187).

6. Try chicken soup made in a pressure cooker to ensure the meat stays tender.

7. Cook grains such as rice, quinoa, or pasta in chicken or beef stock or bone broth.

8. Turkey hamburgers are another great option. Our hamburger recipe on page 159 works just as well with turkey mince.

Fish Fingers
(see recipe on page 57)

tough—literally. Our kids' favorite foods often tend to fall into the easy-to-eat category. Think of white bread and crackers, chocolate, ice cream, soda, French fries, and doughnuts . . . they tend to melt in your mouth and require little chewing. I used to love plain, grilled or pan-fried chicken breasts, lamb chops and beef fillets but since having children I have had to experiment a lot with creating recipes that my children and clients will love.

To get children interested, it makes sense to experiment with different textures and presentations like meat in sauces, in patties, served as kebabs or cut into bite-sized pieces. For toddlers and young children who are okay with mushy textures, slow-cooking meat until it is falling off the bone is your best bet. Choose lean cuts of beef or lamb shanks to make stews, casseroles or roast beef, lamb, or chicken and then shred and freeze into portions.

I always recommend choosing recipes that will fit into the framework of what your child is already eating. If they love chicken nuggets, hamburgers, meatballs, koftas, and bolognaise, experiment with ways to boost their nutritional value (see the recipes at the end of this chapter). Start to increase variety by considering the texture and flavor of their favorite foods and try to vary them slightly. This is also true for fish or any other protein your child may refuse to eat.

IS SOY HEALTHY?

Soy is not an essential part of our diets; however, if your child is following a vegetarian or vegan diet, then eating soy becomes more necessary

Consider this . . .

Researchers from the University of Missouri used fMRI scans to compare the brain activity of teens right before lunch and found that those who had eaten low-protein breakfasts were hungrier by midday than those who had eaten high-protein breakfasts.

ONE MEAL FITS ALL (See Fussy Eating section on page 20 for more info)

DISH	FAMILY MEAL	YOUR YOUNGEST/FUSSIEST
LAMB CUTLETS	Marinated orange Lamb Cutlets over brown rice with sauce and baked vegetables (see recipe on page 165).	Tiny pieces of lamb chopped up (no marinade, only olive oil to cook). Separate plain rice. Vegetables cut up into small pieces on a side plate.
SPAGHETTI BOLOGNAISE	Supercharged Spaghetti Bolognaise with lots of added vegetables. Serve with pasta (see recipe on page 123).	Spaghetti bolognaise pureed so no lumps or bumps. Serve with pasta of choice.
ROAST CHICKEN	Roast chicken with marinade, side of steamed vegetables and baked potato.	Small pieces of roast chicken cut up and removed from bone. Separate from vegetables and potato.
STIR-FRY	Stir-fry strips of beef mixed with julienne vegetables. Full of flavor and different textures. Serve over brown rice.	Plain grilled beef strips, separate plain vegetables, separate brown rice.
SHEPHERD'S PIE	Shepherd's Pie including meat, mash and peas (see recipe on page 169).	Separate mince from mash and offer vegetables on the side.
CHICKEN CASSEROLE	Chicken Drumstick Casserole with quinoa and veggies (see recipe on page 157).	Chicken drumstick removed from casserole, cut into small strips. Separate quinoa and vegetables.
FISH CURRY	Easy Fish Curry served with brown rice, side salad, and yogurt dip (see recipe on page 163).	Fish pieces removed from curry with sauce wiped off, 1–2 vegetables removed from curry with sauce wiped off for 'tasting'. Cut up cucumber/carrot with side of plain brown rice and yogurt dip.

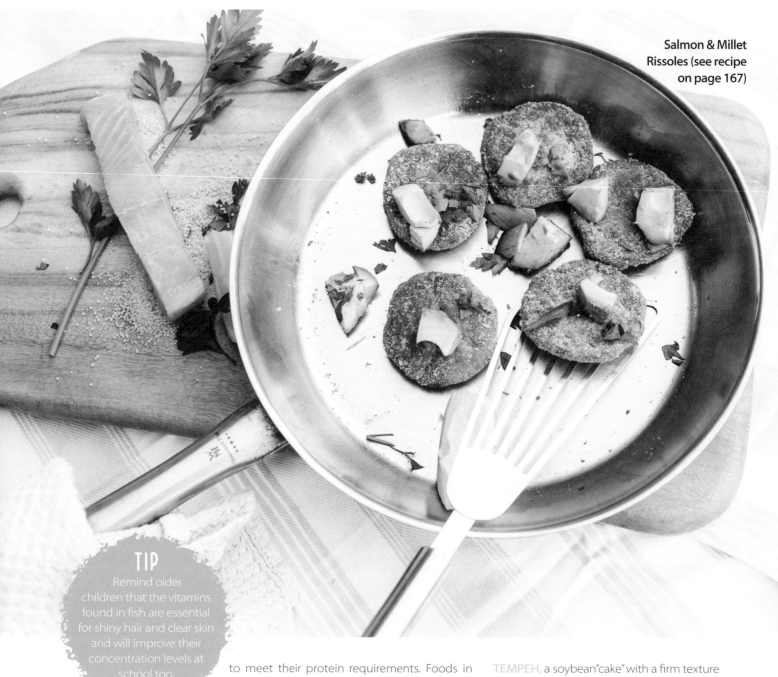

Salmon & Millet Rissoles (see recipe on page 167)

to meet their protein requirements. Foods in the legume family offer the highest source of protein after animal protein. Soybeans are a complete protein, and when cooked, offer approximately 1 oz per cup (edamame have approximately ³/₄ oz of protein per cup).

There is a lot of controversy where soy is concerned. It is a high-pesticide crop and is most often a GM crop too (GM soybeans have been found to contain even more pesticides than conventional or organic soybeans). However, research has also shown that it has beneficial properties. Further investigation is needed to determine the true status of soy and its place in a child's diet. For those reasons, I always recommend choosing organic soybeans wherever possible and also choosing fermented soy products which are easier to digest, such as:

TEMPEH, a soybean"cake" with a firm texture and nutty flavor, has about ¹/₂ oz of protein per half cup.

MISO, a soybean paste with a salty, buttery texture is commonly used in miso soup.

NATTO has a sticky texture and strong, cheese-like flavor.

SOY SAUCE is traditionally made by fermenting soybeans, salt, and enzymes. Make sure to buy a high-quality, wheat-free soy sauce because many varieties are made artificially. Because it is high in sodium it's important to dilute soy sauce for children, as the low-sodium options contain more chemicals.

TAMARI is a version of soy sauce made with little-to-no wheat. Because of the lower wheat level, tamari is made with a greater

MORE IDEAS TO MAKE ONE MEAL THAT EVERYONE WILL EAT

If you're tired of serving different meals to all family members, here are some tips to ensure that one meal serves all, including your fussier eaters.

1. To ensure a child is open to the idea of trying new meals you may need to separate components of the recipe before adding flavor, sauce, onion or garlic.

2. Put aside plain fish, chicken or meat before adding sauce.

3. Offer sauces as a dipping sauce on the side so your child feels in control.

4. Work with your child's ability and acknowledge their textural preferences.

5. If meat, fish or chicken cannot be separated beforehand, scrape off sauce as best as possible before serving to your child.

6. If your child is used to eating chicken nuggets, try crumbing fish or beef and cutting into similar shapes and sizes as your child's preferred nugget.

7. The consistency of fish, chicken and meat varies considerably with cooking style, time, and flavors added. Take your fussiest child's preferences into consideration. This may mean cooking their portion for longer or putting sauces like bolognaise through the blender to make them thinner.

TOP TIPS FOR PREPARING MEAT AND FISH FOR CHILDREN

1. Create crisp and crunchy textures (e.g., homemade chicken or fish nuggets, sausage rolls or fish pies.)

2. Focus on juicy, moist texture by using slow cooking, focusing on casseroles or using homemade marinades.

3. Offer small bites that are easier to chew. Focus on what is eaten and not on what is left over.

4. Crumb your meat or fish with healthy options such as almond meal or rice bread crumbs (see recipe for Salmon & Millet Rissoles on page 167).

5. Offer meat or fish with delicious dips such as homemade ketchup, tzatziki or even pumpkin puree. These work well in masking the smell and flavor.

6. Describe their food with fun, exciting names. Call chicken nuggets "golden nuggets."

7. Try offering meat on skewers. Kids love foods on a stick and it also makes it easier for kids who do not like to touch meat/fish or get the smell on their fingers.

8. If you are worried about bones, choose boneless fillets of pre-packed fish or ask the fishmonger to remove the bones for you.

9. Keep a stock of canned fish such as salmon, pilchards, sardines, and skipjack tuna in your cupboard—these make great sandwich fillings and toppings for baked potatoes and are a good choice when you don't have much time to prepare meals or packed lunches. To reduce salt consumption, opt for those in water or extra virgin olive oil rather than brine.

10. Steam, poach, grill or barbecue chicken or fish rather than frying it to help keep the fat content down.

11. Get children involved in helping you to prepare fish dishes such as sandwich fillings, fishcakes or homemade fish sticks. They'll be more likely to eat it if they've had a hand in making it.

DID YOU KNOW?

Unlike larger fish that are more likely to contain harmful contaminants, wild-caught sardines are free of mercury and PCBs, which means you can serve them frequently. They're also among the best sources of brain-building omega—3s—in fact, one can of sardines boasts roughly 1.9g, even more than a similar portion of salmon.

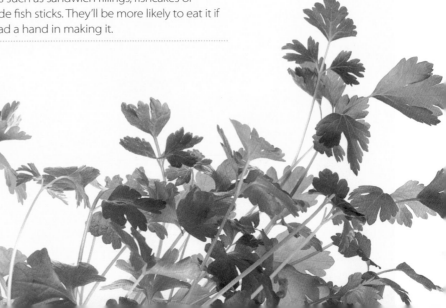

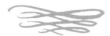

Beans consumed in childhood can lower the risk of developing diabetes and cardiovascular disease in later life because fiber helps balance blood sugar and lower cholesterol. Beans are also good sources of protein, iron, magnesium, potassium, zinc, folate, and vitamin B-6. If you're using dried beans, soak overnight before cooking. Always rinse canned beans under cold water to remove some of the sodium.

concentration of soybeans, adding to its health benefits. Deeper brown in color and slightly thicker than ordinary soy sauce, it provides better flavor for cooking.

NOTE: Tofu is not fermented and can be GM if not organic.

VEGETARIAN BURGERS AND SAUSAGES

These are highly processed soy products that often contain nasty additives, flavorings, and hidden sugars. For these reasons I don't recommend them for children.

WHAT IF MY CHILD IS VEGETARIAN?

While it's easy to ensure that your child is getting all twenty amino acids from a diet that contains meat and fish, the same is not true for children following a vegetarian diet. If your child does not eat animal protein, you will need to ensure they eat food in the correct form and combination to make sure nutrients can be digested and absorbed.

The easiest way to do this is to include eggs and dairy in their diet, along with a variety of plant-based protein-containing foods each day so they get all the amino acids they need. These should include soy protein (preferably fermented), grains (quinoa, oats, and barley), nuts and dried beans, peas, and lentils.

I have consulted for many parents who follow a strict vegetarian diet but struggle to get their children to eat a wide range of proteins due to them being fussy eaters. Many of these kids are underweight and lethargic. Although their parents' belief systems are strong and show

merit—because there are a lot of advantages to vegetarianism—from a nutrition perspective their kids are deficient, and it shows in pale skin, digestive issues, fussiness and disinterest in food.

Once a full range of solid foods have been introduced, young children over the age of one can meet all their amino acid needs through a balanced vegetarian diet, but to be healthy their diet needs to be well thought out and planned ahead. It's important to understand which foods need to be combined for optimal nutrient absorption (e.g., rice with beans), and how to ensure their daily energy, protein, and vitamin requirements are reached.

A vegetarian diet can most certainly be disadvantageous for your child if nutritionally sound food choices are not made. A child is better off eating a low quality diet that still includes meat than a poor quality vegetarian diet. Compare, for example, a child who eats chocolate cereal and milk for breakfast, refined crackers as a snack, a cheese sandwich for lunch, a muffin for afternoon tea, and mac 'n' cheese for dinner with a child who eats oatmeal porridge with milk and crushed seeds and nuts for breakfast, veggie sticks, hummus and trail mix as a mid-morning snack, a wholegrain sandwich with cheese and salad for lunch, a falafel ball with tzatziki for a mid-afternoon snack, and lentil or bean stew and brown rice for dinner.

IS IT OKAY FOR KIDS TO BE VEGAN?

Young children simply cannot thrive on a pure vegan diet without careful consideration and supplementation. Great care needs to be taken, as they are at risk of failure to meet their protein requirements, leading to reduced bone density from a lack of calcium and anaemia from a lack of iron. If your child's diet doesn't include eggs or dairy products they will lack vitamin B12, as it is not found in any plant sources.

It is always important to consult with a pediatrician, dietician, GP or nutritionist to ensure that your child is following a nutritionally adequate diet to support their growth. Along with vitamin B12, vegan children may also lack vitamin D and omega-3s. As most of a vegan child's diet will come from fiber-rich foods such as grains, vegetables and fruit, they will often feel full before their energy requirements are met, so it's important to offer nutrient dense foods such as cashew nut butter, avocado, and bean stews. It is also important to include vitamin C-rich foods with plant-based sources of iron, such as spinach, to enhance absorption.

BEST VEGAN SOURCES OF PROTEINS

1. Hemp seeds contain a whopping 10g of protein in three tablespoons. Chia seeds contain ¼ oz of protein in three tablespoons, sunflower seeds contain ⅕ oz followed by sesame seeds and poppy seeds at ⅐ oz of protein in three tablespoons. Try sunflower butter on sandwiches or in smoothies in place of nut butters

2. Of all the grains, quinoa—technically a seed—contains the highest amount of protein: 8g per cup. It also includes all nine essential amino acids that the body needs for growth and repair, but cannot produce on its own.

3. Except for soybeans, beans are not complete proteins, but they do contain the amino acid lysine, which is usually missing from other plant proteins. As a result, combining beans with other vegetables or brown rice results in a complete protein. The average amount of protein in white, adzuki, pinto, kidney, black, navy, garbanzo, and lima beans is ½ oz per cup. Peas are a good choice too: 1 cup contains ¼ oz, about the same as a cup of milk.

4. Chickpeas contain ¼ oz of protein in just half a cup, and are also high in fiber. Try roasting them to add crunch.

5. Protein powders can be highly beneficial for children whose diets are lacking in protein. However, it's important to consult with a dietician or nutritionist to ensure that the protein powder you are choosing is suitable. I do not advise offering children adult protein powders. The best ones to choose are those that have been specifically formulated for children and are vegan, predigested, and fermented. Avoid protein powders that contain whey protein and instead look for predigested protein blends that contain biofermented pea protein plus amino acids and antioxidants from real food sources.

SEVEN BUDGET-SAVING WAYS TO BUY ORGANIC

For many people concerned about hormones and other harmful additions to meat, chicken, fish or eggs, organic is worth the extra cost. But for others, the cost of organic food is something they simply can't manage. The reality is that organic costs more for good reason. In order to eat organic foods while sticking to a budget, I've

A vegetarian diet must include:

✓ Eggs, dairy products, seeds, legumes, and soy proteins.

✓ Plenty of vegetables and fruit, but do not allow children to fill up on these foods in place of energy-dense foods.

✓ Iron-rich foods to prevent anemia such as lentils, spinach, pumpkin seeds, and sulphite-free dried apricots.

✓ Foods containing vitamin C with foods that are high in iron. For example, offer sliced up red pepper or an orange with baked beans on toast. Vitamin C enhances the absorption of iron.

✓ Vitamin B12 from eggs and dairy products.

✓ Vitamin D and calcium to prevent bone disease.

✓ Suitable fats from non-meat sources (at least 30 percent of their diet must be derived from foods rich in omega-3s, as well as avocado, extra virgin olive oil, butter, ghee, coconut oil, nuts, nut butters and seeds).

✓ Lower energy vegetarian foods, such as vegetables, with higher fat foods, like coconut vegetable fritters (which contain eggs), or high protein Brazil & Cashew Nut patties (see recipe on page 189).

✓ Vegetables served with fats to ensure that fat-soluble vitamins and minerals are readily absorbed.

✓ Six meals through the day (three main meals and three snacks).

✓ Consultation with a qualified practitioner to see if supplementation is required.

devised these seven shopping tips to save you money, while protecting the environment and your health.

1. COMMIT TO BUYING YOUR FAVORITES

If you can't afford to eat a diet that's made up of nearly all organic, you can at least start with your favorite buys. Focus on your family's staples. If you have a little carnivore who is not keen on cheese, choose grass-fed organic meat, but buy conventionally produced cheese. Switching to organic versions of the foods you most commonly eat will greatly reduce your family's exposure to hormones and antibiotics.

2. KNOW WHERE ORGANIC COUNTS

Red meat, pork, chicken, and dairy are the most important proteins to choose organic.

DID YOU KNOW?

Dried beans should be thoroughly cooked to destroy toxins and to help digestion. Undercooking can cause vomiting and diarrhea.

3. USE A GROCERY LIST

Buying only what you need will always save you money, so never hit the shops without a shopping list. Plan all of your meals for the week, list your ingredients, and only buy those products. Alternatively, shop online and avoid the temptation of even entering the store!

4. SHOP IN BULK

Ask your friends and you'll likely discover that they too are wanting to go organic, but fear the costs involved. The good news is that by buying in bulk you can save, and you'll also be cutting down on landfill-bound packaging. If you don't have a friend who can share your shopping items, shop at your local bulk food stores as this can also lead to considerable savings.

5. LOOK OUT FOR DISCOUNTS

Organic meat is often discounted one to two days before the use-by date—if this is purchased from a reputable source, it's perfect to eat and can be frozen and used later as long as it is placed in the freezer before the use-by date.

6. SAVE ON FRESH PRODUCE

Budget-conscious family shoppers should look for discounted produce in health food stores, which may have gotten a few bruises to the skins or need to be eaten within one to two days. Overripe, discounted mangoes and bananas are excellent choices as they can be frozen and used in smoothies. Likewise, use bruised vegetables in soups, sauces or casseroles where even the fussiest of tiny-tastebuds won't know they were in the discount tub at the store

7. CHOOSE CHEMICAL-FREE

Chemical-free fruit and vegetables from a reputable source can be another great wallet-friendly choice, and the quality of products are often just as good as organic. This is because getting a license to certify produce as organic is often too pricey for small, independent growers who are using chemical-free means to farm their produce.

Consider this…

How do you as a family enjoy your spare time? Watching TV, going to see movies or hiking, biking, and kayaking? Just as with good nutrition habits, children learn about being active by example.

GOAL 4: INCREASE EXERCISE

Protein builds healthy muscles, but to be healthy, children also need physical exercise. Aside from junk food, one of the most damaging things to our children's health is inactivity. According to the Australian Bureau of Statistics, in 2012 toddlers and preschoolers (aged two to four years) were spending almost one and a half hours each day watching TV, DVDs or playing computer games.

Growing up, my brother, who suffered from obesity, detested physical activity. These days he is in great shape and he blames his childhood weight problem on his lack of exercise, as well as poor food choices.

I often see young children who are overweight and when I look at their diet, I do not find obvious reasons why. The same food diary could come from a healthy-weight child. Often the differential is lifestyle and inactivity. In inactive children, modest excess food intake can cause disproportionate weight gain.

Dr. Roy Sugarman, a Sydney-based clinical neuropsychologist, points out that in Australia, ten-year-olds spend about thirty-four hours of their free time per week, outside of school, engaged in sedentary activities. By age twelve, this figure increases to forty-one hours and rises again for fourteen-year-olds to forty-five hours (or 6.5 hours per day).

For teenagers living today, this would mean ten thousand hours of sitting by the time they are twenty-one. During continuous sitting, especially in the triple-flexed position we adopt in front of a screen, regulation of lipase (the breakdown of fats) switches off, insulin resistance increases, electrical activity switches off, inflammatory cytokines increase, growth hormones decrease, all of which sets up our children for brain and body ill-health.

Children love anything fun, so engage them in activity-based games and everyday routines to keep their exercise levels high. Work with what interests them and areas they display strength in. Swimming and gymnastics are fantastic for building up core muscle strength. Or, if you can, put a trampoline or a basketball hoop in your outdoor area. And don't forget more simple fun like balloon bashing to motivate a child away from an electronic device.

EXERCISE:

· builds and maintains healthy bones, muscles and joints.

· helps kids sleep better at night.

· controls weight gain.

· increases lean muscle mass and boosts metabolism.

- decreases risk of developing type 2 diabetes, sleep apnoea, and cardiovascular disease.
- strengthens immune system.
- improves mood by boosting serotonin levels.
- is a good outlet for anger.
- increases self–esteem and sense of belonging.
- increases focus and attention span.
- helps kids develop balance, strength, hand-eye coordination and ball skills.
- helps children learn social skills, such as winning, losing, and how to be a team player.
- helps with neuralplasticity (the brains ability to form new neural pathways).

HOW MUCH EXERCISE SHOULD MY CHILD HAVE?

Children under five require three hours of physical activity daily. Over fives should aim for at least one hour daily. This doesn't have to happen in consecutive minutes. You can break it up into thirty-minute sessions or even twenty-minute sessions.

HYDRATE AND RECOVER

As with adults, the harder and longer a child exercises or plays, the more he needs to hydrate. Make sure to replace whatever water they sweat out after each play or sports session. Always offer frequent drinks before, during and after exercise. Choose water or diluted fresh fruit juice—children do not need sports drinks. Recovery eating is equally essential after a child has been involved in an activity such as soccer, basketball, swimming or ballet. Offer a snack with the ratio of 4:1 carbohydrate to protein so that their muscles can repair and break down the lactic acid.

POST-SPORT SNACKS

- Beetroot Bliss Balls (see recipe on page 115)
- Lunch Box Friendly Muesli Bars (see recipe on page 193)
- Peanut butter sandwich on wholegrain sourdough bread
- Veggie sticks with Basic Hummus (see recipe on page 282)
- Trail mix or Quick Homemade Granola (see recipe on page 275)
- Smoothies (see recipes on page 225)
- Malted Chocolate Drink (see recipe on page 275)
- Yogurt with berries (see our Berry & Granola Parfait on page 249)
- Chicken or tuna sandwich on wholegrain bread

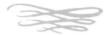

DID YOU KNOW?

If the only protein in the lunch box is in a sandwich while every other option is a carbohydrate, your child may feel hungry again soon after eating. Add protein-rich snacks like trail mix or roasted chickpeas for a better balance.

Exercise Do's and Don'ts

👍 DO...	👎 DON'T...
plan more family fun activities.	leave too many chores for times when you are with your child.
plan three to four afternoon play opportunities per week. Children are naturally active in playgrounds or indoors with friends as long as electronics are not involved.	make outings revolve around eating alone. Even picnics can be more fun with a game of soccer or a running race before lunch.
walk to and from school with younger children. It will benefit your health too.	leave the television on for extended periods or use it as the babysitter.
sign your child up for organized team sports. Many fun activities exist from toddler age on.	force your child to participate in activities that they do not enjoy—this may turn him off exercise for good. Rather find activities he enjoys.
make weekend plans that include hiking, biking, kayaking, swimming, and walking.	make exercise a chore or relate it to weight loss. Children need to think they are doing exercise for fun, not to keep their weight down. Instead talk to children about how exercise helps them get strong or run fast.
ensure that if you are stuck indoors due to rainy weather that you include physical activities such as hide and seek, obstacle course races and treasure hunts.	whine in front of your kid about how difficult is it to get off the couch and exercise. Speak about exercising in a positive light, even if you have to pretend.

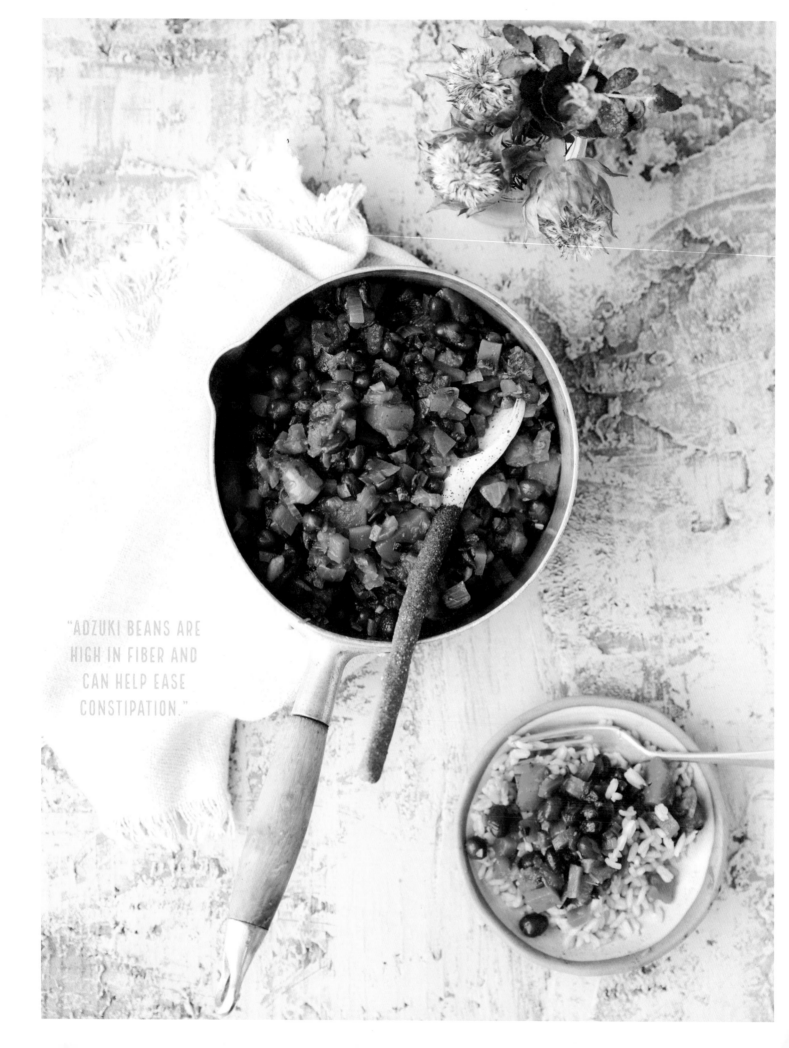

"ADZUKI BEANS ARE HIGH IN FIBER AND CAN HELP EASE CONSTIPATION."

V — Vegan

Gluten Free

Nut Free

Prep time: 15 mins (+ 12 hours soaking time and 1 hour cooking time if using dry beans)
Cooking time: 60 mins
Serves: 8

Adzuki Bean Stew

I learned about adzuki beans when I was studying yoga in my twenties—they're really good for the kidneys. Bean dishes can be hit and miss with kids, but the balance of flavors in this one is perfect and not overpowering.

INGREDIENTS

1–2 tbs extra virgin olive oil

1 yellow onion, finely chopped

2 cloves garlic, finely chopped

2 celery stalks, finely chopped

2 medium-sized carrots, peeled and finely chopped

4 large field mushrooms, finely chopped

½ butternut squash (1 lbs), peeled and cubed

1 tsp ground cinnamon

2 tbs tamari

2 cups (13½ oz) adzuki beans, soaked overnight or for at least 12 hours, rinsed and cooked for 40–60 mins until soft but not mushy, or 1 (14 oz) canned beans, rinsed and drained

2 cups vegetable broth (low sodium)

sea salt, to taste

INSTRUCTIONS

In a large pan or wok, heat oil over medium heat. Sauté onion and garlic until soft, about 5 mins.

Next add celery, carrot, mushroom, squash, cinnamon, and tamari sauce and sauté for 5–10 mins.

Add beans and vegetable broth and allow to simmer for around 30–45 mins. If liquid evaporates before the beans are soft and mushy, add a small amount of stock or filtered water.

Taste and add more sea salt, cinnamon or tamari if necessary.

Allow to cool and serve with brown rice or any whole grain of your choice.

Serving and storing leftovers: Serve immediately. Store in the fridge in an airtight container for up to 4 days or freeze for up to 4 months.

TIP

For children who do not like mixed textures, puree the stew to a smoother consistency to make it more palatable for them.

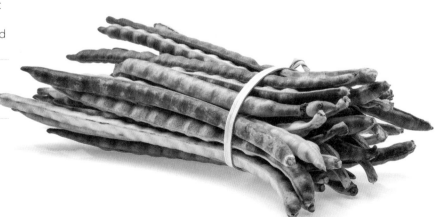

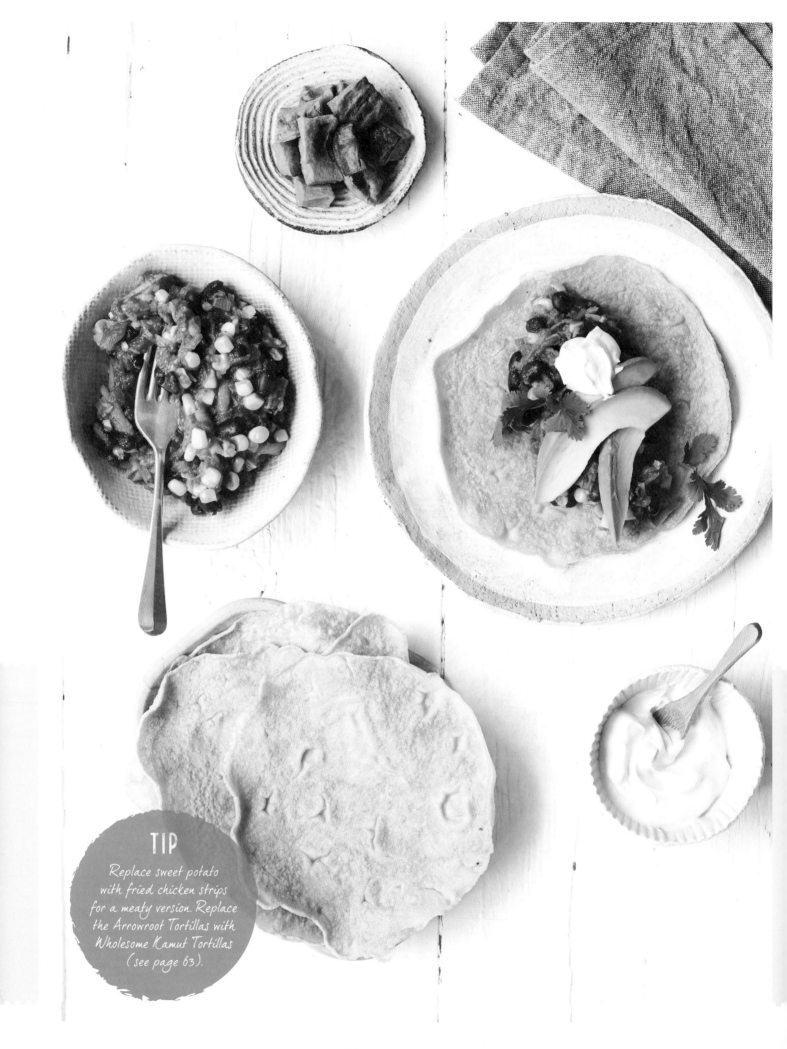

TIP

Replace sweet potato with fried chicken strips for a meaty version. Replace the Arrowroot Tortillas with Wholesome Kamut Tortillas (see page 63).

VEG — Vegetarian | Gluten Free | Nut Free | Egg Free

Prep time: 30 mins
Cooking time: 15–20 mins
Serves: 6–8

Black Bean Tortillas

When I make these I separate the ingredients and let my children make up their own tortillas. They shove as much as they can into their wraps. This is a really unique, tasty combination of ingredients; it's really impressive how it all comes together.

INGREDIENTS

1 medium-sized sweet potato, peeled, finely cubed

1 tbs extra virgin olive oil

½ yellow onion, finely chopped

1 garlic clove, finely diced

2 medium-sized carrots, peeled and grated

1½ cups (9½ oz) cooked black beans or 1 (14 oz) canned beans, rinsed and drained

1⅔ cups (14¾ oz) tomatoes, diced

1 medium-sized red apple, peeled and finely grated

1 cup (6 oz) corn kernels

½ lime, juiced

¼ tsp ground cumin

¼ tsp dried oregano

sea salt and pepper, to taste

1 large avocado, peeled, finely chopped

1 cup (2¾ oz) shredded lettuce

½ cup (4¼ oz) sour cream or natural yogurt

¼ cup (⅙ oz) fresh cilantro

INSTRUCTIONS

Preheat oven to 390°F and line a baking tray with baking paper. Toss the sweet potato cubes with ½ tbs olive oil and bake in the oven for 10–15 mins or until cooked through and browned on the outside.

Meanwhile, heat oil in a large frying pan on medium heat and fry onions and garlic for 3 mins or until soft. Add carrots and fry for another 3 mins. Add beans, tomato, apple, corn, lime juice, and spices and simmer for 10 mins. Season to taste.

Serve black bean mix in Wholesome Kamut Tortilla Wraps (see page 63) or Arrowroot Tortillas (see below) topped with avocado, lettuce, sour cream, and cilantro leaves (optional).

Serving and storing leftovers: Serve immediately. Store in an airtight container in the fridge for up to 4 days or freeze for up to 4 months.

VEG — Vegetarian | Gluten Free | Dairy Free | Nut Free

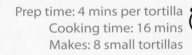

Prep time: 4 mins per tortilla
Cooking time: 16 mins
Makes: 8 small tortillas

Arrowroot Tortillas

INGREDIENTS

4 eggs, beaten

2 tbs coconut cream

½ cup (2⅙ oz) arrowroot

2 tsp coconut flour

½ tsp sea salt

coconut oil, melted (for frying)

INSTRUCTIONS

In a bowl, combine all ingredients (aside from the oil) until a smooth batter forms.

Heat a small frying pan over medium heat and brush with some coconut oil.

Pour ⅛ of the batter into the pan, swirling it to coat the base.

Cook for approximately 1 or 2 mins on each side. Continue with rest of batter.

Keep tortillas warm until ready to serve.

Serving and storing leftovers: Serve immediately, warm. Store in the fridge for up to 4 days.

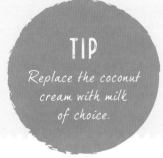

TIP

Replace the coconut cream with milk of choice.

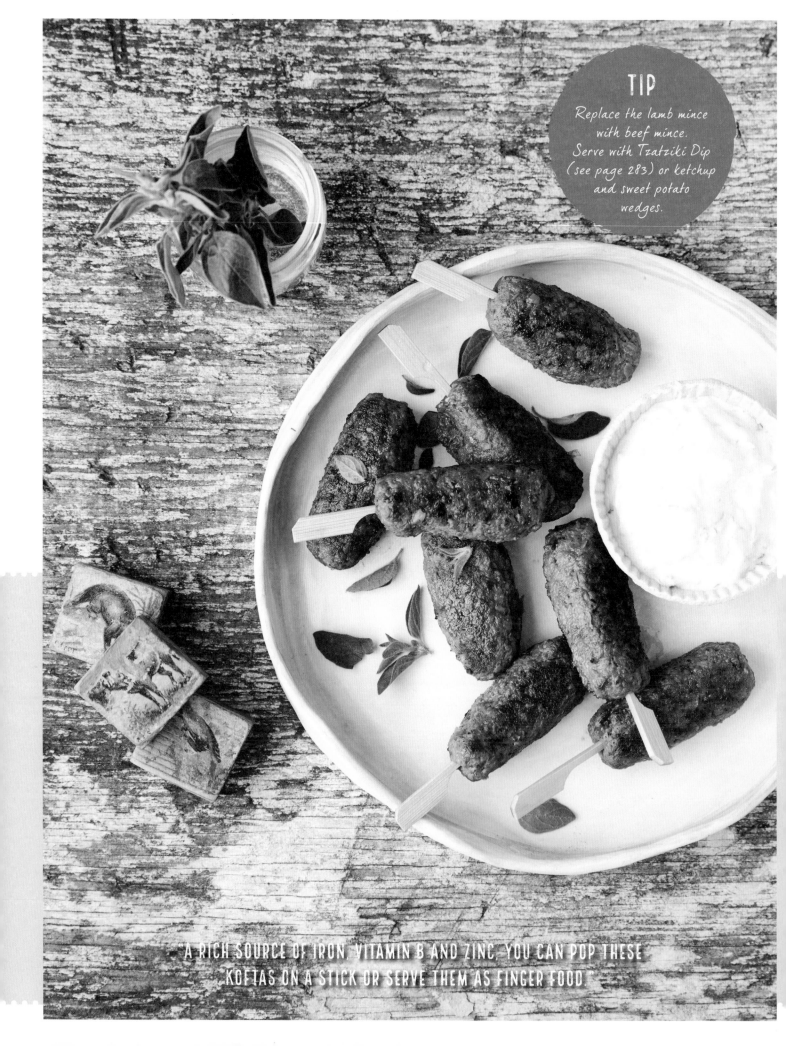

TIP

Replace the lamb mince
with beef mince.
Serve with Tzatziki Dip
(see page 283) or ketchup
and sweet potato
wedges.

"A RICH SOURCE OF IRON, VITAMIN B AND ZINC, YOU CAN POP THESE
KOFTAS ON A STICK OR SERVE THEM AS FINGER FOOD"

Dairy Free
Gluten Free
Nut Free

Prep time: 15 mins
Cooking time: 15–20 mins
Makes: 25–30 koftas (6–8 portions)

Lamb Koftas

This recipe was inspired by a family trip to Greece when my son was one. He was very keen to try kofta, but it was too spicy and salty so I decided to create a healthy version we all could eat. The mix of spices combined with the sweet flavor of dates really makes this dish stand out.

INGREDIENTS

1 leek (5¹⁄₃ oz), finely sliced

1 medium-sized carrot, peeled and grated

2 Medjool dates, pitted

1 garlic clove, crushed

1 lb minced lamb

1 egg (optional)

1 tsp ground cinnamon

¼ tsp ground cumin

sea salt and pepper, to taste

olive oil, macadamia nut oil or coconut oil, for frying (if macadamia nut oil is used this recipe is no longer nut free)

EQUIPMENT

high-speed food processor

INSTRUCTIONS

Place leek, carrot, dates, and garlic in a food processor and blend until smooth.

In a big bowl combine minced lamb with egg, spices, and processed vegetables.

Using your hands, shape the mixture into mini kofta shapes.

Heat oil in a medium-size frying pan and cook koftas in batches for 3–5 mins on each side or until cooked through.

Serving and storing leftovers: Serve immediately, Store in the fridge for up to 3 days or freeze for up to 4 months.

Dairy Free
Gluten Free
Nut Free

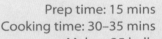
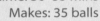

Prep time: 15 mins
Cooking time: 30–35 mins
Makes: 35 balls

Beef & Veggie Meatballs

INGREDIENTS

1 yellow onion, chopped

1–2 cloves garlic

1 medium-sized carrot, peeled and chopped

2 medium-sized zucchinis, chopped

1 egg

1 red apple, peeled, cored and quartered

1 lb beef mince

¼ cup (¾ oz) rice bread crumbs

sea salt and pepper, to taste

2 tsp Italian mixed herbs

INSTRUCTIONS

Preheat oven to 355°F and line a baking tray with baking paper.

Place onion, garlic, carrot, zucchini, egg, and apple in processor and process until smooth.

In a separate bowl add mince—break apart if necessary using a mallet.

Add vegetable mix to mince and combine, using your hands.

Add bread crumbs, salt, pepper, Italian mixed herbs and combine until a smooth consistency is reached.

Take about a ¼ cup of the meat mixture and roll into small balls.

Place on a baking tray and bake for 30–35 mins or until browned on top and cooked through.

Serve with Homemade Ketchup (see page 283), sweet potato mash or brown rice.

Serving and storing leftovers: Serve immediately, store in fridge for up to 3 days or freeze for up to 4 months.

Fry the meatballs instead in olive oil or coconut oil.

CHICKEN IS AN EXCELLENT
SOURCE OF VITAMIN
B12, AND COUPLED WITH
ANTIOXIDANT-RICH VEGETABLES
THIS DISH PACKS A POWERFUL
NUTRITIONAL PUNCH.

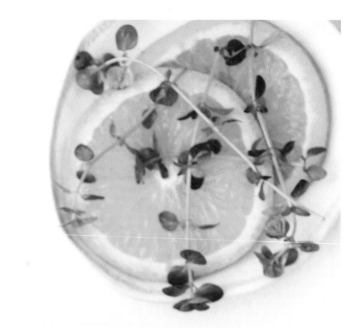

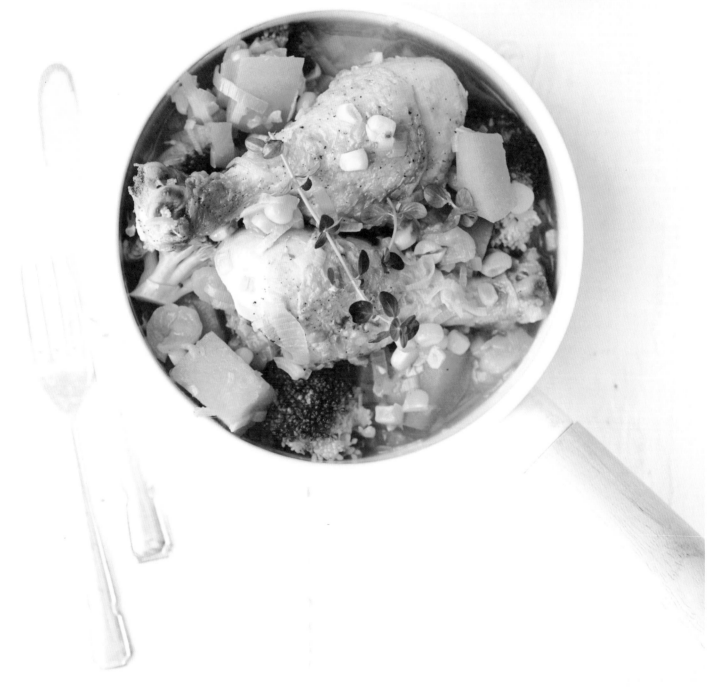

Gluten Free · Dairy Free · Egg Free · Nut Free

Prep time: 10 mins
Cooking time: 50–55 mins
Serves: 3–4

Chicken Drumstick Casserole

The addition of orange juice and apricots give this chicken dish a sweet flavor that children just love. Many conventional sauces use processed sweeteners—this is a much healthier, more natural way of cooking.

INGREDIENTS

2 tbs extra virgin olive oil or coconut oil

1 leek, finely sliced (white part only)

1 clove of garlic, finely minced

2 tsp fresh ginger, grated or chopped finely

8 chicken drumsticks or thighs 1⅓ lbs

1 cup (6 oz) raw corn kernels

½ raw butternut squash (1 lb), peeled and cut into medium-sized slices

1 medium head broccoli, chopped into small pieces

4 dried apricots (sulphur-free), finely sliced

4 sprigs of fresh thyme

juice of two oranges

2 cups chicken stock, low sodium or homemade chicken broth (salt-free for babies)

sea salt to taste

cracked black pepper, to taste

INSTRUCTIONS

Heat oil in large pot or pan.

Add leek, garlic, and ginger and stir-fry for 3 mins until soft.

Add chicken drumsticks and fry for 5 mins each side or until brown on the outside.

Add corn kernels, squash, broccoli, apricots, thyme, orange juice and stock, and bring to boil.

Reduce heat and allow to simmer for 30–40 mins. Add salt and pepper to taste.

Serving and storing leftovers: Serve immediately or store in the fridge for up to 3 days. Freeze for up to 4 months.

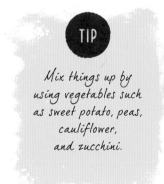

TIP

Mix things up by using vegetables such as sweet potato, peas, cauliflower, and zucchini.

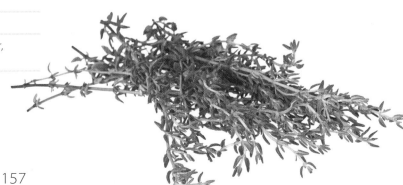

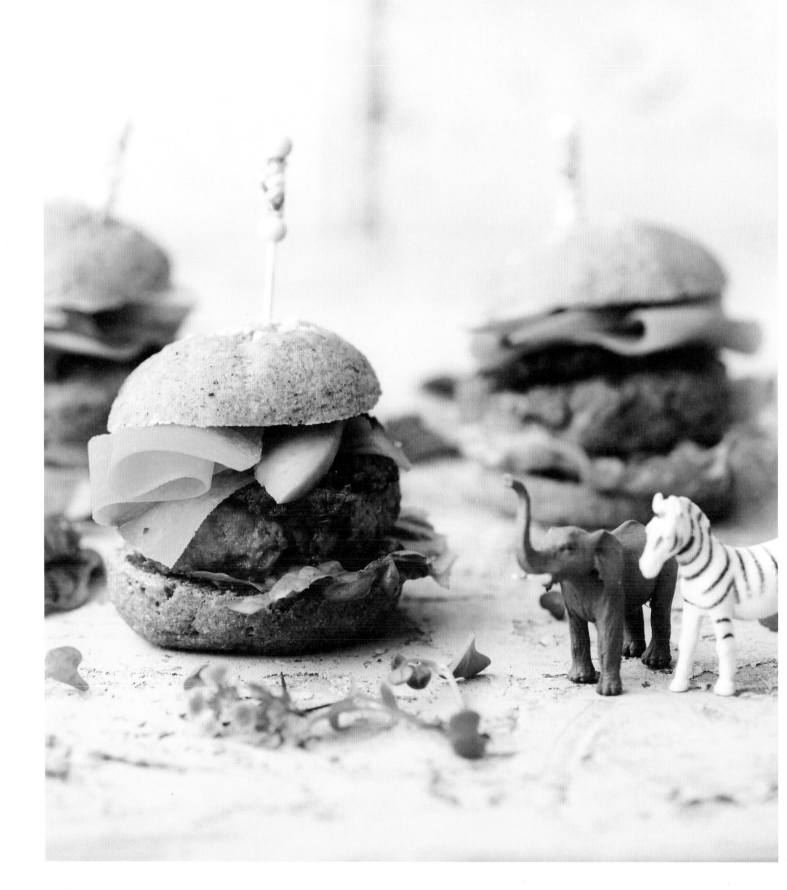

"I OFTEN ADD THESE DELICIOUS PATTIES TO THE SCHOOL LUNCH BOX IN A WRAP AS AN ALTERNATIVE TO PROCESSED MEAT SANDWICHES. THEY'RE HIGH IN ZINC, IRON, VITAMIN B12, AND BETA-CAROTENE."

Gluten Free   Dairy Free   Nut Free

Prep time: 10 mins
Cooking time: 20 mins
Serves: 8

Hamburger Patties

I introduced this recipe to a local daycare menu and the kids gobbled them up! Get creative with how you serve these patties. They can be eaten on their own, in a wrap, in a bun, on a bed of rice or mash, or with plenty of sides.

INGREDIENTS

1 lbs beef mince

¾ cup (6²/₅ oz) sweet potato, steamed and mashed

½ yellow onion, finely chopped

2 egg yolks

1 tbs Dijon mustard

1 tbs tamari or low-sodium soy sauce

pinch of sea salt

pepper, to taste

2 tbs olive oil, coconut oil or avocado oil for frying

INSTRUCTIONS

In a large bowl combine all ingredients (except olive oil), using your hands.

Heat oil in a frying pan on medium heat.

Roll beef mix into patties, and cook for 3–5 mins each side in frying pan in two batches. Alternatively bake in the oven at 355°F for 20 mins, turning once.

Keep warm.

Serving and storing leftovers: Serve immediately in Gluten-free Hamburger Buns (see page 51) with Homemade Ketchup (see page 283), Roasted Garlic Guacamole (see page 191), beetroot and lettuce. Store in the fridge for up to 3 days or freeze for up to 4 months.

Dairy Free   Nut Free   Wheat Free   VEG Vegetarian

Prep time: 15 mins (+ 1 hour refrigeration time)
Cooking time: 20–30 mins
Makes: 30 mini patties

High-protein Veggie Burgers

INGREDIENTS

½ cup (3¹/₅ oz) cooked or canned cannellini beans, rinsed and drained

½ cup (4½ oz) butternut squash, peeled and steamed

½ cup (4½ oz) parsnip, sweet or white potato, peeled and steamed

1 cup (5²/₃ oz) cooked quinoa

1 large egg

¼ cup (1 oz) chickpea flour

¼ cup (1 oz) rolled oats

¼ tsp ground turmeric

2 garlic cloves, crushed

¼ cup (¹/₆ oz) fresh cilantro

sea salt and pepper, to taste

coconut oil for frying

EQUIPMENT

high-speed food processor

INSTRUCTIONS

Place beans, squash, and parsnip into a high-speed food processor and process until smooth.

Add rest of ingredients and pulse to combine.

Place mixture in the fridge for an hour.

Heat oil in a large frying pan and add tablespoons of batter into pan. Fry patties on both sides for 3–4 mins or until golden brown and crispy.

Continue with rest of the batter. Alternatively, bake in oven at 355°F for 25–30 mins, turning halfway.

Serve with a garden salad and sour cream dip on the side.

Serving and storing leftovers:
Serve immediately, store in an airtight container in the fridge for up to 4 days or freeze for up to 4 months.

TIP

For a gluten-free option replace oats with gluten-free oats or 1/4 cup quinoa flakes, 1/4 cup rice crumbs or an extra 1/4 cup chickpea flour.

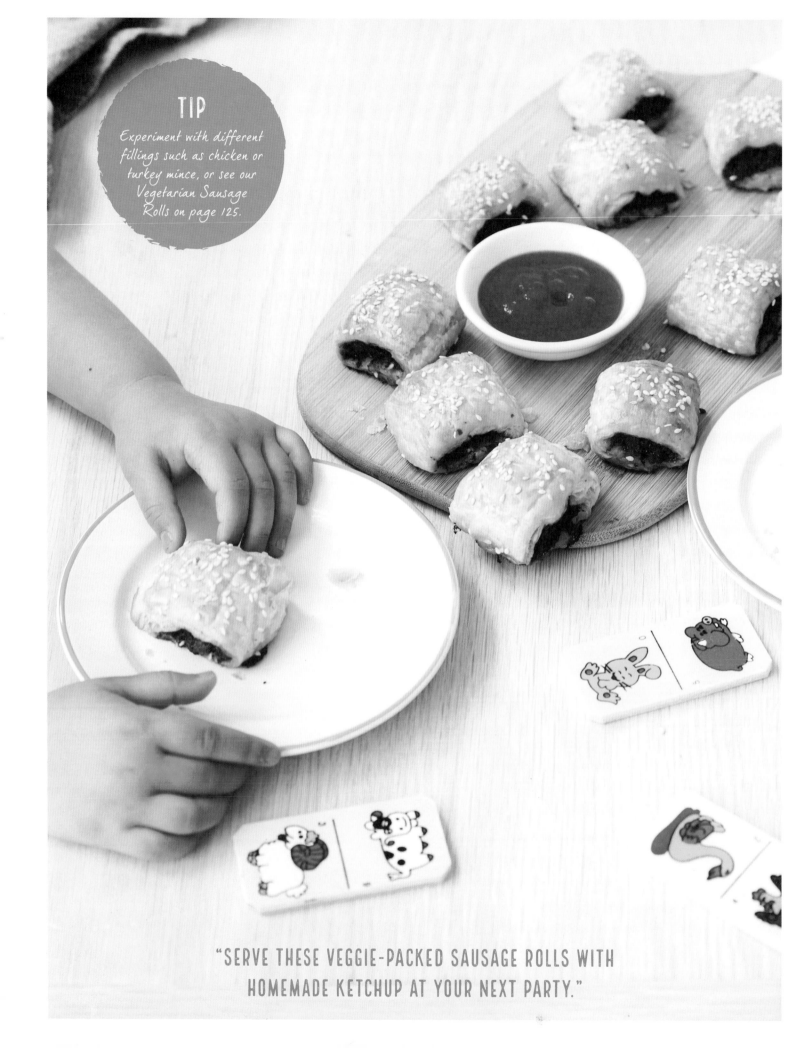

TIP

Experiment with different fillings such as chicken or turkey mince, or see our Vegetarian Sausage Rolls on page 125.

"SERVE THESE VEGGIE-PACKED SAUSAGE ROLLS WITH HOMEMADE KETCHUP AT YOUR NEXT PARTY."

Gluten Free Nut Free

Prep time: 2 hours
Cooking time: 20–30 mins
Makes: 30

Healthy Sausage Rolls

For kids who do not love meat, meat-filled pastry snacks are usually an easy way to encourage them to eat it. Best part is the pastry contains no nasties unlike the store-bought stuff.

INGREDIENTS

PASTRY:

1 cup (5⅓ oz) unsalted butter, cubed and chilled

2½ cups (11½ oz) Wholesome Child gluten-free flour mix (see page 32), plus ⅓ cup for work surface

¾ tsp sea salt

½ cup ice-cold filtered water

1 egg (to glaze the puff pastry)

sesame seeds (optional)

FILLING:

1 yellow onion, finely diced

1 large carrot, grated

1 medium zucchini, grated

½ cup (1¾ oz) brown mushrooms, chopped

¼ cup (1¼ oz) yellow pepper, finely diced

¼ cup (1¼ oz) red pepper, finely diced

2 tbs fresh parsley, finely chopped

1 lb lean organic beef mince

¼ cup (⅞ oz) rice bread crumbs

2 tbs tomato paste

sea salt and pepper, to season

EQUIPMENT

high-speed food processor

INSTRUCTIONS

PASTRY:

Cut ¾ cup (4 oz) butter into small cubes. Place in an even layer on a plate and transfer to freezer to chill.

Place flour and salt together in a high-speed food processor and pulse to combine.

Place remaining butter into a processor and pulse until no visible pieces of butter remain.

Add chilled butter cubes to the flour-butter mixture and pulse twice for three seconds each time.

Add ¼ cup water to the mixture and pulse twice for three seconds each time. Repeat with remaining water, pulsing twice.

Scrape dough from bowl of processor onto a well-floured work surface.

Lightly flour dough and, using your hands, squeeze and shape dough into a cylinder. Press down to flatten into a rectangle.

Roll dough out into a rectangle about ½" thick. Flour under and on top of the dough and roll dough away and back toward you in the length and once in the width.

Fold the two longer ends in toward the middle of the rectangle, leaving a ¾" space in the middle. Starting from the shorter end, roll dough into a snail, then press dough down and wrap in cling wrap. Refrigerate for an hour.

FILLING:

Preheat the oven to 390°F and line a baking tray with baking paper.

Place onion, carrot, zucchini, mushrooms, pepper, and parsley in a food processor and process until smooth.

In a large bowl, place beef mince, rice crumbs, tomato paste, vegetable mix, and seasoning and mix thoroughly, using your hands. Cover and set aside.

Take dough out of the fridge and cut in half.

On a floured surface, roll both halves into rectangles (about ⅙" thick). Cut in half lengthwise.

Shape the filling into a long tube shape and place half along the center of each pastry. Fold pastry over so that the mince mixture is completely covered.

Beat egg lightly then brush over the top of the pastry and sprinkle with sesame seeds.

Cut the sausage roll into ¾" to 1⅕" pieces and place onto the lined baking tray.

Bake in oven for approximately 20–25 mins or until the sausage rolls are golden brown on top.

Serve with Homemade Ketchup (see page 283).

Serving and storing leftovers: Serve immediately. Store in the fridge for up to 3 days or freeze for up to 4 months.

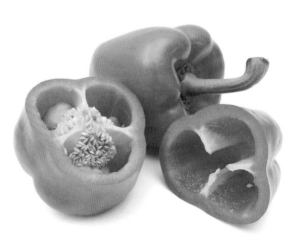

VEG
Vegetarian

Gluten
Free

Dairy
Free

Prep time: 5 mins
Cooking time: 8 mins
Serves: 4

Almond Coconut Waffles

INGREDIENTS

1 cup (4½ oz) almond meal

1 tsp coconut flour

¼ tsp baking powder

pinch sea salt

2 eggs

½ tsp pure vanilla extract

2 tbs maple syrup or
raw honey

2 tbs coconut oil, melted

2 tbs coconut milk

EQUIPMENT

waffle iron

INSTRUCTIONS

Preheat waffle iron.

In a large bowl, mix together almond meal, coconut flour, baking powder, and salt. Set aside.

In a separate bowl, beat the eggs. Stir in the vanilla extract, honey, coconut oil, and coconut milk.

Pour the egg mixture into the dry mixture and whisk until well combined.

Ladle the batter into the preheated waffle iron. Cook the waffles for approximately 4 mins or until golden and crisp.

Serving and storing leftovers: Serve immediately. Store in the fridge for up to 4 days or freeze for up to 4 months.

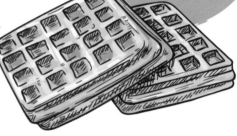

TIP
If you do not have a waffle iron, these will work just as well as pancakes.

Dairy
Free

Gluten
Free

Nut
Free

Prep time: 15 mins
Cooking time: 40 mins
Serves: 6–8

Coconut Lamb Meatloaf

INGREDIENTS

2 medium-sized apples, peeled and cored

½ yellow onion, roughly chopped

1 tomato, halved

½ cup (3⅕ oz) cooked or canned chickpeas, rinsed and drained

2 tbs rice bread crumbs

1 egg

1 tsp ground cinnamon

½ clove garlic

2 tbs coconut milk

1 lb lamb, minced

EQUIPMENT

high-speed food processor

INSTRUCTIONS

Preheat oven to 390°F and line a loaf tin with baking paper.

Place all ingredients (aside from minced lamb) into a processor and blend together. Once a smooth consistency is achieved place into large bowl and add the minced lamb. Mix together using your hands.

Place mince mixture into the loaf tin and bake for 40 mins.

Allow to cool slightly before removing the meatloaf from the tin. Slice thickly and serve.

Serving and storing leftovers: Serve immediately, store in fridge for up to 3 days or freeze for up to 4 months.

Serve with brown rice or sweet potato wedges and steamed vegetables.

Dairy Free Gluten Free Nut Free Egg Free

Prep time: 15 mins
Cooking time: 15 mins
Serves: 4

Easy Fish Curry

INGREDIENTS

1½ tbs coconut oil

3 spring onions, finely sliced

1 garlic clove, crushed

½ tsp ginger, grated

1 tsp curry powder

1 tbs mild tomato paste

1–2 tbs lemon juice

1 medium-sized sweet potato, peeled and cubed

1 medium-sized carrot, grated

1 cup coconut cream/ milk

1 cup low-sodium vegetable broth or filtered water

3–4 white fish fillets (1 lbs to 1⅓ lbs) (snapper, hoki), cubed

1 cup (⅞ oz) baby spinach, chopped (optional)

2 tbs fresh cilantro, finely chopped

sea salt and pepper

INSTRUCTIONS

Heat coconut oil over medium heat in a large frying pan. Add onions, garlic, ginger, curry powder, tomato paste, and lemon juice and cook for 2–3 mins, or until softened.

Add sweet potato and carrot and cook for another 2 mins.

Add coconut cream and broth and let simmer for 5 mins. Then add fish and spinach and cook for another 5 mins.

Season with cilantro, salt and pepper and serve with brown rice or quinoa on the side.

Serving and storing leftovers: Serve immediately or store in the fridge for up to 3 days. Freeze for up to 4 months.

TIP

If you are using frozen fish fillets bake the fish at 390°F for 10-15 mins before adding to the curry to avoid it being too '"fishy" for children.

Dairy Free Gluten Free Nut Free Egg Free

Prep time: 10 mins
Cooking time: 15 mins
Serves: 6–8

Miso Chicken with Vegetables

INGREDIENTS

1 quart filtered water

1⅓ lbs skinless chicken breasts or thighs, cut into strips

2 tbs fresh lemon juice

½ cup (1⅘ oz) carrot, finely diced

½ cup (2½ oz) red pepper, finely diced

1 cup (2 4/5 oz)

broccoli florets, chopped

2 spring onions, finely sliced

3 tbs tamari (or soy sauce)

⅓ cup (3⅕ oz) brown rice miso paste

4 cups (1¾ lbs) cooked brown rice, to serve

INSTRUCTIONS

In a large pot, bring water to the boil.

Add chicken, lemon juice, carrot, pepper, broccoli, spring onions, and tamari and simmer for 15 mins, or until vegetables are soft.

Remove 1 cup of water from the pot and mix with miso paste in a small bowl, then return mixture to pot, stir and cook for another minute.

Serve on top of brown rice in bowls.

Serving and storing leftovers: Serve immediately, store in the fridge for up to 3 days or freeze in covered airtight containers for up to 4 months.

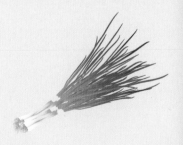

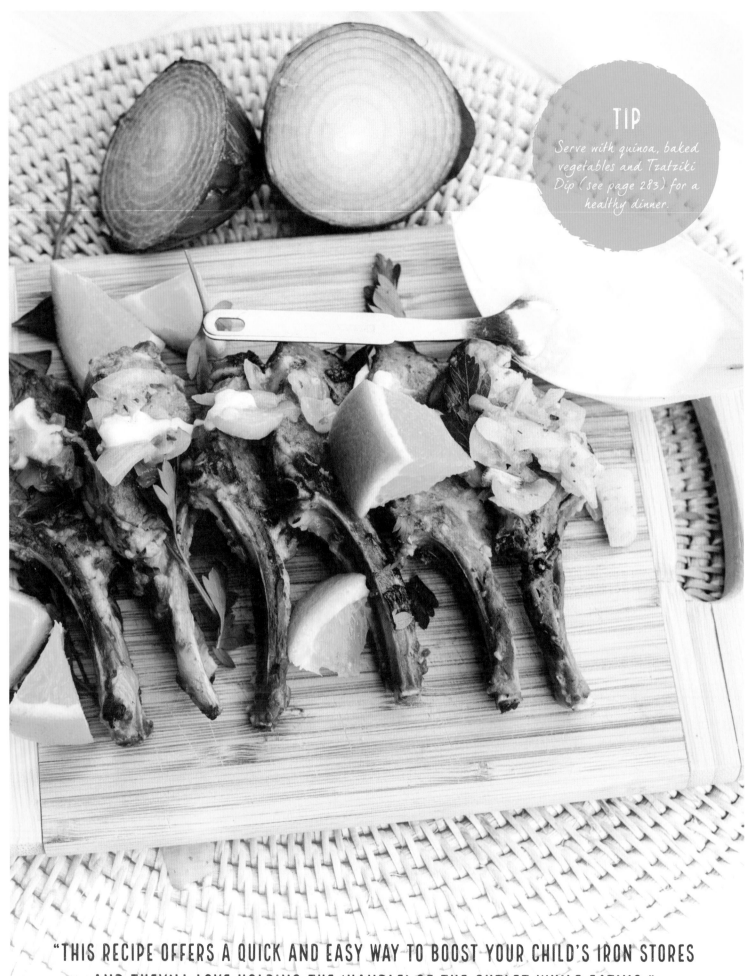

TIP
Serve with quinoa, baked vegetables and Tzatziki Dip (see page 283) for a healthy dinner.

"THIS RECIPE OFFERS A QUICK AND EASY WAY TO BOOST YOUR CHILD'S IRON STORES AND THEY'LL LOVE HOLDING THE 'HANDLE' OF THE CUTLET WHILE EATING."

Dairy Free | Gluten Free | Nut Free | Egg Free

Prep time: 15 mins
Cooking time: 8–10 mins
Serves: 4

Orange Lamb Cutlets

INGREDIENTS

2 garlic cloves, crushed

1 tbs extra virgin olive oil

1 orange, juiced

2 tbs mixed herbs

8 lamb cutlets

1 fresh lemon

sea salt and pepper, to taste

INSTRUCTIONS

Combine garlic, olive oil, orange juice, and mixed herbs in a small bowl. Place lamb cutlets on a plate and pour the mixture over. Cover and leave in the fridge for at least 10 mins but ideally a couple of hours.

Heat a frying pan over medium heat and add the cutlets. Cook the cutlets for 4–5 mins on each side until cooked through. Squeeze lemon over cutlets while cooking. Season to taste.

Serving and storing leftovers: Serve immediately, store in the fridge for up to 3 days or freeze for up to 4 months.

Dairy Free | Gluten Free | Nut Free | Egg Free

Prep time: 10 mins (+ 30 mins to 1 hour marinating time in fridge)
Cooking time: 35–40 mins
Serves: 4

Sticky Chicken Drumsticks with Cauliflower

INGREDIENTS

STICKY DRUMSTICKS:

3 garlic cloves, crushed

pinch sea salt

1/3 cup tamari

1/3 cup raw honey

1 tsp cold pressed sesame oil

zest and juice of 1/2 lemon

8 small chicken drumsticks (1¾ lbs)

CAULIFLOWER:

3/4 cup (4¼ oz) rice flour

3/4 cup (180ml) filtered water

pinch sea salt

pinch garlic powder

1/2 medium-sized cauliflower head, broken into florets

GARNISH

1½ tsp sesame seeds

1 scallion, thinly sliced

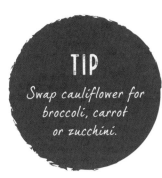

TIP

Swap cauliflower for broccoli, carrot or zucchini.

INSTRUCTIONS

Preheat oven to 390°F and line 2 baking trays with baking paper.

In a bowl, add garlic, salt, tamari, honey, sesame oil, zest and juice of lemon and stir to combine. Reserve 1/4 cup of sticky sauce for the cauliflower.

Place chicken drumsticks in a large bowl, add the sticky sauce and toss to coat. Cover and let sit at room temperature for 30 mins or place in the fridge for an hour to marinate.

In a small bowl, add rice flour, water, salt, and garlic powder and stir to combine.

Dip cauliflower florets in the batter and place on the baking tray. Bake for 10 mins or until batter hardens, then flip over and bake for another 5 mins.

Take the chicken out of the fridge, place on the second baking tray and bake for 35 mins, or until cooked through and golden brown on top.

Brush cauliflower with the reserved sticky sauce and bake for an additional 10–15 mins.

Serve sticky chicken drumsticks and cauliflower with sesame seeds and scallions sprinkled on top..

Serving and storing leftovers: Serve immediately, store in the fridge for up to 3 days or freeze for up to 4 months.

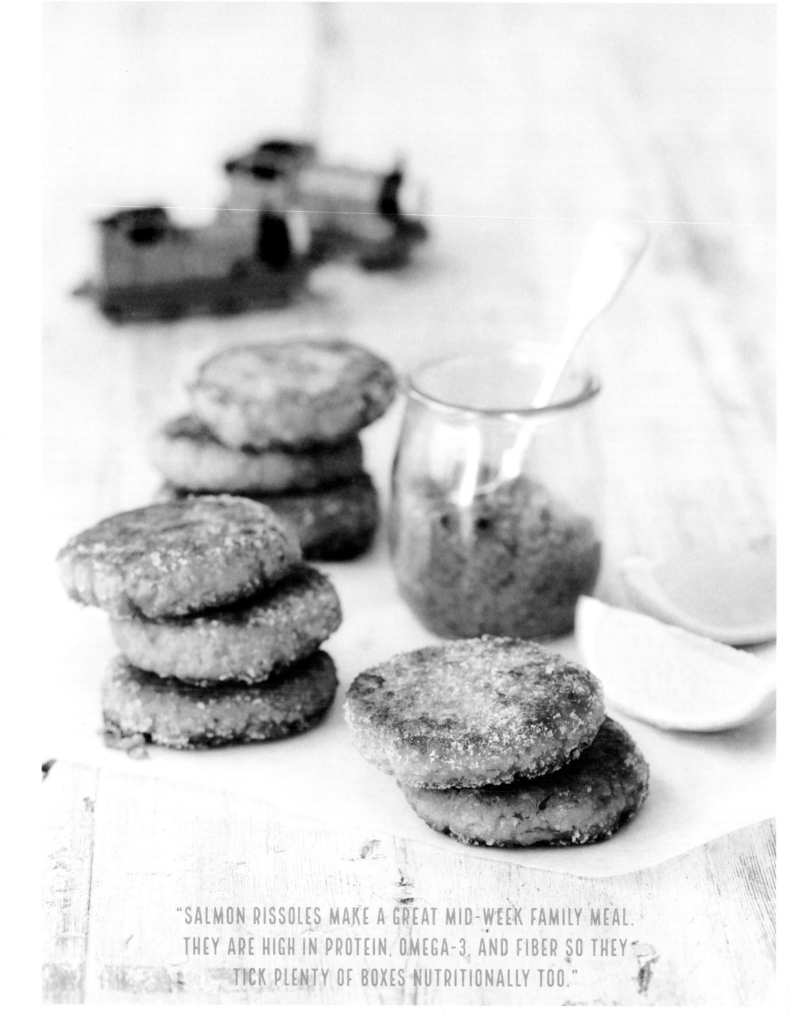

"SALMON RISSOLES MAKE A GREAT MID-WEEK FAMILY MEAL.
THEY ARE HIGH IN PROTEIN, OMEGA-3, AND FIBER SO THEY
TICK PLENTY OF BOXES NUTRITIONALLY TOO."

Gluten Free   Dairy Free   Nut Free

Prep time: 25–30 mins
(+ 30 mins refrigeration time)
Cooking time: 30 mins
Makes: 36 patties

Salmon & Millet Rissoles

My kids enjoy eating salmon but I get bored of serving it grilled or steamed. This delicious alternative tastes great in a burger bun with salad veggies and is great for school lunches.

INGREDIENTS

14 oz raw salmon fillets or 1 (15 oz) can wild salmon, drained

¼ cup (1²/₅ oz) raw corn kernels

¼ cup (⁷/₈ oz) carrot, peeled and grated

1 leek, roughly chopped

2 tbs fresh orange juice

¼ cup (1½ oz) rice flour

½ tsp mixed herbs

½ tsp Himalayan rock salt

½ tbs Dijon mustard (optional)

1 cup (6²/₅ oz) cooked millet

1 cup (3¹/₅ oz) rice bread crumbs, to coat

coconut oil or olive oil (optional)

EQUIPMENT

high-speed processor

INSTRUCTIONS

Preheat oven to 355°F and line a baking tray with baking paper.

Place salmon, corn, carrot, leek, and orange juice in the food processor and process until smooth.

Add rice flour, herbs, salt, and mustard and process again until well combined.

Next, add millet and process on a low speed. Place mixture in refrigerator for 30 mins.

Scoop out 2–3 tbs of mixture and using your hands, shape into mini rissoles. Coat with rice crumbs and place on baking tray. Brush with coconut oil if using and bake in the oven for 30 mins, or until golden brown.

Serving and storing leftovers: Serve immediately. Store in the fridge for up to 3 days or freeze for up to 4 months.

TIP

Replace the rice crumbs with 1 cup almond meal or use 1/2 cup rice crumbs and 1/2 cup almond meal. For a crispier version, pan fry the rissoles instead of baking for 3-4 mins on each side.

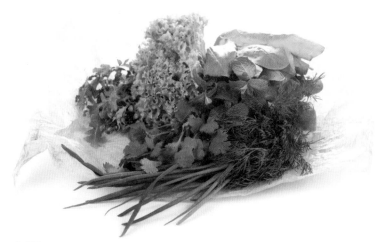

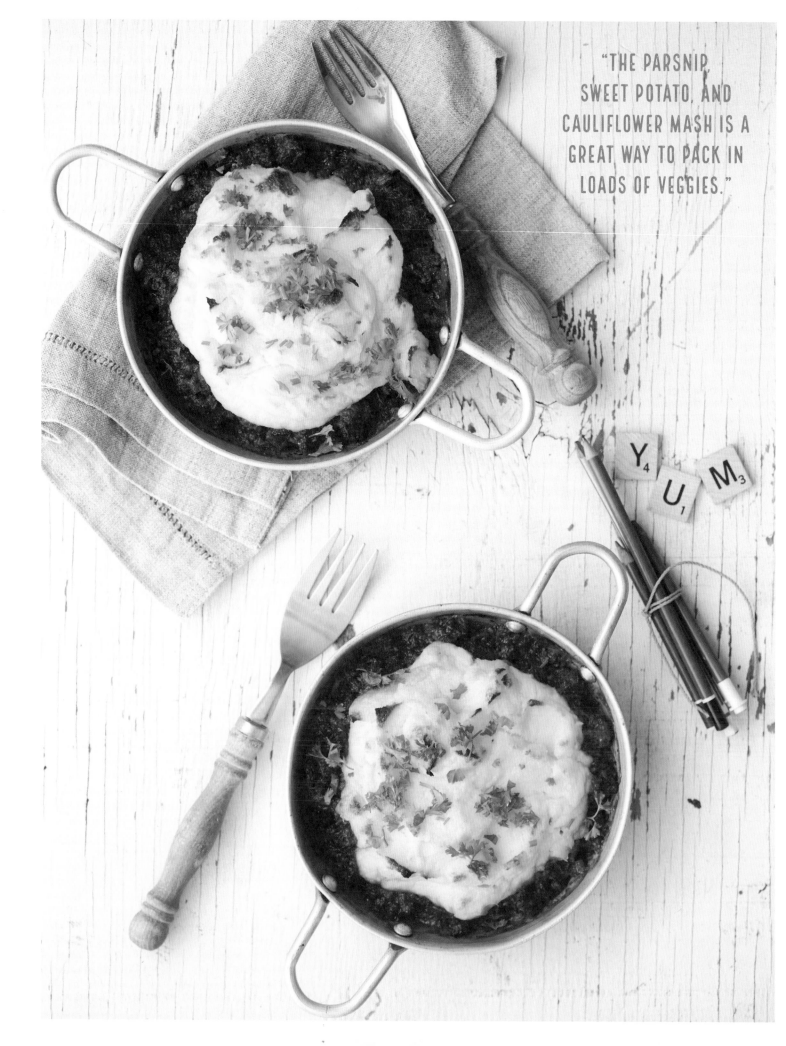

"THE PARSNIP, SWEET POTATO, AND CAULIFLOWER MASH IS A GREAT WAY TO PACK IN LOADS OF VEGGIES."

Gluten Free · Dairy Free · Egg Free · Nut Free

Prep time: 25 mins
Cooking time: 40 mins
Serves: 6

Shepherd's Pie

This versatile family meal is loaded with vegetables and freezes well, so it's a great one to keep on standby for busy days. If you have a small baby, remove a portion of the meat and mash and puree separately before adding the tamari and finishing the pie for the rest of the family to enjoy.

INGREDIENTS

FOR THE MASH:

3 cups (10½ oz) cauliflower florets

1 cup (5⅓ oz) potato or white sweet potato, peeled and chopped

½ cup (2⅞ oz) parsnip, peeled and chopped

1 tbs coconut oil or butter, melted

½ tbs arrowroot

pinch of sea salt

FOR THE MINCE:

1–2 tbs coconut oil or olive oil

½ yellow onion, chopped

1 leek, chopped

2 garlic cloves, crushed

1 medium-sized carrot, chopped

2 celery stalks, chopped

1 lb beef or lamb mince

½ tsp ground cumin

2 tbs mixed herbs

2 tbs tomato paste

1 tbs tamari

1 cup homemade beef broth, or low-sodium beef stock

EQUIPMENT

high-speed food processor

INSTRUCTIONS

Preheat oven to 355°F.

Fill a large pot with water and bring to a boil. Add cauliflower, sweet potato, and parsnip and cook vegetables for about 10–15 mins or until they are soft. Drain, rinse and allow to cool for a few minutes. Place all vegetables and coconut oil into a food processor and process until smooth. Add arrowroot powder and salt and process for another minute. Set aside.

Meanwhile, heat coconut oil in a large pan and cook onion, leek, garlic, carrot, and celery for 3 mins or until they are soft. Transfer into a measurement jar or bowl and blend with a stick blender until smooth. Set aside.

In the same pan, cook the mince for 5–10 mins, or until browned.

Add vegetable mix, cumin, herbs, tomato paste, tamari sauce, and beef stock and let simmer for another 10 mins.

Place the mince mixture into a large deep baking dish, then top with the cauliflower mash and bake uncovered for 20 mins. To brown on top, drizzle with olive oil (it won't brown on top as much as regular mash).

Serving and storing leftovers: Serve immediately, store in the fridge for up to 3 days or freeze for up to 4 months.

TIP

If your children don't mind texture, leave out the step where you blend the onion, leek, garlic, carrot and celery and simply add them to the browned beef.

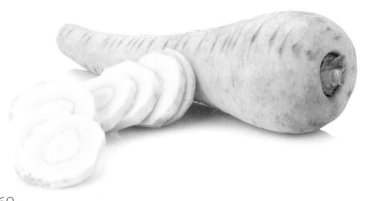

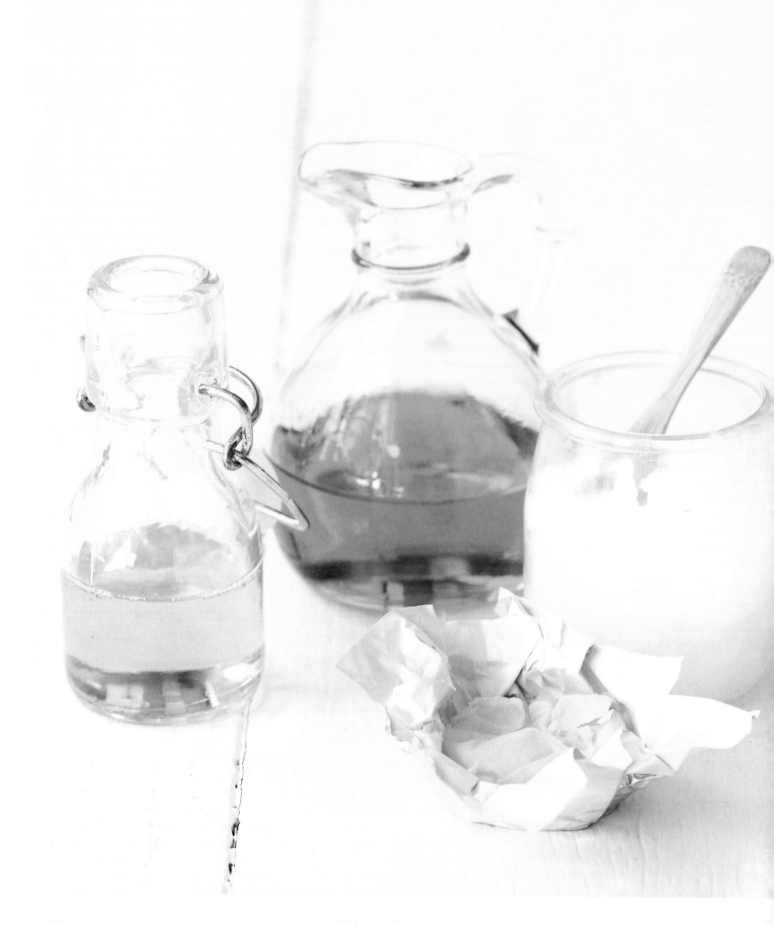

Healthy Fats

STEP 5

FOCUS ON GOOD FATS
AND AVOID PROCESSED
LOW-FAT FOODS

ich, creamy foods satisfy us in a way that other foods cannot. Maybe they remind us of the comforting breast milk or formula that we all began our food journey with; breast milk and infant formula supply 40–50 percent of a baby's energy as fat. Or maybe it's simply the fact that foods containing fats have a better texture and taste. Whatever the reason, these foods tend to be more flavorful and greatly contribute to our eating pleasure.

Despite this, for more than half a century we have thought of fat as the enemy and looked for ways to banish it from our diets wherever possible. It can be quite confusing for a first-time parent who has grown up believing that fat should be avoided to understand that children need healthy fats in their diets for their nerves, brain and skin cells, to protect vital organs in the body, and to help control body temperature. Fat supplies us with essential fatty acids that we can't manufacture ourselves and helps our body absorb vitamins A, D, E and K from food plus it affects the production of hormones and provides us with energy.

HOW HAVE THE FAT FACTS CHANGED?

When I was a teenager low-fat diets were all the rage. We were taught that fat was bad for our waistlines and our hearts. My mother, wanting the best for her kids, packed our pantry and fridge full of low-fat foods. I remember never feeling satisfied after eating and forever looking for something else to snack on, which makes sense when you consider that to compensate for the loss of flavor, manufacturers often end up adding sugar to low-fat products.

In my twenties, I started to incorporate healthy fats back into my diet and I have never looked back. My skin, hormones and overall health improved dramatically. So did my concentration levels. Now research is showing us that abstaining from fat is not a fast track to good health. In fact, while cutting out fats reduces calorie intake it removes the benefits of "good" fats, which are essential to a child's healthy physical development and may also impact cognitive function. From the age of five months, when I introduced solids, my children have been raised on a diet filled with nutritionally beneficial fats and I really believe it's helped them thrive!

Fats with proven health benefits include both monounsaturated and polyunsaturated fats. At the other end of the scale are unnatural trans fats—the actively bad fats that carry the same number of calories as healthier fats but have no nutritional value and are proven to cause disease. Somewhere between the two lies saturated fat, the fat that does raise cholesterol but not necessarily the kind that clogs arteries. There is ongoing debate about optimal fat intake and research is still continuing but it has been accepted that "good" fats are important for all of us, especially growing children who need the nutrients and calories they contain.

EATING HEALTHY FATS WILL:

- ✓ provide essential fatty acids, which have been linked to improved concentration, learning, behavior, and sleep in children.
- ✓ enhance the absorption of fat-soluble vitamins A, D, E and K from food.
- ✓ promote the healthy development of vital organs including brain, eyes, and skin.
- ✓ provide a healthy and satisfying source of calories.
- ✓ help regulate blood sugar.
- ✓ help regulate hormones.

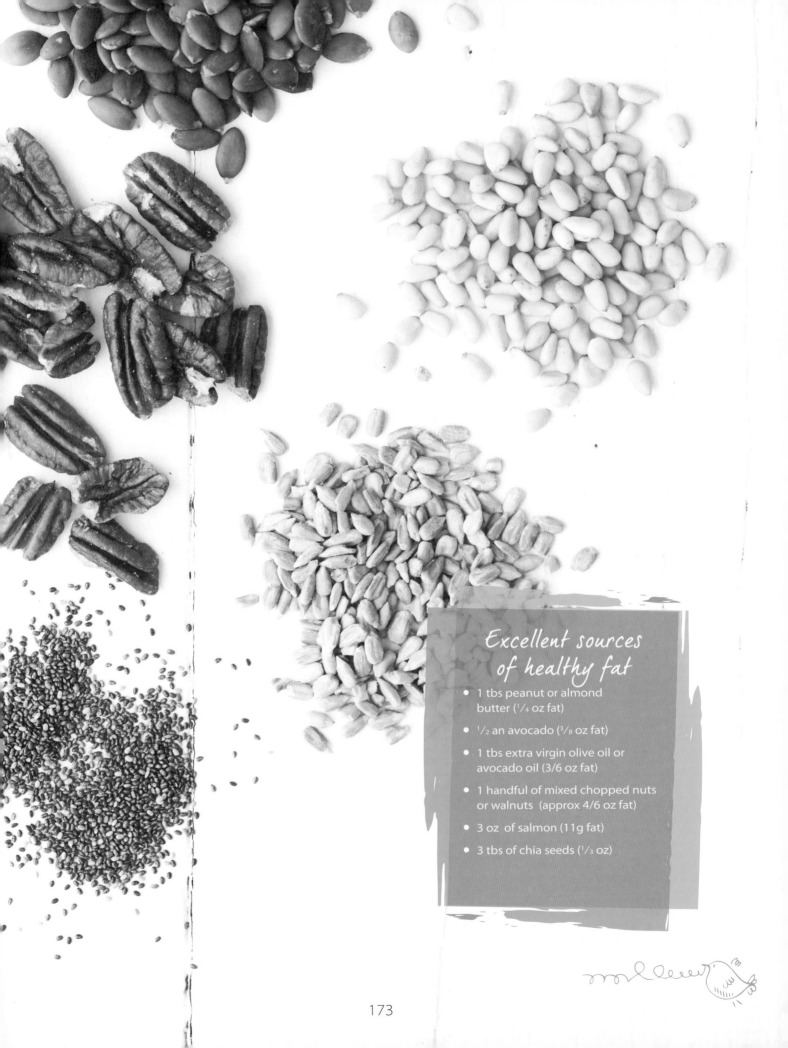

Excellent sources of healthy fat

- 1 tbs peanut or almond butter (¹/₄ oz fat)

- ½ an avocado (³/₈ oz fat)

- 1 tbs extra virgin olive oil or avocado oil (3/6 oz fat)

- 1 handful of mixed chopped nuts or walnuts (approx 4/6 oz fat)

- 3 oz of salmon (11g fat)

- 3 tbs of chia seeds (¹/₃ oz)

FATS: THE GOOD, THE BAD AND THE OKAY IN MODERATION

Not all fats are created equal. Some are beneficial, some are seriously harmful, and others are fine in moderate amounts.

GOOD FATS	BAD FATS	OKAY IN MODERATION FATS
WHAT: Monounsaturated fats	**WHAT:** Trans fats	**WHAT:** Saturated fat
WHY: These are the fats associated with the health benefits of the Mediterranean diet. Reduce bad cholesterol, lower risk of heart disease, normalize insulin levels and stabilize blood sugar levels.	**WHY:** They are the product of hydrogenating vegetable oils which makes them solid at room temperature and prevents them from spoiling. They're universally accepted to be harmful, increasing the danger of heart disease by increasing the amount of harmful LDL cholesterol and decreasing beneficial HDL cholesterol, increasing insulin resistance, type 2 diabetes, and stroke. There's really no debate: Trans fats do not belong in our children's bodies.	**WHY:** There has been a lot of controversy about the role of saturated fat and heart disease. In the 2015–2020 Dietary Guidelines for Americans: One of the key recommendations is to "consume less than 10 percent of calories per day from saturated fats." However, there are also recent findings suggesting that there is no clear evidence that directly links saturated fat to heart disease. In the case of children, saturated fat—when eaten in moderation and obtained from wholefood sources such as grass-fed beef, coconut oil and high quality dairy products—can prove to be a beneficial part of a balanced diet and ensure proper brain health, nerve function, and cell membrane health. Growing children need it as part of a well-balanced diet to help them feel satiated.
BEST SOURCES: Avocado, extra virgin cold-pressed avocado oil, olives, extra virgin cold-pressed olive oil, macadamia nuts, extra virgin cold-pressed macadamia oil.	**SOURCES:** Processed foods, especially baked goods, pastries, shortening, French fries and store-bought cookies. Anything deep-fried, some margarines, vegetable shortening, and snack foods like French fries. A very small amount of trans fats can occur naturally in meat and dairy products too.	**SOURCES:** Coconut oil, pasture-fed beef, lamb, organic chicken, turkey and eggs, whole dairy products. Feeding your children saturated fats from these sources as opposed to grain-fed beef or processed sausages will make a key difference.
WHAT: Omega-3 (polyunsaturated fat)		
WHY: Omega-3s are known as essential fatty acids because they are essential to vital biological processes in the body. We are not able to manufacture them ourselves so we must include them in our diet to reduce bad cholesterol, decrease the risk of heart disease, stroke and type 2 diabetes. Deficiency can cause dry skin, eczema, lethargy, weakened immune system, hormonal imbalances and depression. A lack of these fats can also impact performance on reading tests and working memory and may add to symptoms of attention-deficit/hyperactivity disorder (ADHD) in children. A diet rich in these protective fats may also help to prevent heart disease, arrhythmias, stroke, and reduce blood pressure.		
BEST SOURCES Oily fish such as salmon, trout, sardines and mackerel, flaxseeds, chia seeds, walnuts, egg yolks, and dark green leafy vegetables. Ensuring your meat is grass fed and grass finished (i.e., not grain fed just prior to being slaughtered) will help too.		
WHAT: Omega-6 (polyunsaturated fat)		
WHY: As with omega-3s, our bodies are unable to make this essential fatty acid and consuming it in the right quantity can help to protect against heart disease, eczema, ADHD, and certain allergies.		
BEST SOURCES: Meat, poultry, eggs, sesame seeds, walnuts, pumpkin seeds, linseed, green leafy vegetables, borage and evening primrose oils.		

SO HOW MUCH FAT SHOULD MY CHILD BE EATING?

Ages 1–3: It's recommended that fats contribute toward 30–40 percent of young children's total calorie intake. Fat provides 9 calories per gram. Therefore, a toddler who consumes 1000 calories would require 1 1/6 oz to 1 4/6 oz of fat each day. It is recommended that toddlers consume 700 milligrams of omega-3s each day, some of which can be achieved from eating foods such as oily fish or a handful of chopped walnuts. If you're struggling to get your child to eat omega-3 rich foods, ask your pediatrician, nutritionist, or GP about purified omega-3 oils for children.

Age 4+: Fats should contribute 25–35 percent of their total calories. Depending on the level of activity and gender, children aged four to eight need 1200 to 2000 calories and kids aged nine to thirteen require 1600 to 3200 calories. Based on these calorie guidelines, children aged four to eight need 1 1/6 oz to 2 4/5 oz grams of fat daily and kids aged between nine and thirteen need 45g (25 percent) to 125g (35 percent) fat daily. Individualized fat requirements for your child vary by age, gender, and specific calorie needs. It is recommended that children over four consume 900 milligrams of omega-3s each day. Children ages nine to thirteen should consume 1000 mg for girls and 1200 mg for boys each day.

BUT WON'T FAT MAKE MY CHILD FAT?

Healthy children will not gain weight if they eat fat from the correct sources. During the 1990s when low-fat diets were all the rage, many parents, following on from their own diets, offered their kids foods like low-fat cottage cheese, 99% fat-free yogurt, and used spray oils in canisters to further limit their intake of fats. Fuelled by an increasing fear of overweight and obese children, and told that limiting fats could prevent heart disease, parents understandably came to believe that restricting dietary fats could keep children from becoming fat. However, a child's energy demands are much higher than an adult's, so low-fat diets do not provide an adequate supply of nutrients and can even disrupt a child's normal rate of growth and development.

FAT, SATIETY, AND METABOLISM

In contrast to low-fat foods, whole foods leave children more satiated, reducing cravings for bigger portion sizes and unhealthy snacks.

Although fat has more calories per gram than carbohydrates or protein, eating the right type of fat can cause your body to burn more energy and, importantly, can signal to your child when they are full, as fat causes satiety.

In my practice, I see a lot of children on carb-intense diets. Multiple crackers, especially rice cakes or corn cakes, are a staple part of their snack routine. If you add a layer of fat to crackers in the form of almond butter, coconut oil, avocado, mashed eggs or unsalted butter, a child will tend to feel more satisfied.

Often I see kids who complain to their parents that they are hungry just thirty minutes after a meal and this can often be solved by increasing the good fats offered at mealtimes. For example, if a child is eating porridge with honey and milk, adding a tsp of unsalted butter or crushed almonds, chia seeds or flaxseeds will help them to feel satiated for longer. Vegetables, too, need fat to ensure their fat-soluble vitamins and minerals are absorbed, so go ahead and add a drizzle of extra virgin olive oil or unsalted butter.

DO YOU NEED TO WATCH YOUR CHILD'S CHOLESTEROL?

In infancy, cholesterol is one of the most important fats as it has a huge part to play in the development of cognitive health as well as proper hormone and sexual function and development. Good cholesterol or high-density lipoprotein (HDL) works to lower bad cholesterol or low-density lipoprotein (LDL). Foods such as olive oil, flaxseeds, chia seeds, chopped nuts, fiber and legumes can all help to lower LDL. Even from a young age, it's important to focus on sources that help to raise good cholesterol.

OMEGA-6 VS OMEGA-3: WHAT'S THE DIFFERENCE?

Both are beneficial, but if there is too much omega-6 in a child's diet and not enough omega-3, it can increase the risk of inflammation and disease. An ideal ratio is between 2:1 or 4:1—two to four times as much omega-6 as omega-3. The average Western diet has a ratio of 20:1. To correct the balance, try to focus on avoiding processed foods containing vegetable oils and

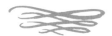

DID YOU KNOW?

Breast milk is 40%–50% saturated fat and cholesterol—nature knows best when it comes to what infants need to grow and develop.

Consider this...

Some studies have shown that people who ate high-fat diets had a faster metabolism. Low-fat, high-carb diets, on the other hand, spiked insulin, subsequently slowing metabolism and storing belly fat.

Five Ways to Reduce Trans Fats

1. Choose healthier cooking methods such as baking, steaming, sautéing, and grilling over deep-frying.

2. Cut back on processed and commercial foods such as cookies, pastries, doughnuts, and cakes.

3. When buying potato chips, choose those containing 100% high oleic sunflower oil.

4. When eating out, choose dishes that are not deep-fried. Choose grilled or pan-fried fish over deep-fried battered fish.

5. Read labels and choose products that do not contain trans fats.

THE IMPORTANCE OF AVOCADOS

Nutrient-dense and delicious, avocados contain mostly monounsaturated and some polyunsaturated fats, and are sodium-free. Most babies, when they are weaned, enjoy avocado straight up. It's an easy on-the-go meal—just peel, mush and serve. Many parents, however, lament that while their kids loved it as babies, they won't touch avocado now that they are toddlers or older. Here are my fave go-to ways to get your kids to eat their avos:

1. Throw half an avocado in a smoothie—it adds a creamy, rich texture and leaves your child feeling fuller for longer (see our Omega-3 Smoothie on page 197).

2. Add it to a homemade chocolate mousse.

3. Use it in a frosting (see our recipe for Chocolate Avo Frosting on page 93).

4. Serve it with a sprinkle of sea salt, apple cider or balsamic vinegar, and olive oil.

5. Spread avocado on toast and cover with a slice of cheese or add a sprinkling of sea salt and pepper.

6. Use avocado oil in cooking.

upping omega-3-rich foods. This will help you manage your child's overall intake of omega-6s and avoid it in its worst most processed forms. It's best to ensure your child gets their omega-6s from fresh chopped nuts and seeds, green leafy vegetables, and eggs.

Media attention has been focused on the health benefits of omega-3s recently, especially DHA and EPA, which are most easily obtained from oily fish such as trout, salmon, mackerel, sardines, and herring. Vegetarians can rely on non-animal sources such as flaxseeds, walnuts and, in smaller amounts, green leafy vegetables that contain ALA (alpha linolenic acid) that the body can convert into DHA and EPA. Unfortunately, however, the conversion process is not as stable or reliable as eating food that contains DHA and EPA directly.

Lots of the kids I see in my practice who do not like oily fish show signs of fatty acid deficiency such as eczema or an inability to concentrate. It's important to take every opportunity to include these types of fats in our children's diets through eating fish, walnuts, and linseeds. If your child is not eating low mercury oily fish 2–3 times a week then it may be appropriate to supplement their diet with a pure omega-3 supplement.

WHAT'S THE PROBLEM WITH VEGETABLE OILS?

In the past we were told that vegetable oils, which are made up of long-chain polyunsaturated fats, were healthy. And while they may contain omega-6s which are beneficial in moderation, we now know that many vegetable oils are extracted through processing methods that involve heating, highly toxic solvents, and various industrial chemicals.

The polyunsaturated fats in vegetable oils tend to react with oxygen and turn rancid fairly quickly. To prevent the fats from degenerating, they are often heat treated or hydrogenated (a process that causes vegetable oils to turn solid at room temperature). Unfortunately, these processes turn them into harmful trans fats. If you need to use vegetable oils for cooking, look for organic cold-pressed options wherever possible (as this avoids the dangers of heat-damaged vegetable oils) and use in moderation.

IS COCONUT OIL A BETTER CHOICE?

Coconut oil has more saturated fat than butter, yet studies show it is one of the most stable oils at high heat (more on this below), it is satiating and when used in moderation, has numerous health benefits for children.

Natural and unprocessed, coconut oil is one of the richest sources of Lauric acid, a healthy medium chain-triglyceride (MCT) found in breast milk. When Lauric acid is digested, it forms a substance called Monolaurin. Both Lauric acid and Monolaurin can help kill harmful pathogens like bacteria, viruses, and fungi. Coconut oil also contains Capric and Caprylic acid—more beneficial saturated fats, with antibacterial properties.

COOKING WITH OILS

When vegetable oils are used at high heats, they begin to smoke and the fumes can contain dangerous carcinogenic compounds which may contribute to cancer. In order to minimize your child's exposure to these harmful and carcinogenic compounds, it is essential to cook only with fats that are stable in high heat (see chart on next page).

THE PROPERTIES OF COOKING OILS THAT MATTER MOST

1. **Smoke point:** The temperature at which the fats begin to break down and turn into smoke.

2. **Oxidative stability:** How resistant the fats are to reacting with oxygen.

TOP TIPS FOR COOKING WITH OILS

- Never reuse oil.

- Never overheat oil. Yellow onions, for example, slowly on medium heat and cook for longer.

- Do not put anything wet into hot oil as it can splatter, which is especially dangerous if children are nearby.

- Always turn handles away from the edge of the stove to avoid a child pulling a pan off the stove.

- If you or your child get a burn, run it under cold water rather than applying ice and seek medical attention.

- Ensure when a hot pan with oil is removed from the stove top to cool down, it's out of reach of children.

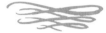

DID YOU KNOW?

With every 2% of calories from trans fat consumed daily, the risk of heart disease rises by 23%.

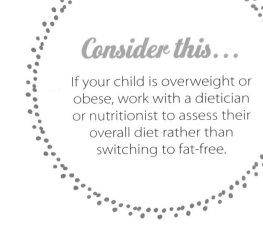

Consider this…

If your child is overweight or obese, work with a dietician or nutritionist to assess their overall diet rather than switching to fat-free.

Healthy Fats

OLIVE OIL	COCONUT OIL	MACADAMIA NUT OIL	GHEE/CLARIFIED BUTTER

What is it?
Derived from the first pressing of the olives, cold-pressed extra virgin olive oil contains the most bioactive substances, including powerful antioxidants and vitamin E. As olive oil becomes more refined it loses some of its antioxidants and vitamins.

PROS
Cold-pressed extra virgin olive oil is rich in monounsaturated fats which are stable, making it a healthier choice for most cooking methods than vegetable oils, which are high in polyunsaturated fat and not stable at higher heat points.

CONS
There has been a lot of concern about cooking with cold-pressed extra virgin olive oil due to its moderate heat threshold. More refined versions of this oil tend to be more heat stable but then they do not have all the health benefits. A better bet is to choose cold-pressed extra virgin olive oil and keep temperatures medium to low on a stovetop or in an oven and cook for longer.

What is it?
Extracted from coconut flesh, it's semi-hard at room temperature and is not prone to oxidization. Virgin coconut oil is the best option, as it has not undergone any processing.

PROS
High in lauric acid. Medium heat threshold. It can add a nutty flavor to foods and bring out the sweetness in baked goods.

CONS
Some people don't like the flavor in savory foods. Refined coconut oil will often have a stronger flavor and virgin coconut oils vary in flavor. There are many different versions on the market so shop around until you find one that has a flavor that your family can enjoy.

What is it?
Made from macadamia nuts. Always choose cold-pressed extra virgin macadamia oil.

PROS
High in monounsaturated fat and low in omega-6. Medium to high smoke point.

CONS
Not school-friendly due to potential allergies. May not work with all dishes as it has a subtle nutty flavor.

What is it?
Made from gently melted and separated butter.

PROS
High in conjugated linolenic acid (CLA) and rich in antioxidants with a high smoke point.

CONS
Cannot be used in dairy-free cooking and baking. It can take time getting used to the rich flavor.

How to use it
GOOD FOR
Sautéing, light frying, sauces, braising, stewing, baking at lower heats, finishing dishes. Do not use for deep frying.

SMOKE POINT
Extra Virgin is 160°C/320°F, Virgin is 216°C/420°F, Pomace is 238°C/460°F, Extra light is 242°C/468°F (Medium to high heat).

How to use it
Stir-frying, pan-frying, grilling, braising, in raw treats, as a spread, or in baking.

SMOKE POINT
177°C/350°F (Medium heat).

How to use it
Sautéing, grilling, light frying, baking, sauces.

SMOKE POINT
210°C/413°F (Medium to high heat).

How to use it
Frying at high heats, baking, and in sauces.

SMOKE POINT
252°C /485°F (Medium heat).

Wholesome Child's favorite fats and oils

LARD	SESAME SEED OIL	BUTTER	AVOCADO OIL	FLAXSEED OIL
What is it? Rendered animal fat, usually from pigs.	**What is it?** Derived from sesame seeds, it provides a rich, nutty flavor. Often used in Asian dishes.	**What is it?** Churned milk.	**What is it?** Pressed from avocado.	**What is it?** Pressed from flax seeds, sometimes with chemical assistance. Best choice is organic cold-pressed flaxseed oil.
PROS Gives a crispy finish to fried vegetables and makes a crumbly pastry.	**PROS** Cold-pressed sesame oil contains high levels of natural antioxidants and vitamin E, and is rich in both polyunaturated fat and monounsaturated fat. It is also loaded with B-complex vitamins, including thiamin, riboflavin, niacin, pantothenic acid, pyridoxine, and folic acid.	**PROS** Not only a delicious flavor, grass-fed butter contains vitamin D, high levels of easy-to-absorb vitamin A and lecithin necessary for cholesterol metabolism.	**PROS** It has a high smoke point and is high in monounsaturated fats, vitamin E, and antioxidants. It may also have anti-inflammatory benefits.	**PROS** Contains both omega-3 and omega-6 fatty acids, the essential fatty acid alpha-linolenic acid (ALA), which the body converts into eicosapentaenoic acid (EPA), and docosahexaenoic acid (DHA). Can be a beneficial source of omega-3s for children who do not eat fish.
CONS High in saturated fat and may also be high in polyunsaturated fat depending on the diet of the animal. Unsuitable for vegetarians.	**CONS** Because it has high omega-6 levels, I would recommend consuming in very small amounts. If your child has an allergy to sesame seeds, do not use this oil, as it may cause an allergic reaction.	**CONS** Only a moderately high smoke point. Can be high in sodium so always choose unsalted.	**CONS** Avocado oil is very thick, so avoid using on salads if you prefer a light oil. May give some fried foods a yellow tinge and can have a noticeable odour.	**CONS** Not suitable for cooking.
How to use it Frying, as a spread, or for greasing cookware. Use sparingly.	**How to use it** Stir-frying, grilling, sauteeing, marinades, dressings.	**How to use it** Yellow onions or leeks with it, make omelettes, use in baking and sauces or as a spread.	**How to use it** Choose cold-pressed unrefined avocado oil to keep all the benefits and use to fry meats and vegetables, sauté spinach or add to sauces.	**How to use it** Use cold in salad dressings or add to smoothies.
SMOKE POINT 182°C/370°F (Medium heat).	**SMOKE POINT** 210°C/410°F (Medium to high heat).	**SMOKE POINT** 150°C/302°F (Medium heat).	**DO NOT USE FOR** Deep frying. **SMOKE POINT** 270°C/520°F (High heat).	**SMOKE POINT** N/A—Cold use only.

Wholesome Child

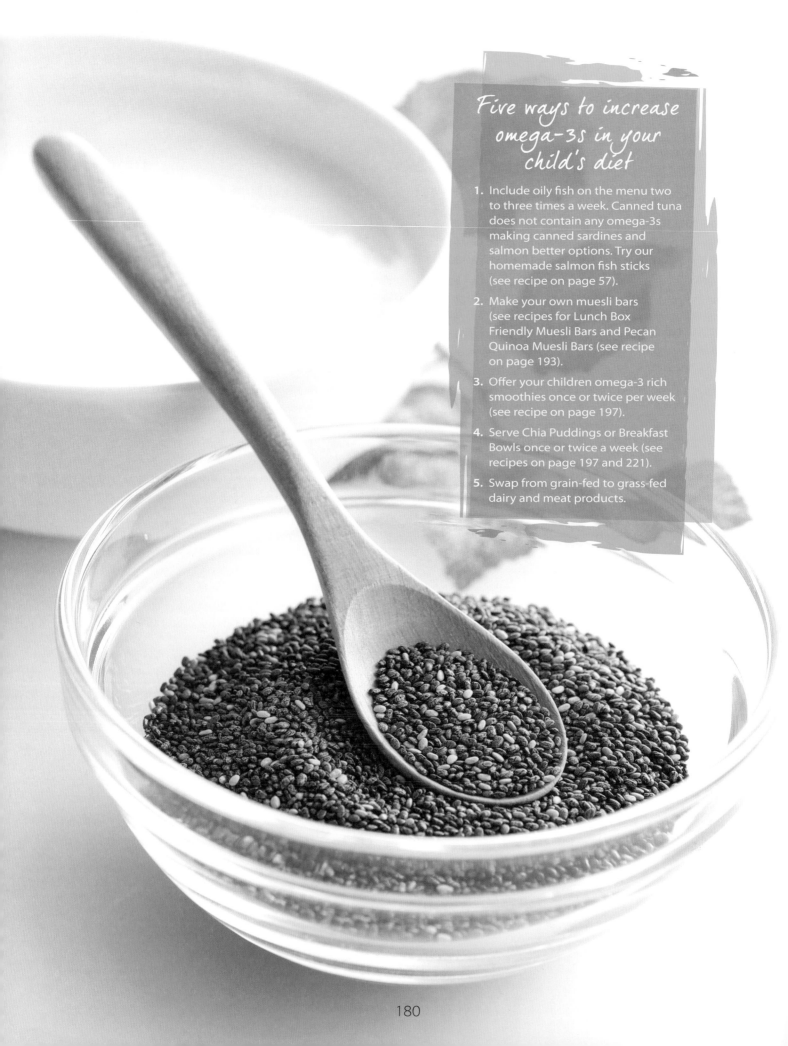

Five ways to increase omega-3s in your child's diet

1. Include oily fish on the menu two to three times a week. Canned tuna does not contain any omega-3s making canned sardines and salmon better options. Try our homemade salmon fish sticks (see recipe on page 57).

2. Make your own muesli bars (see recipes for Lunch Box Friendly Muesli Bars and Pecan Quinoa Muesli Bars (see recipe on page 193).

3. Offer your children omega-3 rich smoothies once or twice per week (see recipe on page 197).

4. Serve Chia Puddings or Breakfast Bowls once or twice a week (see recipes on page 197 and 221).

5. Swap from grain-fed to grass-fed dairy and meat products.

GOAL 5: LEARN HOW TO SPEAK TO YOUR CHILD ABOUT FOOD

Children learn attitudes to food and their bodies from their parents and caregivers every day, so it goes without saying that passing on a fear of gaining weight can negatively impact a child's body image and their relationship with food.

The most important thing I learned when I helped develop MEND, a program to empower overweight and obese children and their parents, is that improving a family's health takes more than simply swapping out junk food for healthier options and enrolling in extra physical activities. It also involves changing ingrained unhealthy behaviors and attitudes towards foods for healthier ones.

Often families struggle to adopt long-lasting healthy lifestyle behaviors because of the underlying issues that cause them to overeat or rely on comfort foods in the first place. It's very difficult to expect a child to switch to healthy food if they are mimicking a parent's unhealthy food behaviors and attitudes, or if they are relying on food as a way to combat boredom, depression, anxiety or other negative feelings. Depression and low self-esteem can also be the root cause of overeating and dislike of physical activity in children. Children are impressionable and this can in turn cause them to reject their own bodies.

One of the things my brother remembers affecting him most negatively when he was a child was being told by our parents or his teachers that he had to lose weight. Instead of inspiring him, this threw him into a spiral of self-disgust and depression which caused him to eat more. My younger brother, who played competitive tennis, was super-fit so while he was drinking sports drinks and going for ice cream after a match, my older brother was not allowed to eat these things. Of course he felt like he was being punished as a result of being overweight. This led to him eating in secret.

The ethos behind the MEND program, which I helped my brother to develop, was that we treat the whole family, not just the child. MEND (which was recently adopted by the YMCA across the US) has been so successful because it enables children to feel safe and secure through building up their self-esteem. The word diet is never used. Rather it focuses on how eating healthy foods will help them run faster and work harder.

On the flip side, after obesity and asthma, eating disorders like anorexia nervosa and bulimia are the third most common chronic illness in young people. Often children as young as six have already developed an active dislike for the overweight body shape and research indicates that 50 percent of teenagers begin dieting before the age of fifteen, whether they need to or not.

Potential warning signs of an eating disorder include noticing your child begin cutting their food into small pieces (after they have reached an age where this is no longer necessary), cutting out food they usually enjoy, avoiding family meals, making excuses for missing meals, or suddenly having an increased interest in food preparation.

A CLINICAL PSYCHOLOGIST'S PERSPECTIVE

I recently reconnected with a childhood friend, Romy Kunitz, who is a clinical and developmental psychologist. I love what she has to say about the relationship between a parent's self esteem and attitude toward food, and their child's attitude toward food and how they perceive their own body.

She shared three insightful tips:

1 "Don't talk about your own weight. From my clinical experience, I have seen children as young as nine experience much anxiety around gaining weight. A nine-year-old that was seeing me for play therapy commented that she worried that she would 'become fat' and was considering restricting her food intake. This appeared to emanate from overhearing her mother telling a friend that she had started a strict diet to 'get rid of her big bottom'. Research has revealed that the children of parents who place an emphasis on food intake and weight gain and of mothers who diet regularly are far more susceptible to developing an eating disorder."

Consider this...

According to the American Association of Pediatrics, three parenting practices have been shown to be associated with excess weight gain: feeding in response to emotional distress, using food as a reward, and excessive prompting to eat.

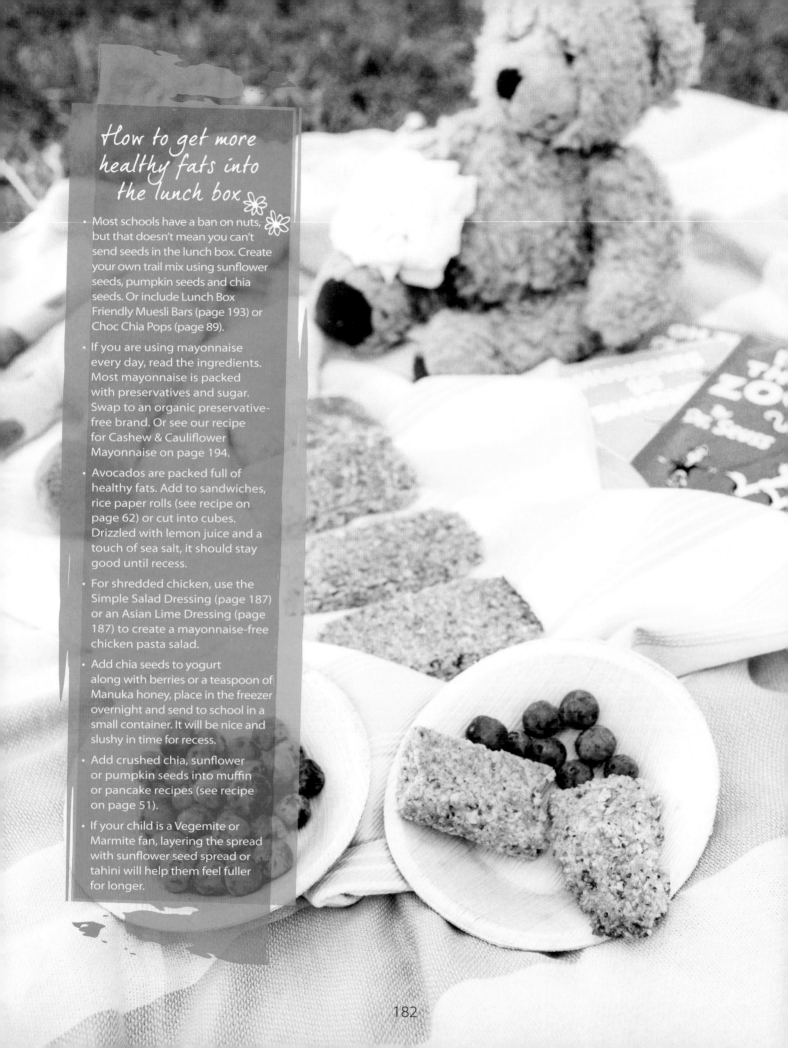

How to get more healthy fats into the lunch box ✿

- Most schools have a ban on nuts, but that doesn't mean you can't send seeds in the lunch box. Create your own trail mix using sunflower seeds, pumpkin seeds and chia seeds. Or include Lunch Box Friendly Muesli Bars (page 193) or Choc Chia Pops (page 89).

- If you are using mayonnaise every day, read the ingredients. Most mayonnaise is packed with preservatives and sugar. Swap to an organic preservative-free brand. Or see our recipe for Cashew & Cauliflower Mayonnaise on page 194.

- Avocados are packed full of healthy fats. Add to sandwiches, rice paper rolls (see recipe on page 62) or cut into cubes. Drizzled with lemon juice and a touch of sea salt, it should stay good until recess.

- For shredded chicken, use the Simple Salad Dressing (page 187) or an Asian Lime Dressing (page 187) to create a mayonnaise-free chicken pasta salad.

- Add chia seeds to yogurt along with berries or a teaspoon of Manuka honey, place in the freezer overnight and send to school in a small container. It will be nice and slushy in time for recess.

- Add crushed chia, sunflower or pumpkin seeds into muffin or pancake recipes (see recipe on page 51).

- If your child is a Vegemite or Marmite fan, layering the spread with sunflower seed spread or tahini will help them feel fuller for longer.

❷ "If your child has a sore stomach and refuses their meal, instead of talking about the food, talk about their feelings. A lot of the time children express their feelings through food and parents, caregivers and teachers need to be sensitive to how they deal with this. A sore tummy is most often where a child's feelings are expressed. When this happens and it seems clear to you that the tummy ache isn't due to constipation/diarrhea or something he has eaten, attempt to talk about what the sore tummy looks like or feels like. Ask your child to draw what he is feeling, for example, and then make the association for him that maybe he is feeling angry, sad or anxious. Also, read books about feelings at bedtime."

❸ "As parent, you can help children to avoid comforting themselves with food. An example from my clinical practice is one child who experienced an awful day at school where he had been bullied. That night, he asked his mother for ice cream. Mom didn't think anything of it, but the child wanted more and more ice cream and mom began to get angry.

However, she was sensitive enough to think about what could really be going on. At bedtime, she lay in bed with him and spoke about the day's events, and he told her about the struggles he'd had at school. She was able to make the link for him about his difficult day and his need to fill the gap with something sweet, like the ice cream, to make him feel better inside. She spoke about how normal that is, but also explained that the ice cream doesn't take his bad feelings away. She continued the next day to get him to open up about his feelings, resisting his requests to give him ice cream as an alternative. This approach obviously requires a lot of patience. You need to listen and help your child understand what he is feeling, rather than simply refusing the food or allowing it, even though it's hard when your child is distressed."

DID YOU KNOW?

An Australian study found evidence of body dissatisfaction in 70% of adolescent girls.

Consider this...

Your fat choices can harm the environment as well as your health, so it's best to avoid palm oil from non-sustainable sources; choose coconut oil instead.

How to encourage healthy eating behaviors

👍 DO...	👎 DON'T...
speak about healthy and unhealthy attributes of food. For example, fish will make your skin glow, carrots can ensure good eyesight, and doughnuts may upset your tummy. For older kids you can explain this in more detail.	speak negatively about food in terms of high and low calories.
speak about your body in terms of strength.	speak negatively about your own weight or body dissatisfaction in front of children.
help children to learn productive ways to deal with unpleasant emotions when they arise.	let your child eat out of boredom or when they're thirsty (thirst often presents as hunger).
teach children to identify when they are hungry and when they are full.	keep keep junk food in the house and prohibit it for one child only.
remove unwanted triggers—like junk food—from the pantry.	teach your child to eat when unpleasant emotions arise.
constantly praise your child for making healthy choices.	make your child feel guilty for their food choices.

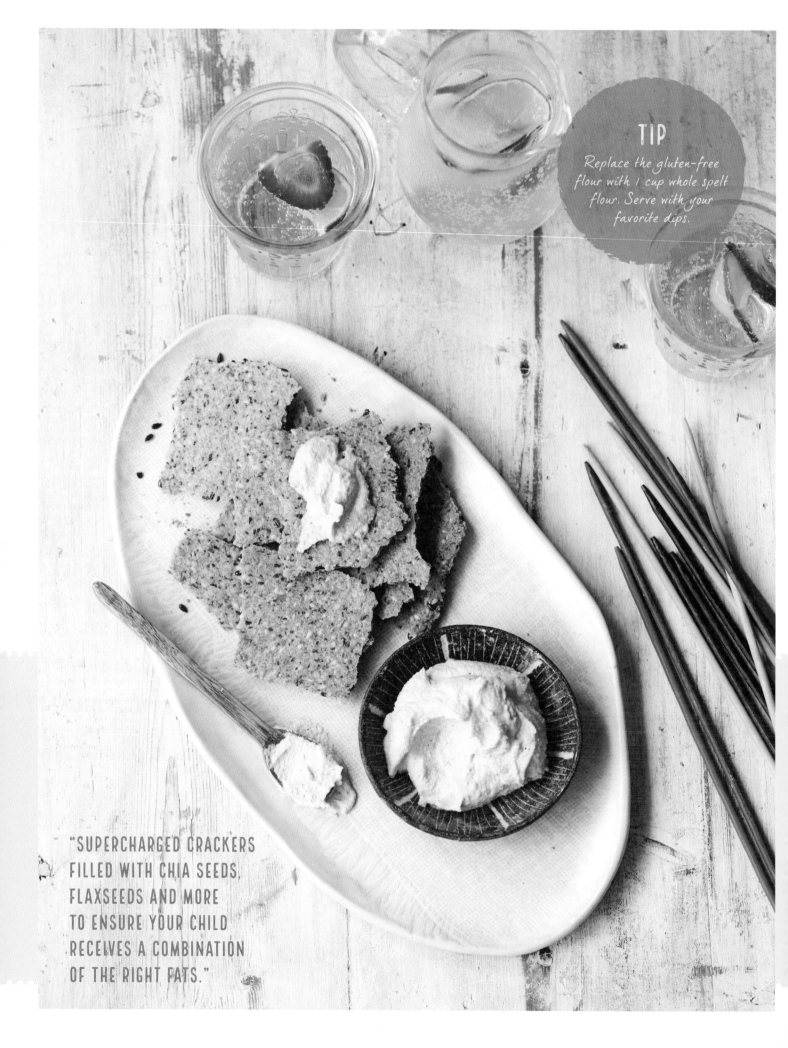

TIP

Replace the gluten-free flour with 1 cup whole spelt flour. Serve with your favorite dips.

"SUPERCHARGED CRACKERS FILLED WITH CHIA SEEDS, FLAXSEEDS AND MORE TO ENSURE YOUR CHILD RECEIVES A COMBINATION OF THE RIGHT FATS."

Vegan · Gluten Free · Nut Free

Prep time: 10 mins
Cooking time: 20 mins
Makes: 50 crackers

Flaxseed Crackers

My all-time favorite crackers; they fill the gap between meals and combine so well with hummus or vegan cashew cheese. There are many variations to choose from. Combine with your child's favorite dip and send to school in the lunch box.

INGREDIENTS

¼ cup (1⁴/₅ oz) flaxseeds

¼ cup (1²/₅ oz) pumpkin seeds

¼ cup (1²/₅ oz) sunflower seeds

¼ cup (1³/₄ oz) chia seeds

¼ cup (1²/₅ oz) sesame seeds

½–1 tsp sea salt

1 cup (4³/₅ oz) Wholesome Child gluten-free flour mix

½ cup filtered water

¼ cup extra virgin olive oil

EQUIPMENT

high-speed food processor

INSTRUCTIONS

Preheat oven to 325°F.

Place all seeds into a food processor and pulse until smooth. If you don't want them to become meal consistency then just give them a few pulses.

Add remaining ingredients and process until just combined.

Place in between two sheets of baking paper and roll to 4/32" to 6/32" thick. Remove top sheet of baking paper and transfer to baking tray. Bake for 20 mins or until golden and crisp.

Allow to cool on a wire rack then break into pieces to serve.

Serving and storing leftovers: Serve immediately or store in an airtight container for up to 14 days.

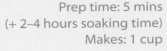

Vegan · Gluten Free

Prep time: 5 mins
(+ 2–4 hours soaking time)
Makes: 1 cup

Vegan Cashew Cheese

INGREDIENTS

1 cup (5 2/3 oz) cashews

2¼ cups filtered water

2 tbs nutritional yeast

1–2 tbs lemon juice

1 garlic clove

1 tbs Dijon mustard

1 tbs fresh dill, roughly chopped

sea salt and pepper, to taste

EQUIPMENT

blender

INSTRUCTIONS

Place the cashew nuts in a small bowl, cover with 2 cups of water, and allow to soak for 2–4 hours. Rinse and drain.

Place soaked cashews, ¼ cup of water, nutritional yeast, lemon juice, garlic, mustard, dill, salt and pepper into a blender and blend until smooth and creamy.

Transfer cashew cheese to a glass jar and keep in the fridge.

Serving and storing leftovers: Serve immediately or store in the fridge for up to 5–7 days.

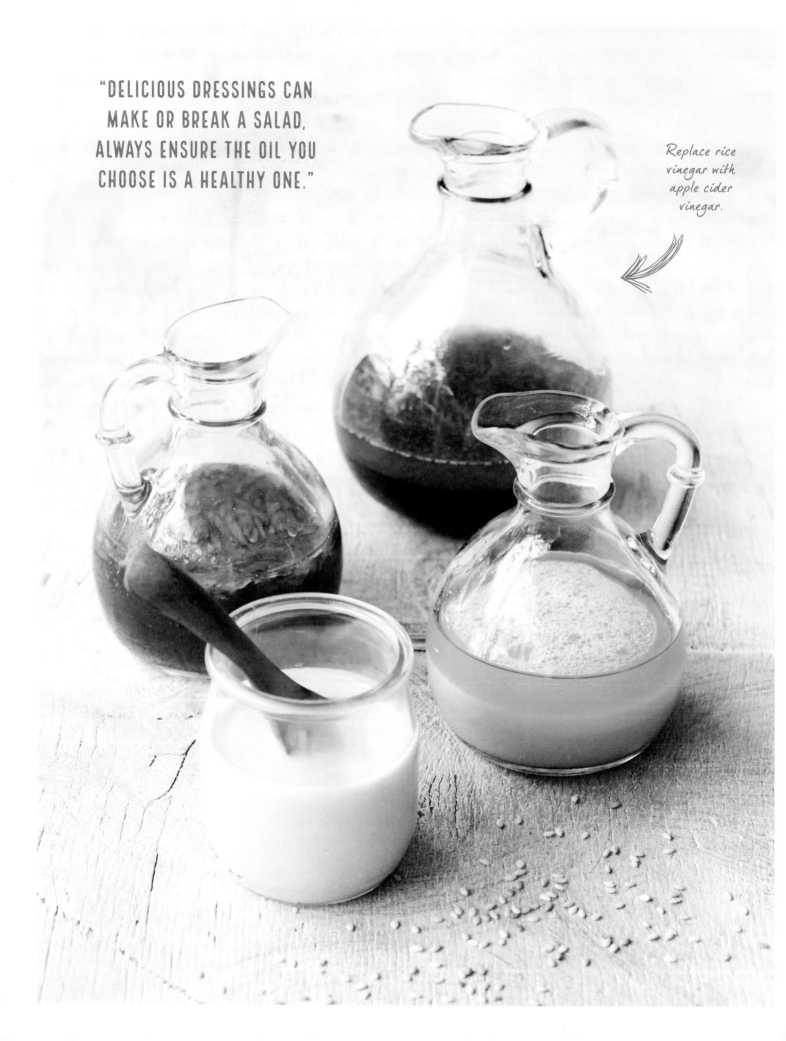

"DELICIOUS DRESSINGS CAN MAKE OR BREAK A SALAD, ALWAYS ENSURE THE OIL YOU CHOOSE IS A HEALTHY ONE."

Replace rice vinegar with apple cider vinegar.

Vegan · Gluten Free · Nut Free

Prep time: 5 mins
Serves: 12

Asian Lime Dressing

INGREDIENTS

2 tbs rice vinegar

1 tbs tamari

juice and zest of 1 lime

1 clove garlic, crushed

1 tbs coconut sugar

1 tbs cold pressed sesame oil

1 tbs fresh cilantro, finely chopped

1 tbs fresh mint, chopped

½ cup filtered water

INSTRUCTIONS

Combine all ingredients in a small jar, put lid on top and shake vigorously.

Pour over salad of choice.

Serving and storing leftovers: Serve immediately or store in an airtight container in the fridge for up to 2 weeks.

Vegan · Nut Free · Gluten Free

Prep time: 5 mins
Serves: 12

Simple Salad Dressing

INGREDIENTS

¼ cup apple cider vinegar

1 tbs Dijon mustard

1 garlic clove, crushed

1–2 tsp maple syrup or raw honey

¼ cup extra virgin olive oil

¼ cup filtered water

INSTRUCTIONS

Combine all ingredients in a small jar, put lid on top and shake vigorously.

Pour over salad.

Serving and storing leftovers: Serve immediately or store in a jar in the fridge for up to 2 weeks.

> **TIP**
> Add finely chopped fresh herbs if your kids like them. Replace the apple cider vinegar with balsamic vinegar if the flavor is too strong.

Vegan · Nut Free · Gluten Free

Prep time: 5 mins
Serves: 16

Miso & Tahini Dressing

INGREDIENTS

¼ cup (2⅓ oz) white miso paste

1–2 tbs maple syrup or raw honey

⅓ cup (3⅕ oz) tahini

2 tbs cold-pressed organic sesame oil 1 tbs lemon juice

½ cup filtered water

¼ tsp fresh ginger, grated (optional)

INSTRUCTIONS

Blend all ingredients in a bowl. Add more water if too thick. Serve over steamed veggies and brown rice.

Serving and storing leftovers: Serve immediately or store in an airtight container in the fridge for up to 2 weeks.

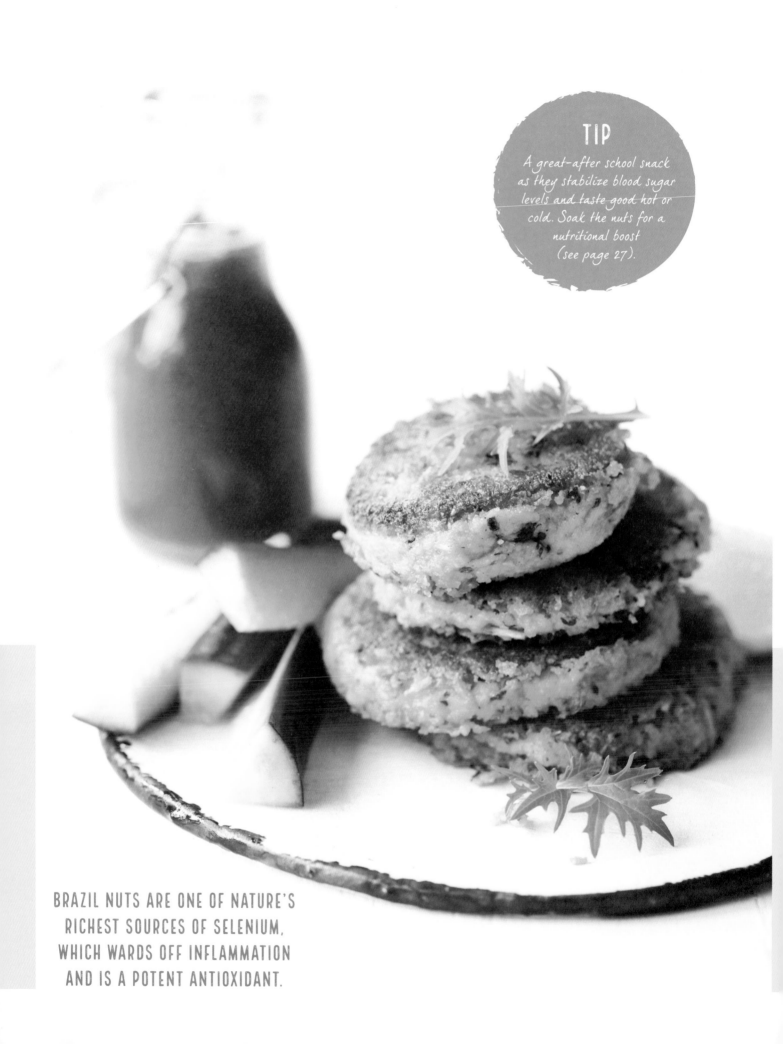

TIP

A great-after school snack as they stabilize blood sugar levels and taste good hot or cold. Soak the nuts for a nutritional boost (see page 27).

BRAZIL NUTS ARE ONE OF NATURE'S RICHEST SOURCES OF SELENIUM, WHICH WARDS OFF INFLAMMATION AND IS A POTENT ANTIOXIDANT.

VEG — Vegetarian | Gluten Free | Dairy Free

Prep time: 15 mins (+ 1 hour refrigeration time)
Cooking time: 20 mins
Makes: 15–20 patties

Brazil & Cashew Nut Patties

Brazil nuts are not popular among kids, so I decided to create this nut burger to include in their diets. My son loves preparing these with me and tasting the ingredients. My daughter and husband loved them too.

INGREDIENTS

¼ cup (1²/₅ oz) brazil nuts

¼ cup (1²/₅ oz) cashews

½ yellow onion, roughly chopped

2 spring onions, roughly chopped

2 garlic cloves, crushed

2 tbs fresh cilantro

1 small egg

¾ cup (6²/₅ oz) butternut squash, peeled and steamed

¼ cup (2/3 oz) rice bread crumbs

2 tbs almond meal

sea salt and pepper, to taste

coconut oil, for frying

EQUIPMENT

high-speed food processor

INSTRUCTIONS

Place brazil and cashew nuts in a high-speed food processor and process until the mixture reaches a fine consistency.

Add onion, spring onion, garlic, cilantro, and egg and process until smooth.

Add squash, rice crumbs, almond meal, salt and pepper and pulse to combine.

Refrigerate for an hour.

Heat coconut oil in a large frying pan over medium heat. Form small patties using your hands or scoop spoonfuls directly into the pan and fry for 3–4 mins on each side, or until golden brown and crisp. Be careful when flipping patties over, as they are quite soft.

Allow to cool for 10 mins before serving.

Serving and storing leftovers: Serve immediately, store in an airtight container in the fridge for up to 4 days or freeze for up to 4 months.

V — Vegan | Gluten Free

Prep time: 5 mins
Makes: 1 cup

Peanut Butter Satay Sauce

INGREDIENTS

⅓ cup (3²/₅ oz) peanut butter, no added sugar

¼ cup coconut milk

½–1 tbs tamari

½ tbs maple syrup or raw honey

juice of 1 lime

1 garlic clove

½ tsp fresh ginger

1–2 tbs fresh cilantro

pinch of pepper

EQUIPMENT

blender

INSTRUCTIONS

Place all ingredients into a blender and blend until smooth and creamy.

Drizzle over roasted vegetables, fried chicken, and salads or simply use as a dip for veggie sticks.

Serving and storing leftovers: Serve immediately or store in the fridge for up to 2 weeks.

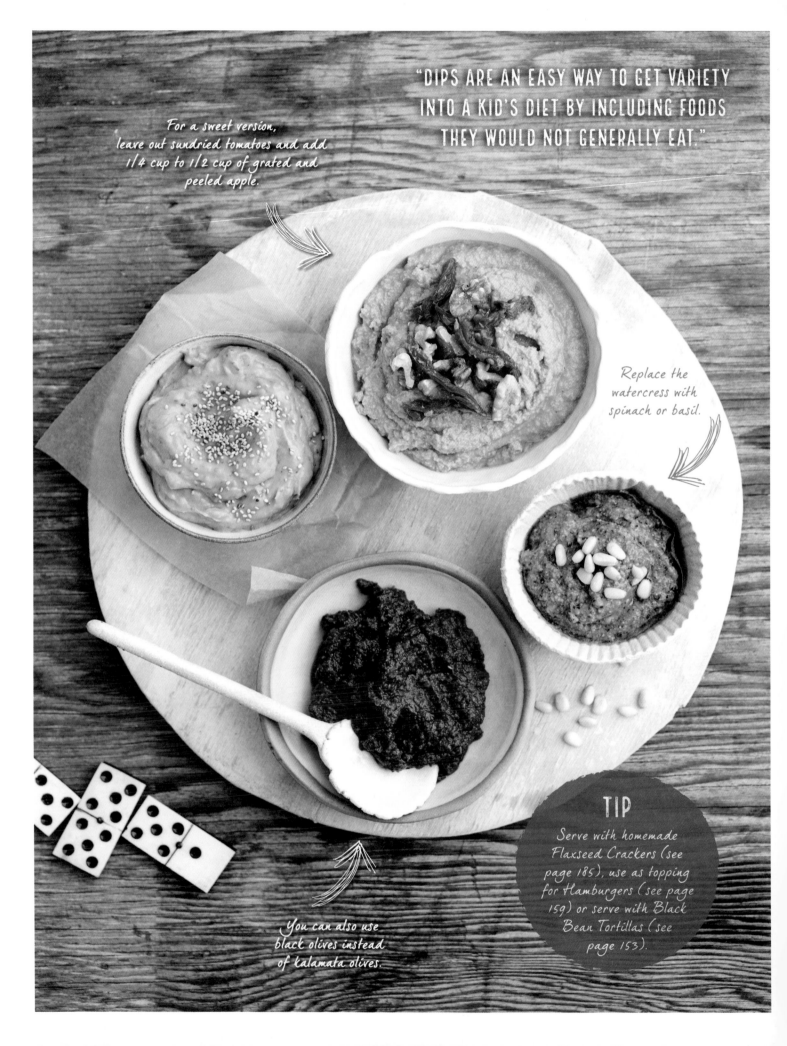

For a sweet version,
leave out sundried tomatoes and add
1/4 cup to 1/2 cup of grated and
peeled apple.

"DIPS ARE AN EASY WAY TO GET VARIETY
INTO A KID'S DIET BY INCLUDING FOODS
THEY WOULD NOT GENERALLY EAT."

Replace the
watercress with
spinach or basil.

You can also use
black olives instead
of kalamata olives.

TIP

Serve with homemade
Flaxseed Crackers (see
page 185), use as topping
for Hamburgers (see page
159) or serve with Black
Bean Tortillas (see
page 153).

VEG Vegetarian | **Gluten Free** | **Egg Free**

 Prep time: 5 mins
Makes: 1 cup

Basil & Pine Nut Pesto

INGREDIENTS

¹⁄₃ cup (1⁷⁄₈ oz) pine nuts, lightly toasted

1 clove garlic

1 cup (⁷⁄₈ oz) fresh basil

1 cup (⁷⁄₈ oz) fresh parsley

¹⁄₂ cup (1²⁄₅ oz) parmesan cheese, grated

¹⁄₄ cup cold-pressed avocado oil or extra virgin olive oil

squeeze of lemon juice

sea salt and pepper, to taste

EQUIPMENT
blender

INSTRUCTIONS

Heat a small frying pan over medium heat, add pine nuts, and toast lightly for 2–4 mins. Allow to cool.

Place all ingredients into a blender and blend until smooth and creamy.

Serving and storing leftovers:
Serve immediately, store in an airtight container in the fridge for up to 7 days or freeze portions in ice cube trays for up to 4 months.

Egg Free | **Nut Free** | **Gluten Free** | **VEG** Vegetarian

 Prep time: 5 mins
Makes: 1¹⁄₄ cups

Olive Tapenade

INGREDIENTS

1 cup (7 oz) kalamata olives, pitted

2 tbs sundried tomatoes, sulphur free

3–4 tbs extra virgin olive oil

1 clove garlic

1 tbs lemon juice

1 tbs fresh basil

2 tbs parmesan cheese (optional)

pinch pepper

EQUIPMENT
blender

INSTRUCTIONS

Place all ingredients into a blender and blend until desired consistency is reached.

Use as a dip for Teff & Parmesan Crackers (see recipe on page 62) or raw vegetable sticks.

Serving and storing leftovers: Serve immediately. Store in the fridge for up to 7 days or freeze for up to 4 months.

V Vegan | **Gluten Free**

 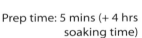 Prep time: 5 mins (+ 4 hrs soaking time)
Makes: 2¹⁄₂ cups

Walnut Hummus

INGREDIENTS

1¹⁄₂ cups (9¹⁄₂ oz) cooked chickpeas or 1 x 14 oz can chickpeas, rinsed, drained

¹⁄₂ cup filtered water

1 tbs tahini

1¹⁄₂ tbs lemon juice

¹⁄₃ cup (1¹⁄₅ oz) walnuts, soaked in filtered water for 4 hours

1–2 tbs sundried tomatoes, sulphur free, finely sliced

1 tbs extra virgin olive oil

¹⁄₂ clove garlic (optional)

sea salt and pepper, to taste

EQUIPMENT
blender

INSTRUCTIONS

Place all ingredients into a blender and blend until smooth and creamy.

Use as a dip for raw veggie sticks, salads, sandwiches or serve with the Cheesy Cauliflower Falafel Patties (page 117).

Serving and storing leftovers: Serve immediately or store in a jar or airtight container in the fridge for up to 4 days.

V Vegan | **Gluten Free** | **Nut Free**

 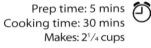 Prep time: 5 mins
Cooking time: 30 mins
Makes: 2¹⁄₄ cups

Roasted Garlic Guacamole

INGREDIENTS

1 bulb garlic

1 tsp extra virgin olive oil

3 ripe medium avocados, peeled and pitted

juice and zest of 1 lime

1–2 tsp chia seeds

¹⁄₂ cup (¹⁄₂ oz) fresh cilantro, finely chopped (optional)

sea salt and pepper, to taste

EQUIPMENT
blender

INSTRUCTIONS

Preheat oven to 390°F.

Cut off top of garlic bulb, drizzle olive oil over it, wrap in baking paper, and roast in the oven for 30 mins.

Allow to cool, remove skin, and place with all the other ingredients in a blender and blend until smooth and creamy.

Serving and storing leftovers: Serve immediately or store in an airtight container in the fridge for up to 2 days.

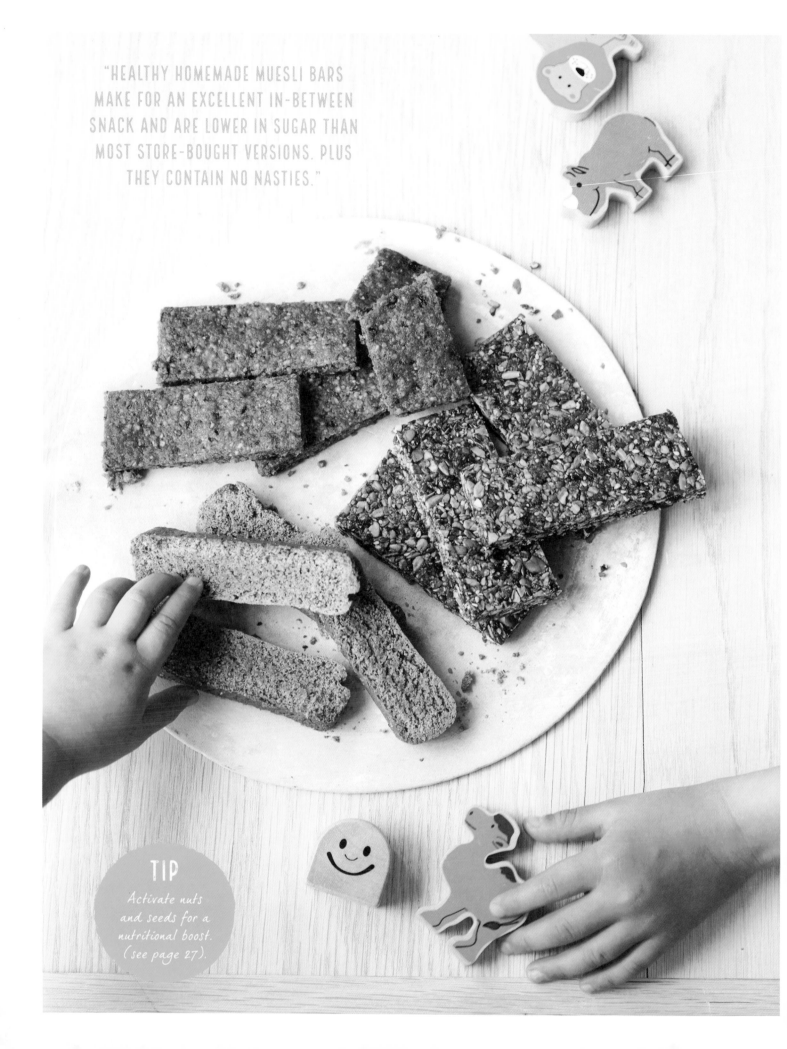

"HEALTHY HOMEMADE MUESLI BARS
MAKE FOR AN EXCELLENT IN-BETWEEN
SNACK AND ARE LOWER IN SUGAR THAN
MOST STORE-BOUGHT VERSIONS. PLUS
THEY CONTAIN NO NASTIES."

TIP
Activate nuts
and seeds for a
nutritional boost.
(see page 27).

Prep time: 10 mins
Cooking time: 20–25 mins
Makes: 10 bars

V
Vegan

Nut
Free

Wheat
Free

Lunch Box-friendly Muesli Bars

INGREDIENTS

2 cups (8^1/$_2$ oz) rolled oats

2 tbs chia seeds

^{1}/$_4$ cup (1^2/$_5$ oz) pumpkin seeds

^{1}/$_2$ cup (^{1}/$_3$ oz) puffed quinoa

^{1}/$_3$ cup (1^1/$_5$ oz) oat meal

pinch sea salt

^{1}/$_2$ tsp baking soda

1 tsp pure vanilla extract

^{1}/$_4$ cup coconut oil, melted

^{1}/$_3$–^{1}/$_2$ cup maple syrup

INSTRUCTIONS

Preheat oven to 325°F and line a 8" x 11^3/$_4$" baking dish with baking paper.

Place oats and seeds in a food processor and process until a fine consistency is achieved. Add remaining ingredients and process until it forms a gooey mixture.

Place mixture into the prepared baking dish, press down firmly and evenly over the base of the dish.

Bake for approximately 20–25 mins or until golden brown. The mixture will harden as it cools. Cut into slices and serve.

Serving and storing leftovers: Serve immediately, store in an airtight container for up to 4 days, refrigerate for up to 14 days or freeze for up to 4 months.

Prep time: 10 mins
Cooking time: 30–35 mins
Makes: 14 bars

V
Vegan

Gluten
Free

Nut
Free

Superseed Bars

INGREDIENTS

1 cup (8^1/$_2$ oz) Medjool dates, pitted, chopped

1 cup (5 2/3 oz) sunflower seeds

1 cup (5 2/3 oz) pumpkin seeds

2 tbs maple syrup

1 tsp pure vanilla extract

1 tsp ground cinnamon

pinch sea salt

EQUIPMENT

high-speed food processor

INSTRUCTIONS

Preheat oven to 325°F and line a 8" x 11^3/$_4$" baking tin with baking paper.

Place all ingredients into a food processor and mix until well combined.

Press mixture firmly into the prepared tin and bake in the oven for 30–35 mins, or until golden brown and crisp on top.

Allow to cool completely on a wire rack. Cut into bars.

Serving and storing leftovers: Serve immediately, store in a container for up to 4 days, refrigerate for up to 14 days or freeze for up to 4 months.

Prep time: 10 mins
Cooking time: 35–40 mins
Makes: 16 bars

V
Vegan

Gluten
Free

Pecan Quinoa Muesli Bars

INGREDIENTS

1 cup (2/3 oz) puffed quinoa

^{1}/$_2$ cup (2^1/$_3$ oz) Wholesome Child gluten-free flour mix

^{1}/$_2$ cup (1^7/$_8$ oz) pecans

^{1}/$_4$ cup (^{7}/$_8$ oz) goji berries or golden raisins

^{1}/$_2$ cup (1^2/$_5$ oz) coconut flakes

^{1}/$_4$ cup (1^2/$_5$ oz) pumpkin seeds

^{1}/$_2$ cup (4^1/$_4$ oz) Medjool dates, pitted

^{1}/$_2$ cup coconut oil, melted

^{1}/$_4$ cup maple syrup

1 tsp ground cinnamon

pinch sea salt

EQUIPMENT

high-speed food processor

INSTRUCTIONS

Preheat oven to 325°F and line a 8" x 11^3/$_4$" baking tin with baking paper.

Place all ingredients into a food processor and process until well combined and until the consistency is fine but still a bit crumbly.

Press mixture firmly into tin and bake for 35–40 mins, or until golden brown on top.

Allow to cool in the baking tin before moving on to a wire rack to cool completely. Cut into bars.

Serving and storing leftovers: Serve immediately, store in an airtight container for up to 4 days, refrigerate for up to 14 days or freeze for up to 4 months.

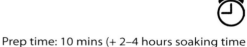

Prep time: 10 mins (+ 2–4 hours soaking time
and 1 hour refrigeration time)
Makes: 1¹/₂ cups

Cashew & Cauliflower Mayonnaise

INGREDIENTS

1 cup (5²/₃ oz) cashews, soaked for 2–4 hours, rinsed, drained

¹/₂ cup (1³/₄ oz) raw cauliflower florets, roughly chopped

¹/₃ cup filtered water

¹/₃ cup extra virgin olive oil or cold-pressed macadamia oil

1 tbs lemon juice

1 tsp apple cider vinegar

¹/₄ tsp Dijon mustard

sea salt, to taste

pinch pepper

EQUIPMENT

high-powered blender or high-speed food processor

INSTRUCTIONS

Soak the cashew nuts for 2–4 hours for creamiest outcome. Rinse nuts and place with all other ingredients into a blender or food processor.

Process until smooth and creamy for about 5 mins (depends on what processor you are using).

Refrigerate for an hour before serving.

Serving and storing leftovers: Serve immediately or store in the fridge for up to 1 week.

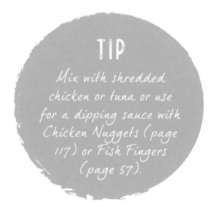

TIP

Mix with shredded chicken or tuna or use for a dipping sauce with Chicken Nuggets (page 117) or Fish Fingers (page 57).

VEG
Vegetarian

Gluten
Free

Nut
Free

Egg
Free

Prep time: 10 mins
Makes: ¹/₄ cup

Ghee Garlic Spread

INGREDIENTS

¹/₄ cup (2¹/₆ oz) ghee, room temperature

2 garlic cloves, crushed

1 tbs fresh herbs (dill/parsley/cilantro/sage/oregano)

sea salt and pepper, to taste

INSTRUCTIONS

In a small bowl, mix all ingredients together until well combined.

Use on homemade Naan Bread (see recipe on page 283) or on grilled meat and vegetables.

Serving and storing leftovers: Serve immediately, store in the fridge for up to 1 month or freeze for up to 4 months.

If your child doesn't like "green" foods, leave out the herbs or use dried herbs instead. You can substitute unsalted butter for ghee.

Gluten Free   Nut Free   Dairy Free   Egg Free

Prep time: 10 mins (+ 4–5 hours refrigeration time)
Cooking time: 15 mins
Makes: 1½ cups

Chicken Liver Paté

INGREDIENTS

¼ cup coconut oil, butter or ghee

1 medium shallot, diced

1 garlic clove, crushed

1 small apple, peeled and diced

7 oz organic chicken livers, rinsed and patted dry

1 tsp fresh sage, diced

¼ cup coconut milk

sea salt, to taste

pinch pepper

pinch nutmeg

EQUIPMENT
blender

INSTRUCTIONS

Heat oil in a large frying pan over medium heat.

Add shallot and garlic and cook slowly for 5 mins.

Add apple and sauté for another 2 mins. Transfer to a small bowl and wipe the pan clean with some paper towel.

Add chicken livers and sage and lightly fry for 5 mins or until browned on both sides but still a bit pink inside (otherwise they become grainy).

Place in a blender with onion-apple mixture, coconut milk and seasonings and blend until smooth and creamy.

Transfer to a glass jar with lid and place in the fridge for 4–5 hours before serving.

Serving and storing leftovers: Serve immediately or store in the fridge for up to 3 days or freeze for up to 3–4 months.

VEG   Vegetarian   Gluten Free   Egg Free

Prep time: 5 mins (+ 2–4 hours soaking time)
Makes: 1¼ cups

Watercress & Cashew Pesto

INGREDIENTS

¼ cup (⅙ oz) fresh watercress, rinsed, drained

2 cups (1¾ oz) baby spinach, rinsed, drained

1 ripe avocado

¼ cup (⅙ oz) fresh parsley

1 tbs fresh cilantro

¼ cup extra virgin olive oil

¼ cup (1²⁄₅ oz) pine nuts, toasted

¼ cup (1²⁄₅ oz) cashews (soaked for 2–4 hrs, optional)

1 garlic clove

1 tbs lemon juice

1 tbs parmesan cheese (optional)

EQUIPMENT
blender

INSTRUCTIONS

Place all ingredients in a blender and blend until smooth and creamy.

Use as a dip for homemade seeded crackers (see page 185) or serve with cooked wholegrain pasta as a main dish.

Serving and storing leftovers: Serve immediately, store in the fridge for 7 days or in freezer for 4 months.

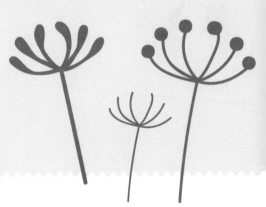

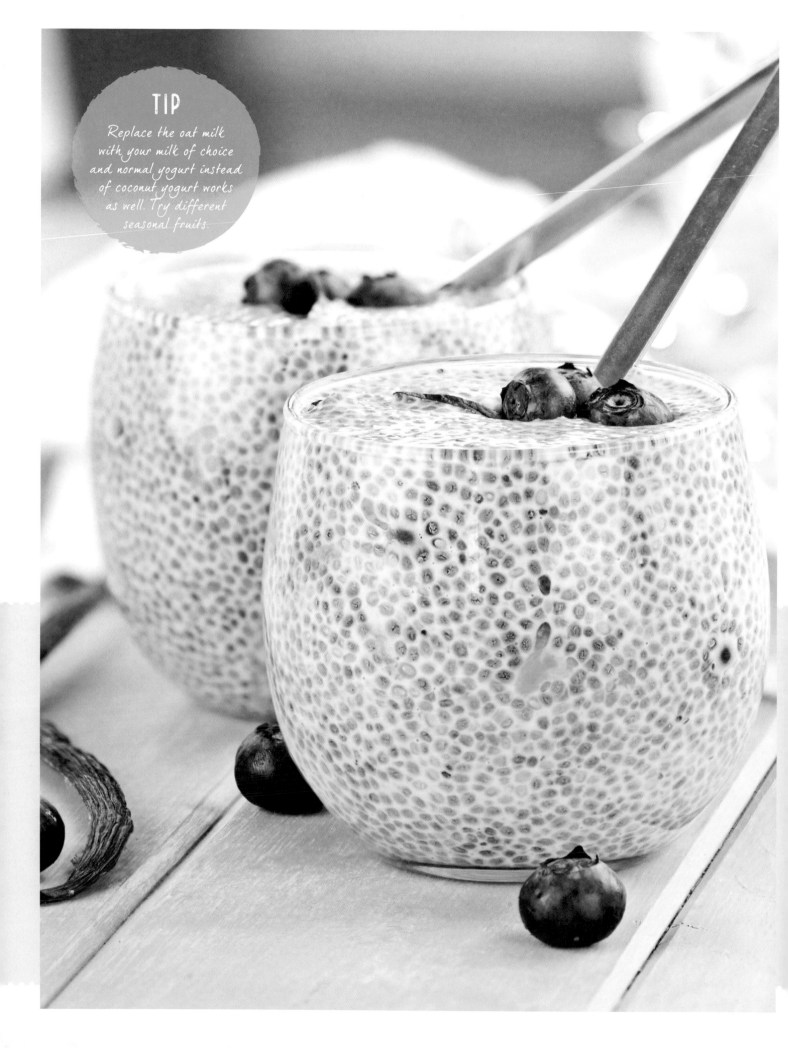

TIP

Replace the oat milk
with your milk of choice
and normal yogurt instead
of coconut yogurt works
as well. Try different
seasonal fruits.

Vegan Gluten Nut
        Free   Free

Prep time: 5 mins (+ 6–8 hours refrigeration time)
Serves: 2

Mango Chia Pudding

Chia pudding is a great breakfast choice as it's packed with nutrients such as calcium, omega-3s and protein. The sweetness of the mango helps to make it more palatable for little tastebuds.

INGREDIENTS

1 cup oat milk

4 tbs chia seeds

½ tbs maple syrup or pinch stevia (optional)

2 tbs coconut yogurt

½ mango, diced

fresh blueberries

INSTRUCTIONS

Place all ingredients into a bowl or glass jar and stir until well combined.

Cover and let set in the fridge overnight or for 6–8 hours. Top with blueberries before serving.

Serving and storing leftovers: Serve immediately or store in the fridge for up to 4 days.

VEG Gluten Egg   Dairy
Vegetarian Free Free Free

Prep time: 8 mins (+ 4–8 hours soaking time)
Serves: 3–4

Omega-3 Smoothie

INGREDIENTS

1 ripe banana, frozen

1 medium ripe avocado

¼ cup (1 oz) walnuts, soaked in filtered water for 4–8 hours or overnight

1 tbs chia seeds

1 tbs flaxseed meal

2 cups almond milk, or milk of choice

½ cup filtered water, plus 4 large ice cubes

2 tsp manuka or raw honey (optional)

1 tbs cacao powder (optional)

1 tbs carob powder (optional)

EQUIPMENT

blender

INSTRUCTIONS

Place all ingredients into a blender and blend until smooth and creamy.

Serving and storing leftovers: Serve immediately, store in the fridge for up to 24 hours or freeze for up to 6 months.

TIP

If your child is not used to smoothies, slowly build up to the full recipe. Leave out any of the following: avocado, walnuts, chia seeds or flaxseed meal.

"HIGH IN FIBER AND PROTEIN, THESE HEALTHY MACARONS
ARE A GUILT-FREE TREAT FOR THE WHOLE FAMILY."

TIP

For a school-friendly
version omit almond meal and
add 1/4 cup of coconut flakes
or seed meal. Replace the
honey with stevia for a
low-sugar option.

VEG
Vegetarian

Gluten Free

Dairy Free

Prep time: 15 mins (+ 30 mins refrigeration time)
Cooking time: 10 mins
Makes: 20

Coconut Macarons

When my dinosaur-obsessed son begged me for dinosaur cookies I made these dinosaur rocks instead. He helped me make them and took them to school the next day to show his classmates.

TIP

For an extra treat, drizzle some melted dark chocolate on top or make a macaroon sandwich by placing the Chocolate Avo Frosting (see page 93) or Healthy Chocolate Spread in the middle of two macaroons (see page 275).

INGREDIENTS

4 egg whites

4–6 tbs raw honey

2¹⁄₃ cups (6³⁄₅ oz) coconut flakes

¹⁄₃ cup (1²⁄₅ oz) almond meal

pinch sea salt

pinch ground cinnamon

EQUIPMENT

electric hand mixer

INSTRUCTIONS

Preheat oven to 355°F and line a baking tray with baking paper.

In a small bowl, beat egg whites until stiff. Add honey and beat until well incorporated.

In another bowl, combine coconut, almond meal, salt, and cinnamon. Fold in egg mixture, cover, and refrigerate for at least 30 mins.

Using your hands, form tablespoon-sized balls and place them on baking tray, flattening them slightly.

Bake for 10 mins, remove from oven, and allow to cool completely on a wire rack before serving. Macarons will harden once cooled.

Serving and storing leftovers: Serve immediately, store in an airtight container for up to 1 week or freeze for up to 4 months.

  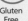

V
Vegan

Gluten Free

Egg Free

Dairy Free

Prep time: 10 mins
Cooking time: 10–15 mins
Makes: 4 cups

Paleo Granola

INGREDIENTS

1 cup (5 2/3 oz) almonds

1 cup (3⁷⁄₈ oz) pecans

¹⁄₄ cup (1²⁄₅ oz) sunflower seeds

¹⁄₄ cup (1²⁄₅ oz) pumpkin seeds

1 cup (2³⁄₄ oz) shredded coconut

¹⁄₄ cup (1⁴⁄₅ oz) flaxseeds

¹⁄₂ cup (4¹⁄₄ oz) dates, pitted and chopped

1 tsp ground cinnamon

pinch Himalayan rock salt

¹⁄₄ cup maple syrup or raw honey

2 tbs coconut oil, melted

1 tsp pure vanilla extract

EQUIPMENT

high-speed food processor

INSTRUCTIONS

Preheat oven to 355°F and line a baking tray with baking paper.

Place nuts and seeds in a high-speed food processor and process for 5 seconds or until they have broken apart a little bit, but don't turn it into a meal.

Place nut and seed mixture in a large bowl and combine with all the other ingredients until everything is well combined.

Spread mixture onto the baking tray and roast in the oven for 10–15 mins, stirring halfway.

Allow granola to cool completely—the air will help the granola obtain a crunchy texture.

Serving and storing leftovers: Serve immediately, store in a glass jar or airtight container in a cool, dry spot for up to 1 month or freeze in an airtight container for up to 6 months.

Use golden raisins or dried sulphur-free apricots instead of the dates. Or replace the pecans with cashews or macadamias.

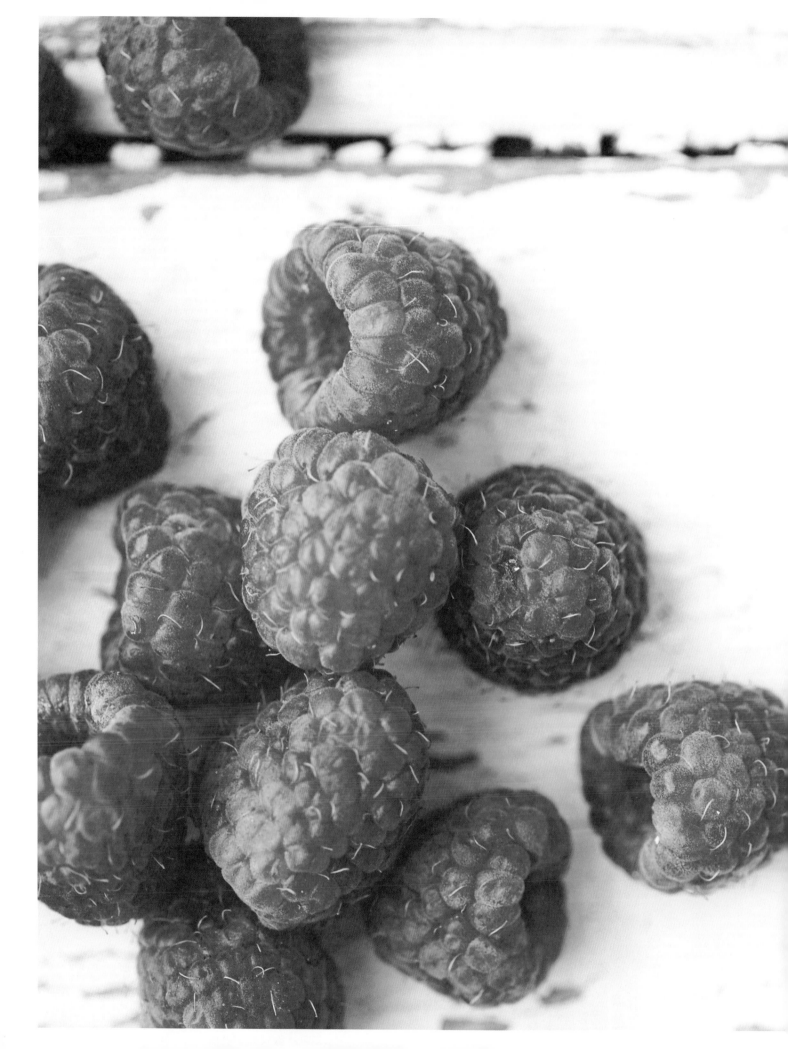

Balance
Fruit

IN THE RECOMMENDED
AMOUNTS, IT'S A HEALTHY
PART OF A CHILD'S DIET

*I*f there's ever a food group battle that most parents don't have to fight, it's getting their children to eat enough fruit. Thanks to the sweetness inherent in many fruits, most children are fans. But while fruit is packed full of vitamins and antioxidants, there is such a thing as eating too much of it, especially if it starts to replace other foods in the diet.

One client of mine, aged four, loved fruit almost to the exclusion of everything else. This petite little girl nagged her mother throughout the day for fruit. She could easily eat a pint of blueberries, an apple, and a banana in one sitting. And while that may sound healthy it isn't, especially when replacing other important food choices. While fruit is a great source of carbohydrates, fiber, minerals and vitamins A, B and C, unfortunately it has little protein and virtually no fat, both essential for a growing child.

Consider this...

Apples are a great fiber source if you don't peel them. The skin contains quercetin, an antioxidant with antihistamine and anti-inflammatory power that may help protect us from heart disease and possibly allergic reactions.

EATING FRUIT WILL:

✓ add fiber to your child's diet, keeping him fuller for longer and keeping him regular.

✓ build the immune system thanks to antioxidants.

✓ help fight off high blood pressure and heart disease in later life.

✓ prevent some types of cancer.

✓ lower the risk of eye and digestive problems.

✓ have a positive effect on your child's brain and memory, helping him recall information easier and faster.

SO WHAT'S THE DEAL WITH FRUIT?

Thanks to the anti-sugar crowd, fruit often gets lumped with other high-sugar foods. It is true that fruit contains the intrinsic sugar fructose and that some fruits contain more fructose than others, yet many fruits have a low Glycemic index. When it comes to giving children fruit as a snack or dessert, I'm all for it, especially if replacing a refined sugar treat.

When kids eat candy or a chocolate bar, they tend to immediately crave more. However, when they eat fruit, they ingest the fructose along with fiber and other nutrients which slow down sugar absorption and prevent spikes in insulin. In most cases it is very unlikely that a child will go completely overboard on the natural sugars that come from fruit, but like anything else it's all about balance.

Remember, it isn't just about how much fruit your child eats, but what he eats it with. Pairing fruit with a protein and healthy fat will keep your child satiated longer. Try apple slices with some nut butter, berries with yogurt or ricotta cheese, or half a banana with a handful of sunflower seeds. Our bodies are designed to metabolize the amount of fructose contained in 2–3 servings of fruit a day but if your child has eaten a lot of foods containing added sugar, it may be wise to lower their fruit consumption on that day.

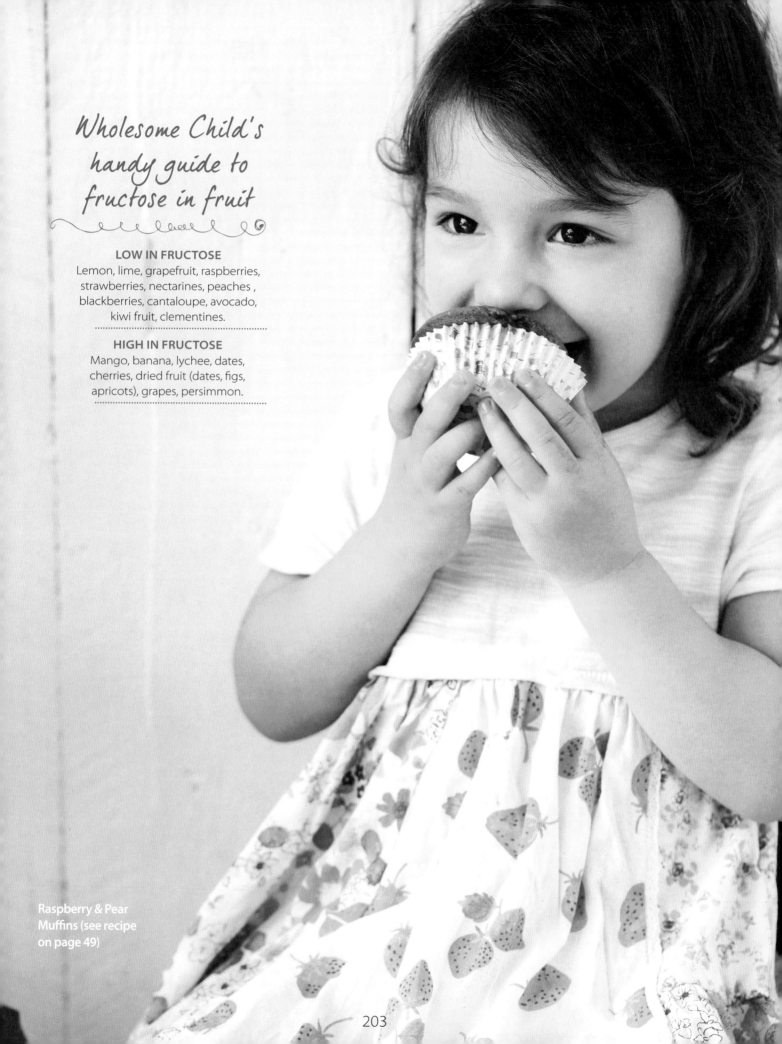

Wholesome Child's handy guide to fructose in fruit

LOW IN FRUCTOSE
Lemon, lime, grapefruit, raspberries, strawberries, nectarines, peaches , blackberries, cantaloupe, avocado, kiwi fruit, clementines.

HIGH IN FRUCTOSE
Mango, banana, lychee, dates, cherries, dried fruit (dates, figs, apricots), grapes, persimmon.

Raspberry & Pear Muffins (see recipe on page 49)

WHAT DOES ONE SERVING OF FRUIT LOOK LIKE?

FRUIT	SERVING
apple, banana, orange or pear	1 medium
berries	½ cup
apricots, kiwis or plums	2 small
fresh squeezed juice	½ cup
mixed fruit salad	½ cup
homemade popsicles (see recipes on page 217)	1
melon	½ cup or 1 medium-sized wedge
grapes	½ cup
dried fruit or freeze-dried fruit	1½ tbs
diced or canned fruit (with no added sugar)	½ cup

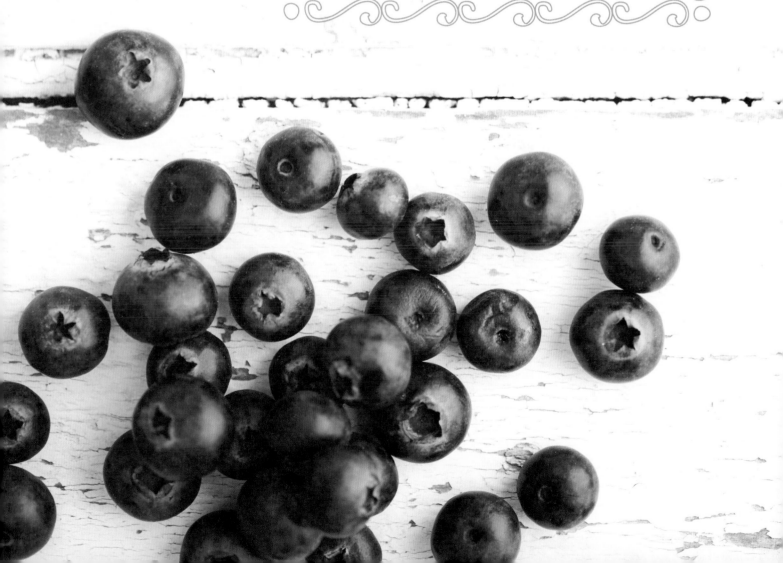

HOW MUCH FRUIT SHOULD MY CHILD BE EATING?

The recommended guidelines for children are 1.5 to 2 servings of fruit per day. However, for children who are active and play sports, I recommend an extra serving of fruit as long as that fruit does not replace other foods in the diet. One serving of fruit is around 5⅓ oz and a serving of dried fruit is 1 oz.

ORGANIC VS NON-ORGANIC

Studies have shown that when children are switched to an organic diet there is a reduced amount of pesticide in their urine. When fruit is labeled organic it typically means that it has been grown in soil that has been free of most synthetic fertilizers or pesticides for at least three years.

Children tend to consume more fruit than adults per body weight, so if you can afford to buy organic it makes sense to do so, especially when it comes to fruit that tends to have the highest concentrations of pesticide residue (typically those not peeled before eating).

When out shopping, take a copy of the Environmental Working Group's "Dirty Dozen" list of fruit and vegetables that contain the most pesticides and the "Clean Fifteen" list of those with the lowest pesticide load (hint: they all have a thick skin). And remember if you are peeling non-organic fruits, you are losing important nutrients, like fiber, contained in the skin.

BUY ORGANIC:
1. Strawberries
2. Apples
3. Peaches
4. Grapes
5. Cherries
6. Tomatoes
7. Cucumbers

BUY CONVENTIONAL:
1. Avocados
2. Pineapples
3. Mangos
4. Onions
5. Cauliflower
6. Honeydew melon
7. Grapefruit
8. Asparagus

THE PROS AND CONS OF DRIED FRUIT

In its purest form (i.e., without any added sugar), dried fruit is just fresh fruit with the water removed. Drying, in fact, causes some nutrients to become more concentrated.

One study found that antioxidants in dried cranberries, grapes, and plums are twice as potent as those in the fresh fruits. Of course along with more potent antioxidants comes more concentrated sugar.

Also, take note of the ingredient list: only the fruit should be listed. Watch for added sweeteners (sugar, corn syrup), particularly in tart fruits, like cherries and cranberries. Look for packages that say "no sulphites," a preservative that maintains color. While it might not look as appealing, brown and shriveled sun-dried fruit is healthier.

PROS
- Concentrated form of fiber, vitamins, minerals, and antioxidants.
- Can help ward off constipation. I've often seen young babies and children on laxatives and by introducing Apricot & Pear Compote, mild cases are easily resolved (see recipe on page 222).
- Raisins, apricots, peaches, sun-dried tomatoes, and figs provide iron for fussy eaters who refuse to eat meat or for vegetarians.
- Figs, dates, apricots and prunes are a good source of calcium.

CONS
- Contributes to dental cavities more than chocolate by sticking to teeth.
- It's not as filling as whole fruit as the water has been lost.
- Vitamin C and folate content can be diminished.
- High in concentrated sugars or fructose.

BE SMART WITH DRIED FRUIT

Kids can easily scoff raisins by the handful, whereas it's more difficult to eat too many grapes without feeling full. One small packet of raisins (1½ oz) contains 1 oz of sugar, or six teaspoons! Avoid buying packaged portions and offer dried fruit in small amounts: four apricot halves or 1 oz of dried mango without added sugar.

DID YOU KNOW?

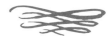

A banana is made up of around 25% sugar making it an average choice for breakfast as it will give your child an initial energy boost followed by a mid-morning crash. Serving a banana with porridge or plain yogurt will slow down the release of sugar into the blood, making it a great choice.

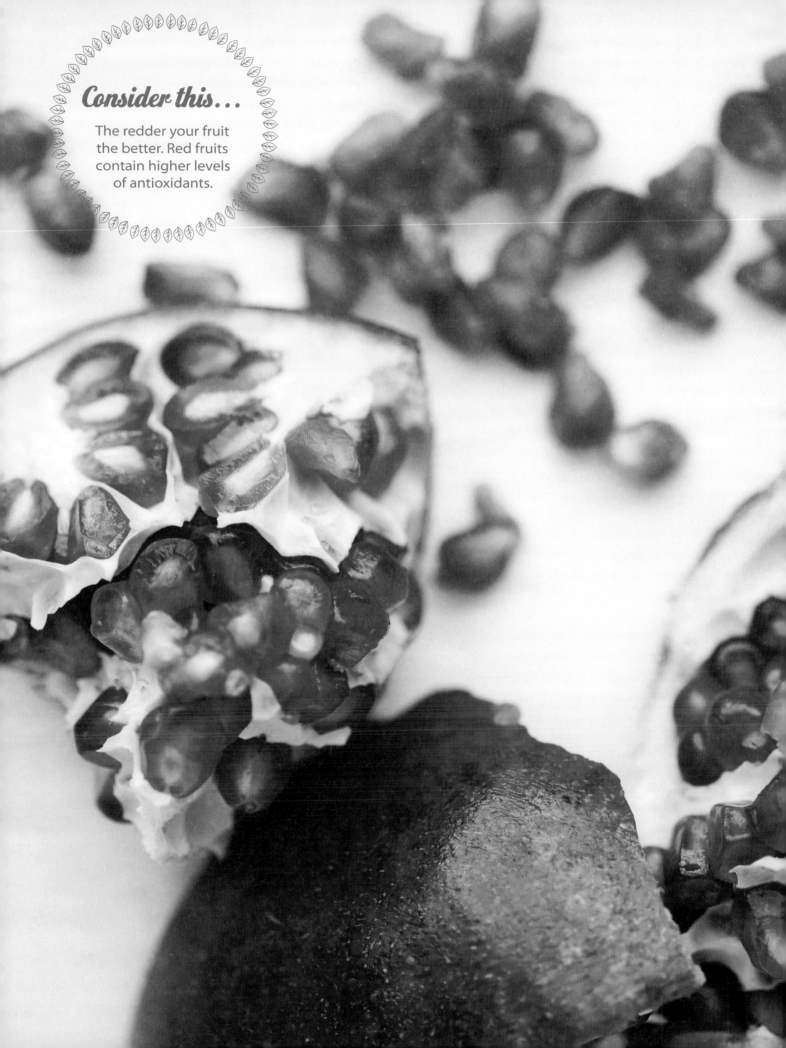

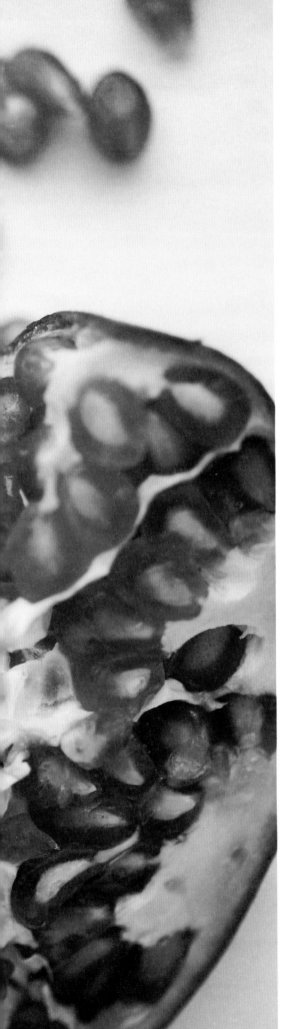

Fresh juice vs smoothies: What's the healthier choice?

FRUIT JUICE

With freshly squeezed juices readily available at juice bars and restaurants, many parents opt for it over water as it appears to be a healthy drink for kids. And while freshly squeezed juice is certainly healthier than store-bought juices that often contain as much added sugar as fizzy drinks, juice doesn't contain the fiber or filling qualities of whole fruit. Juicing extracts the liquid content of the whole fruit. The fiber is discarded.

Still, fresh juice can offer amazing nutritional benefits if you use a ratio of 1:4 fruit to vegetables and choose blended juices that keep the flesh rather than pure juices that discard the fiber. Juices made at home using the Nutribullet or Vitamix are good options. Remember, half a cup of freshly squeezed juice counts as one serve of fruit, so offer it in small portions and water it down. It's best when kids eat their calories, not drink them. Also, freshly squeezed juice has a high acid content that can erode tooth enamel.

IF YOUR CHILD LOVES
FRUIT JUICE:

- Start by diluting juice to water by ratios of 1:3, then 1:4.

- Offer juice on special occasions or out of the home so it's not the expected norm.

- Lunch boxes can contain fruit but skip the fruit juice.

SMOOTHIES

Unlike juicing, blending uses the whole fruit. That's why smoothies are a step up from freshly squeezed juices. Because they contain the fiber, they are far more filling than juice. But be aware that smoothies on the menu in restaurants may contain ice cream, or frozen or flavored yogurts that are high in added sugar. It's always best to check and even better to make your own so you really know what's in it. A healthy smoothie is usually a combination of milk (almond, rice, soy, coconut or regular), ice, and a blend of fruit and vegetables.

IF YOUR CHILD LOVES
SMOOTHIES:

- Ensure they contain protein from plain unsweetened yogurt, soaked cashew nuts or almonds or nut butter.

- Ensure they contain healthy fats from sources like chia seeds, pumpkin seeds, flaxseeds, walnuts, avocado or coconut flesh.

- Great additions to smoothies include easily disguised vegetables like spinach, kale or beetroot.

- If you need to sweeten the smoothie, use a little raw or Manuka honey.

- Don't discard any leftover homemade smoothies. Freeze any leftovers in popsicle molds. These make great mid-afternoon snacks.

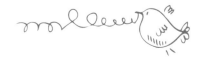

Superfruits

GOJI BERRIES	ACAI BERRIES	BLUEBERRIES, RASPBERRIES, STRAWBERRIES	CHERRIES	CRANBERRIES	CITRUS FRUITS
Benefits	**Benefits**	**Benefits**	**Benefits**	**Benefits**	**Benefits**
Goji berries are composed of 18 essential amino acids, 21 trace minerals, vitamins B1, B2, B6, and E, linoleic acid, selenium, germanium, and more betacarotene than the common carrot. A study from the *Chinese Journal of Oncology* found that patients with cancer responded better to treatment when goji berries were added to their daily diet. Gojis help the body kick infections and are beneficial for children's eyesight.	These deep purple berries contain excellent amounts of iron, calcium, fiber and vitamin A. They also contain anthocyanin compounds which not only give fruits and vegetables their distinct color, but also team up with flavonoids to defend the body against harmful free radicals. Rich in antioxidants, amino acids and fiber, they're an excellent immune booster and can increase your child's energy and combat fatigue.	Several studies have linked the high flavonoid levels in blueberries with a better memory, making them a great addition to the school lunch box. Just half a cup of raspberries will give your child four grams of fiber and 25 percent of his recommended intake of vitamin C and manganese. Strawberries are high in vitamin C and folic acid too, which can help prevent colds and flu and protect the heart. Blackberries are rich in polyphenols, which may help prevent cardiovascular disease, cancers and osteoporosis in later life.	High in a disease-fighting antioxidant called anthocyanin, which can reduce inflammation and lower triglyceride and cholesterol levels, cherries are an excellent fruit choice for young children. They're also rich in melatonin which helps children sleep better and may calm the nervous system and reduce irritability.	They're rich in vitamins C and A and antioxidants such as proanthocyanidins which work to kill bacteria helping fight off urinary-tract infections. One study also found that cranberries may slow the growth of some cancer cells.	Oranges, grapefruits, lemons, limes, mandarins, and tangerines are full of vitamin C, fiber, and disease-fighting chemicals such as naringenin and d-limonene which can stimulate the liver to burn excess fat, reduce blood sugar, lower cholesterol and fight cancer. Vitamin C may help to reduce the length of the common cold, help with wound healing and minor scars, and keep kids gums and teeth healthy. Lemon is excellent for promoting healthy digestion. Just a squeeze in water can do wonders for your child's liver.
How to use them	**How to use them**	**How to use them**	**How to use them**	**How to use them**	**How to use them**
Grab a handful for the lunch box, create a trail mix or add them to muesli bars. See recipe for our Pecan Quinoa Muesli Bar on page 193.	Use in homemade ice cream, add to smoothies, and sprinkle over porridge. See recipe for our Acai Breakfast Bowl on page 221.	Serve fresh with plain, unsweetened yogurt and muesli to make a yogurt parfait, add into smoothies or bake into muffins. See our recipe for Berry & Granola Parfait on page 249.	They're delicious on their own (mind the pits), or added to yogurt, porridge, smoothies or muffins.	Most commonly eaten in their dried form, they can be added to granola, trail mix, used in muesli bars or bliss balls. Look for cranberries with no added sugar or preservatives.	Add orange and lemon slices to a jug of water and drink through the day, squeeze lemon juice in water or over fish fingers. Add zest in baking and lemon to salad dressings. See recipe for Chicken Drumstick Casserole on page 157 or Salad Dressing on page 187.

Wholesome Child's top 12 vitamin and antioxidant-packed fruits for kids

KIWI	BANANA	GRAPES	PAPAYA	WATERMELON	DRAGON FRUIT
Benefits	**Benefits**	**Benefits**	**Benefits**	**Benefits**	**Benefits**
High in fiber and pre-biotic complex carbohydrates, kiwi fruit is your go-to for constipation relief. One kiwi fruit also provides children with their daily quota of vitamin C and can work to reduce bouts of wheezing and coughing.	Among the most popular and favorite fruit for children, bananas are loaded with fiber, potassium, antioxidants, and magnesium. Potassium is essential for heart health and one banana a day supplies on average 400mg of potassium, which is nearly one quarter of your child's recommended intake. The World Health Organization (WHO) advises that children increase their intake of potassium-rich food to effectively control their blood pressure.	The antioxidant resveratrol keeps hearts healthy. Studies have also found that compounds found in grape seed extract can also fight certain cancers (at least in the laboratory).	Papaya is rich in papain, an enzyme that helps to digest proteins, making it an excellent remedy for constipation. It's also loaded with vitamin C and a good source of vitamins A and E, two powerful antioxidants that may help protect against heart disease and colon cancer.	Packed with vitamins A and C and twice as much disease-fighting lycopene as a fresh tomato, watermelon can help improve the body's immune system as well as reduce the risk of asthma and cardiovascular disease.	Children love this fruit, especially when they hear the name. The seeds are packed with essential fatty acids like oleic acid, which helps lower bad cholesterol and raise good cholesterol.
How to use them	**How to use them**	**How to use them**	**How to use them**	**How to use them**	**How to use them**
Grab a spoon and eat them fresh. Add to smoothies and frozen ice blocks. See our delicious Kiwi & Coconut Popsicles on page 217.	Add to smoothies and porridge, use to sweeten muffins or cakes or make healthy ice cream. See our recipe for Banana Split Trio on page 227.	Grapes are best eaten fresh. Kids love them added to lunch boxes or as on-the-go snacks but remember grapes are a choking hazard for young children so always slit them lengthways. You can also freeze them and eat frozen.	Cut lengthways, discard seeds and spoon out the flesh, add to smoothies (along with a tablespoon of the seeds) or to fruit salads. Green papaya is a great addition to salads too.	Cut into slices and serve on an ice cream stick. On summer days, place in the freezer and serve frozen as a granita.	Cut in half and spoon out the flesh. Add to smoothies and chia pudding or take your fruit salad up a notch with striking black and white chunks of dragon fruit.

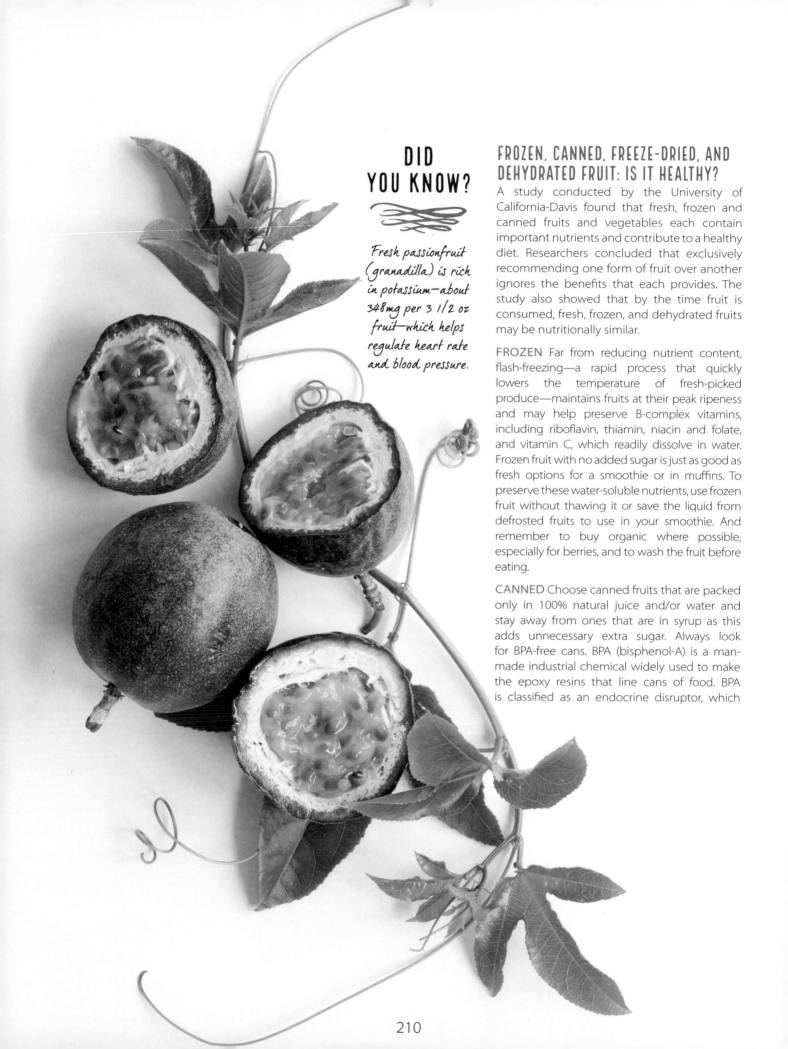

DID YOU KNOW?

Fresh passionfruit (granadilla) is rich in potassium—about 348mg per 3 1/2 oz fruit—which helps regulate heart rate and blood pressure.

FROZEN, CANNED, FREEZE-DRIED, AND DEHYDRATED FRUIT: IS IT HEALTHY?

A study conducted by the University of California-Davis found that fresh, frozen and canned fruits and vegetables each contain important nutrients and contribute to a healthy diet. Researchers concluded that exclusively recommending one form of fruit over another ignores the benefits that each provides. The study also showed that by the time fruit is consumed, fresh, frozen, and dehydrated fruits may be nutritionally similar.

FROZEN Far from reducing nutrient content, flash-freezing—a rapid process that quickly lowers the temperature of fresh-picked produce—maintains fruits at their peak ripeness and may help preserve B-complex vitamins, including riboflavin, thiamin, niacin and folate, and vitamin C, which readily dissolve in water. Frozen fruit with no added sugar is just as good as fresh options for a smoothie or in muffins. To preserve these water-soluble nutrients, use frozen fruit without thawing it or save the liquid from defrosted fruits to use in your smoothie. And remember to buy organic where possible, especially for berries, and to wash the fruit before eating.

CANNED Choose canned fruits that are packed only in 100% natural juice and/or water and stay away from ones that are in syrup as this adds unnecessary extra sugar. Always look for BPA-free cans. BPA (bisphenol-A) is a man-made industrial chemical widely used to make the epoxy resins that line cans of food. BPA is classified as an endocrine disruptor, which means it can interfere with our hormones. It's especially important to avoid acidic fruit, like tomatoes, in cans as this speeds up erosion and the BPA is able to leach into the food. Wherever possible, choose fruit preserved in glass bottles over cans.

DEHYDRATED You can go the whole hog and buy a dehydrator or simply slow-cook fruit in the oven. Thinly sliced apple slices take two hours or less in the oven to transform into crisp, sweet chips free of the additives you often find in store-bought versions.

FREEZE-DRIED Freeze-drying preserves fruit by removing 98 percent of its water content. This prevents fruit from spoiling, while still maintaining most of its flavor, color, texture, and nutritional value, plus it adds delicious crunch. Research has shown that while freeze-dried fruits contain slightly lower amounts of certain vitamins, they are rich in antioxidants and fiber. Because freeze-dried fruits lack water, like dried fruits they are highly concentrated, which means they contain more fructose, so use sparingly to sprinkle on yogurt or oatmeal.

IS IT OKAY TO EAT FRUIT AT NIGHT?

Giving your child a piece of fruit after dinner can have nutritional benefits. Fresh fruits are low-calorie options that supply nutrients like fiber and potassium. A bowl of fresh berries or a banana, loaded with satiating fiber and relaxing tryptophan, are both good choices. Cherries contain melatonin, an important natural chemical related to healthy sleep rhythms. However, be aware that fruit can make kids pee, so encourage them to go before they get into bed.

GOAL 6: COOK WITH YOUR KIDS

Children learn through play and experience and there is no better way to expand a child's repertoire than by cooking delicious meals with mom, dad or another grown-up. Not only is it a fun and engaging experience, it is also an important teaching and development tool for all ages. For time-poor parents, it's also an excellent way to combine play with the daily routine of meals. For the fussy eaters I see in my practice, preparing meals together is an essential part of their journey toward healthy eating. However, I truly recommend it for all kids, no matter their age and interest in food.

In my house, Sunday mornings are the best quality family time. My kids love preparing a special family breakfast with me. My son's favorite part is tasting—whether sucking on limes, trying cacao powder or sampling sweet potato puree, he taste-tests all of my ingredients. It always surprises me how adventurous he'll be when he has his chef's apron on. I think this is partly due to the fact that we started cooking together when he was very young. These days he also knows the difference between ½ cup and ⅓ cup and how many ¼ cup make a whole cup. My three-year-old daughter is fast becoming a fan of cooking too. The rule in my kitchen is that once the food is prepared we all have to taste it, but no one is forced to eat it if they don't want to. Often, one kid loves something while the other rejects it but because they feel safe and there are no expectations, they are eager to cook with me.

Children also learn to accept new foods through role-modeling, repetition and exposure and there is no better way to expose children to a variety of ingredients than by choosing a recipe that you and your child would like to prepare together. Children love to eat what they've helped to make.

HERE'S HOW TO GET STARTED:

Make a list of ingredients. Depending on the age of your child, they can either write the words or draw little pictures of what is needed. Go to the grocery store together or, if you are a working parent and this is not possible, choose your ingredients together online. Either way let your child pick ingredients off supermarket shelves or unpack a box that arrives at your doorstep. All this time you are exposing your child to these ingredients—and exposure and repetition are key. Kids love picking vegetables, fruit or herbs and seeing them transform into a dish. Grow your own if you are fortunate enough to have a backyard where you can grow a veggie patch. If you do not have space for vegetables, a few pot plants with herbs on a windowsill or balcony will do the trick.

COOKING WITH YOUR CHILD WILL:

✓ develop fine motor skills.

✓ help him learn about nutrition.

✓ help with desensitization.

✓ add to his food appreciation.

✓ develop his vocabulary.

✓ develop self-esteem.

✓ encourage learning about math.

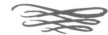

DID YOU KNOW?

Fructose takes a little longer to digest compared to other natural dietary sugars such as glucose or sucrose, so it has less impact on insulin and blood-sugar levels.

HAVE ON HAND:

✓ a sturdy stepping stool

✓ an apron and oven gloves (always supervise when dealing with anything hot)

✓ wooden spoons

✓ metal, plastic or silicone measuring spoons and cups (glass ones can break)

✓ egg separator

✓ spatula

✓ whisk

✓ vegetable peeler

✓ small rolling pin

✓ kid-friendly knife and fork

✓ cookie cutters in different shapes

✓ a set of small bowls

✓ mini muffin pans

✓ salad spinners

✓ cheese grater

✓ knife designed for young cooks or small adult knife (recommended from age four or five)

✓ a child-friendly apron and cooking utensils in colors they like so that your child can help to prepare all aspects of the dishes

KITCHEN SAFETY 101

Safety in the kitchen is something you can never overlook. Teaching children to respect the kitchen environment from a young age will ensure they are responsible and less likely to hurt themselves.

❶ Ensure that all possible hazards are out of reach from young hands. Pot handles need to be turned the other way. Sharp knives should be out of reach.

❷ Never allow children to handle hot food or liquids, sharp utensils, or cleaning products.

❸ Ensure that children wash hands before they start cooking and afterwards as raw food like eggs, meat or fish can contain salmonella or other bacteria.

COOKING WITH UNDER THREES

From the time your child can sit unassisted they will love banging on pots, splashing, and putting (or throwing) veggies or fruit into a bowl or playing with plastic storage containers. From as young as eighteen months they will be ready to assist in more kitchen activities including:

• Washing vegetables. This is an excellent way to expose kids to as many and varied veggies as possible. Peel veggies such as carrots or cucumbers before your little one washes them as this will allow more of the aroma to escape and they will get some of the taste and juice on their hands—all helping to familiarize all their senses to these vegetables.

Cooking Do's and Don'ts

👍 DO...	👎 DON'T...
encourage your child to cook with you on a weekly basis.	talk negatively about food even if you're baking something you don't like or that is high in calories.
create a safe environment for your child.	shout at them for slip-ups or accidents, like eggshells in the batter or spills. Accept that they're bound to happen.
create healthy versions of their favorite foods.	force them to make something. Allowing children to help in choosing what to cook helps them to feel in control.
allow them to get their hands messy.	prepare something that is too sophisticated or does not contain any familiar ingredients (unless your child is an adventurous eater).
praise them for their help (even if it's messy and inaccurate).	force them to eat what you have prepared together.
encourage them to taste the ingredients.	leave young children unattended for even a moment in a kitchen.
taste the food, once prepared, along with them (role modeling).	leave sharp knives within reach.

Do this outdoors when possible as it tends to get very messy.

- Mixing ingredients with a large wooden spoon (always make sure these are at room temperature). Encourage them to hold the bowl with one hand.

- Mashing potatoes with a fork or a potato masher (always make sure the potatoes are at room temperature).

- Playing with raw cookie batter, pizza dough, or bliss ball mix and trying to make balls or other shapes.

- Placing all the ingredients in measuring cups (assisted) into a big bowl.

- Cracking eggs on the side of a bowl with your help (always wash their hands afterwards).

MY TOP RECIPES FOR UNDER THREES:
- Choc Chia Pops, without the chocolate topping (see page 89)
- Tropical Turmeric Smoothie (see page 225)
- Scroll Dough (see page 251)
- Healthy Gingerbread Cookies (see page 92)
- Banana Pancakes (see page 227)

COOKING WITH OVER THREES

As your child gets older, let him take on more responsibilities. All children develop at a different pace, but by the age of three or four, he'll probably have the ability to use basic numeracy (1, 2, 3 teaspoons) and follow instructions. He'll also be able to perform a wider range of tasks like weighing ingredients or using measuring spoons and cups. Also try:

- Washing fruit and veggies with a scrubbing brush over the kitchen sink. This should be a less messy exercise now.

- Cutting and chopping with a kid-friendly knife. Choose soft food such as bananas, dates, cheese or strawberries.

- Mixing ingredients with a spoon or his hands.

- Kneading dough. Let him start the process and take over to ensure the desired outcome.

- Rolling and cutting cookie dough—choose plastic cutters and a small rolling pin.

- Tearing herbs and lettuce or squashing fruit.

- Straining. This can become messy so it's best to teach your child to balance the sieve over a bowl and tap it rather than shake it around.

- Crumbing. When making fish fingers or chicken nuggets, set up three stations with flour, beaten egg, and breadcrumb/almond meal mixture.

- Using a pestle and mortar to crush spices. A light wooden one is a better choice than a heavy stone or marble one.

- Child-friendly scissors. Always consider the ability of your children before handing them sharp tools. If you do think they can manage then still always keep an eye on them as it's very easy to slip, even for adults.

MY TOP RECIPES FOR OVER THREES:
- Chocolate Spelt Cookies (see page 95)
- Homemade Sweet Potato Pizza (see page 131)
- Fish Fingers (see page 57)
- Smoothies (see page 225)

COOKING WITH OVER FIVES

By age five, your child should be becoming adept at more fine motor skills. Always exercise caution while giving him tasks that involve sharp utensils.

- Measuring. This is a great opportunity for them to use their developing reading and math skills, and to portion out the ingredients.

- Cutting. Snipping herbs is a great place to start and children's scissors work just as well as larger kitchen scissors.

- Chopping. Using a small knife, teach your child to form his other hand into a claw to keep fingertips out of danger. Stay close.

- Grating. Buy a standing grater with a handle and keep watch to ensure your child doesn't get too close to the end of whatever he's grating. Fingers can easily be cut this way.

- Folding. Show children how to fold an egg white into a cake mixture.

- Greasing a cake pan or tray with butter or lining with wax paper.

- Peeling. Children can peel hard-boiled eggs with their fingers—just run them under the cold tap first. They should be more deft with vegetable peelers too, but stay close when they're using these.

- Setting the dinner table. Make family meals a cherished time by handing over this responsibility to your children.

MY TOP RECIPES FOR OVER FIVES:
- Salmon & Millet Rissoles (see page 167)
- Rich Chocolate Black Bean Brownies (see page 119)
- Lamb Koftas (see page 155)
- Cheese Scrolls (see page 251)
- Veggie Pasta Sauce (see page 121)

DID YOU KNOW?

Studies have found that eating whole fruits—especially blueberries, grapes, and apples—is associated with a lower risk of type 2 diabetes.

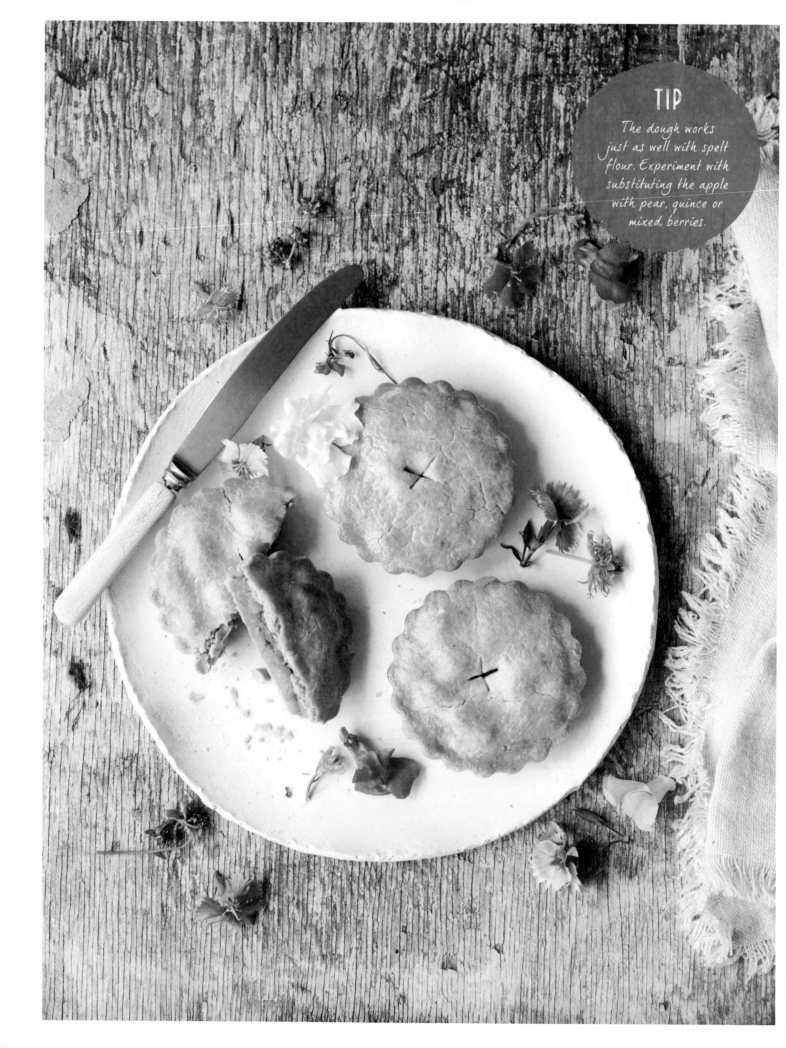

TIP
The dough works just as well with spelt flour. Experiment with substituting the apple with pear, quince or mixed berries.

Prep time: 30 mins
Cooking time: 45 mins
Makes: 6 mini apple pies 3 5/32"
or 1 large pie 8"

Gluten-free Apple Pies

This one was inspired by the grandparents—a delicious dessert that everyone can enjoy without the nasties often found in store-bought pies.

INGREDIENTS

CRUST

2¼ cups (11½ oz) Wholesome Child gluten-free flour mix (see page 32) or 2½ cups (12¼ oz) whole spelt flour

1–2 tbs coconut sugar

¼ tsp sea salt

1 cup (5⅓ oz) cold unsalted butter, diced, plus extra for greasing tin

2 eggs

squeeze lemon juice

pinch lemon zest

FILLING

5–7 red apples, peeled, cored and diced

1–2 tbs coconut sugar (optional)

½ tsp ground cinnamon

2 tbs lemon juice

½ cup (2¾ oz) raisins

2 tbs almond meal or rice crumbs

INSTRUCTIONS

Preheat the oven to 355°F. Grease 6 mini pie tins or one large pie tin with unsalted butter.

To make the crust, mix the dry ingredients together in a large bowl. Add the diced butter and use your fingertips to gently work the butter into the flour and sugar until the mixture resembles bread crumbs.

Crack one egg into the bowl, add lemon juice and zest and gently mix with your hands until the dough comes together. Wrap it in cling wrap and place in the fridge.

Meanwhile, add the apple to a medium-sized pan with the coconut sugar, cinnamon, and lemon juice and place over a medium heat.

Simmer gently for 5 mins or until the apples are just tender. Remove from the heat and add raisins and almond meal. Leave to cool.

Dust a clean work surface and rolling pin with gluten-free flour. Divide pastry dough into two and roll out one half until ⅙" thick.

If making mini apple pies, divide dough into six 4" squares and carefully ease the pastry into the pie tins. If you are making one large apple pie, roll pastry around the rolling pin, then unroll carefully over a 8" pie dish.

Pour apple filling into the dish.

Roll out the other pastry half until 6/32" thick. Divide into six 4" squares and place each square on top of the pie. If making a large pie carefully roll the pastry around the rolling pin, then unroll it over the top of the pie.

Fold the excess pastry back in then pinch and crimp the edges together using your finger and thumb and cut away excess.

Brush the top with the remaining egg, then using a small sharp knife, make small incisions in the center of the pies to let steam escape as it cooks.

Bake for 30–40 mins or until golden brown.

Allow to cool. Serve with homemade coconut custard or macadamia nut ice cream.

Serving and storing leftovers: Serve immediately, store in the fridge for up to 4 days or freeze for up to 4 months.

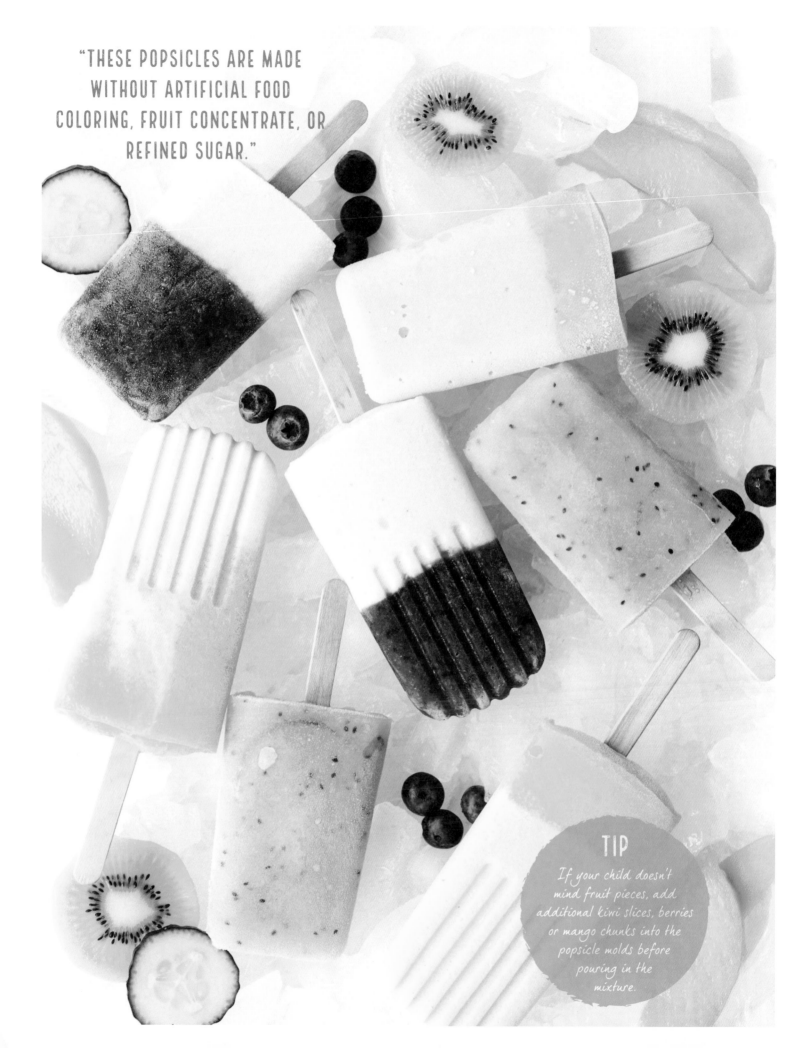

"THESE POPSICLES ARE MADE WITHOUT ARTIFICIAL FOOD COLORING, FRUIT CONCENTRATE, OR REFINED SUGAR."

TIP

If your child doesn't mind fruit pieces, add additional kiwi slices, berries or mango chunks into the popsicle molds before pouring in the mixture.

Prep time: 10 mins
(+ 4 hours freezing time)
Makes: 4

Vegan Gluten Free Nut Free

Kiwi & Coconut Popsicles

INGREDIENTS

2 very ripe kiwis

1 medium-sized cucumber, peeled and chopped

1/4 tsp lemon juice

1 cup coconut water

1 tbs maple syrup (optional)

EQUIPMENT

4 popsicle molds

INSTRUCTIONS

Place all ingredients in a blender and blend until smooth and creamy.

Pour into popsicle molds and freeze for at least 4 hours before serving.

Serving and storing leftovers: Serve immediately or store in the freezer for up to 4 months.

Prep time: 10 mins
(+ 4½ hours freezing time)
Makes: 4

Vegan Gluten Free

Berry & Pineapple Popsicles

INGREDIENTS

FIRST LAYER:
1/2 cup (2⁴/₅ oz) mixed berries, frozen

1/4 cup coconut milk

1 tsp maple syrup (optional)

SECOND LAYER:
1/2 cup (2⁴/₅ oz) pineapple, frozen

1/2 cup coconut cream

1/4 cup (1²/₅ oz) cashews, soaked for 2 hours, rinsed and drained

EQUIPMENT

4 popsicle molds

INSTRUCTIONS

To make the first layer, place all ingredients into a blender and blend until smooth and creamy. Pour mixture into popsicle molds, leaving room for the second layer. Place in the freezer for 30 mins to set.

To make the second layer, place all ingredients into a blender and blend until smooth and creamy. Remove molds from freezer and pour mixture on top of the first layer. Freeze for at least 4 hours before serving.

Serving and storing leftovers: Serve immediately or store in freezer for up to 4 months.

Prep time: 10 mins
(+ 4½ hours freezing time)
Makes: 6

Vegan Gluten Free Nut Free

Mango Popsicles

INGREDIENTS

FIRST LAYER:
1/2 cup (2⁴/₅ oz) mango, frozen

1/4 cup coconut cream

1/4 cup (2¹/₃ oz) coconut yogurt

1/4 tsp pure vanilla extract

1/2 tbs maple syrup (optional)

SECOND LAYER:
1 cup (5 2/3 oz) mango, frozen

1/2 cup filtered water

1/2 tbs maple syrup

EQUIPMENT

6 popsicle molds

INSTRUCTIONS

To make the first layer, place all ingredients into a blender and blend until smooth and creamy. Pour mixture into popsicle molds, leaving room for the second layer. Place in the freezer for 30 mins to set.

To make the second layer, place all ingredients into a blender and blend until smooth and creamy.

Remove molds from freezer and pour mixture on top of the first layer. Freeze for at least 4 hours before serving.

Serving and storing leftovers: Serve immediately or store in freezer for up to 4 months.

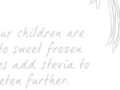

If your children are used to sweet frozen popsicles add stevia to sweeten further.

TIP

For a dairy-free version, try whipped coconut cream or our Coconut Cream Frosting (see page 281), or simply top with berries.

"WATERMELONS ARE HIGH IN POTASSIUM, VITAMIN C, AND PHYTONUTRIENTS INCLUDING LYCOPENE."

VEG
Vegetarian

Gluten
Free

Nut
Free

Egg
Free

Prep time: 15 mins
Makes: 16 pieces

Watermelon Cake

When my daughter turned two and started daycare we served a watermelon cake for her birthday. The kids loved it, the teachers thought it was the best idea ever, and parents were amazed at how quickly it disappeared!

INGREDIENTS

1 large seedless watermelon (15½ lbs to 19¾ lbs)

1–2 cups whipping cream (depends on the size of your watermelon)

½ tsp pure vanilla extract (optional)

seasonal fresh fruit (for topping)

EQUIPMENT

electric hand mixer

INSTRUCTIONS

Remove the top and bottom from the watermelon as well as the rind from the middle section. You should be left with a cake-shaped piece of watermelon.

Pat the outside of the watermelon dry with paper towels. This is a very important step as it helps the whipped cream adhere to the watermelon.

In a large bowl, whip the cream until firm and creamy. Add vanilla extract, if using, and whip to combine.

Frost the watermelon cake with the whipped cream and top with your favorite fruits and berries or serve without.

Serving and storing leftovers: Serve immediately or store in the fridge for up to 3 days.

VEG
Vegetarian

Gluten
Free

Nut
Free

Egg
Free

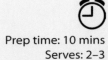

Prep time: 10 mins
Serves: 2–3

Watermelon & Feta Salad

INGREDIENTS

¼ seedless watermelon (approx 4½ lbs)

¾ cup (3¾ oz) sheep's feta cheese, crumbled

juice of 2 limes or lemons

¼ cup (⅙ oz) fresh mint, finely chopped

sea salt and pepper, to taste

INSTRUCTIONS

Cut rind off watermelon then chop into small cubes and place in a medium-sized bowl. Add feta, lime juice, and mint and season with a pinch of salt and pepper.

Serving and storing leftovers: Serve immediately or store in the fridge for up to 4 days.

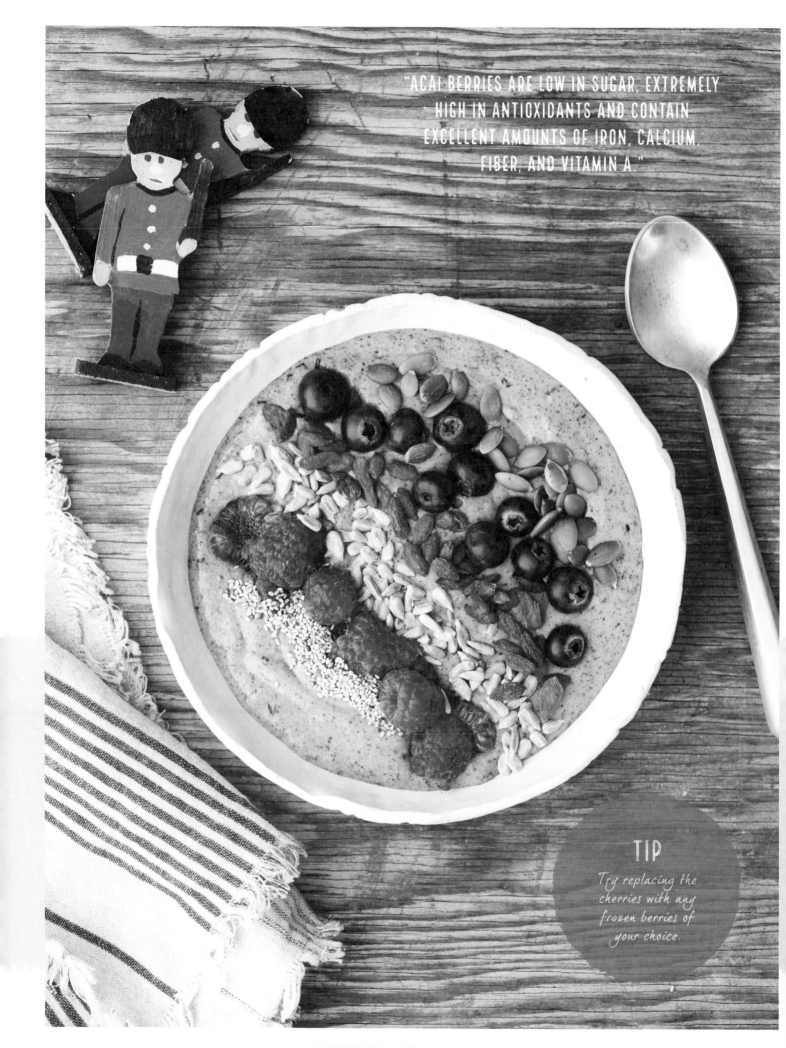

"ACAI BERRIES ARE LOW IN SUGAR, EXTREMELY
HIGH IN ANTIOXIDANTS AND CONTAIN
EXCELLENT AMOUNTS OF IRON, CALCIUM,
FIBER, AND VITAMIN A."

TIP
Try replacing the
cherries with any
frozen berries of
your choice.

Prep time: 5 mins
Serves: 2

Acai Breakfast Bowl

My daughter and I call this a princess bowl and decorate it with pink and purple fruits—her favorite colors. Packed with antioxidants, it's a great way to start the day.

INGREDIENTS

1 large ripe banana

1 cup (5 2/3 oz) frozen cherries

1 cup coconut milk

2 tbs acai powder

2 tbs chia seeds

5 cashews, soaked, or 1 tbs nut butter

2 Medjool dates, pitted

optional toppings: banana slices, berries, nuts, seeds

EQUIPMENT

blender

INSTRUCTIONS

Place all ingredients into a blender and blend until smooth and creamy. Place in a bowl and add favorite toppings.

Serving and storing leftovers: Serve immediately or store in the freezer for up to 4 months. Alternatively, place leftovers in popsicle molds and freeze for 4 hours before serving.

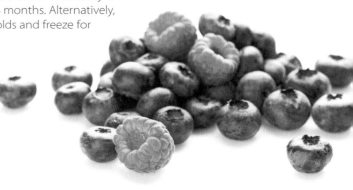

Prep time: 10 mins
Serves: 2

Carrot, Walnut & Apple Salad

INGREDIENTS

4 medium-sized carrots, peeled and grated

2 medium-sized green apples, peeled and grated

1/3 cup (1 3/4 oz) golden raisins

1/3 cup (1 4/5 oz) walnuts, crushed

juice of 1 lemon

1/2 tbs maple syrup or raw honey (optional)

2 tbs extra virgin olive oil

1/4 cup (2 1/3 oz) natural yogurt

sea salt and pepper, to taste

INSTRUCTIONS

In a medium-sized bowl, add carrot, apple, golden raisins, and walnuts and stir well to combine.

Mix remaining ingredients well and use as dressing.

Serving and storing leftovers: Serve immediately or store in the fridge for up to 4 days.

Prep time: 5 mins. Cooking time: 45 mins.
Makes: 3 cups

Prep time: 5 mins. Cooking time: 30 mins.
Makes: 1 cup

Apricot & Pear Compote

INGREDIENTS

4 large pears, peeled and cored

1⅓ cup (7½ oz) dried apricots (sulphur-free)

½ tsp ground cinnamon

1 vanilla pod, insides scraped out or ½ tsp pure vanilla extract

filtered water

EQUIPMENT

blender

INSTRUCTIONS

Place all the ingredients in a medium-sized pot and cover with filtered water, then place on a medium heat.

Bring to a boil, reduce heat and cover with a lid. Simmer until water has evaporated. Add more water if necessary. The more you reduce the compote the more intense the flavor and thicker the consistency.

Transfer compote to a blender and blend until smooth.

Fig Jam

INGREDIENTS

12 dried figs, stems removed & chopped

1 tbs lemon juice

2 tbs fresh orange juice

½ tsp fresh thyme

1½ cups filtered water

1 tbs chia seeds

1 tsp coconut sugar (optional)

EQUIPMENT

blender

INSTRUCTIONS

Add all ingredients to a small pot, place over medium heat and bring to a boil. Simmer until water is evaporated and figs are soft.

Place mixture into a blender and blend until smooth.

Serve with yogurt, porridge or on its own.

Our fig jam is high in iron, calcium, fiber, and omega-3s thanks to the added chia seeds.

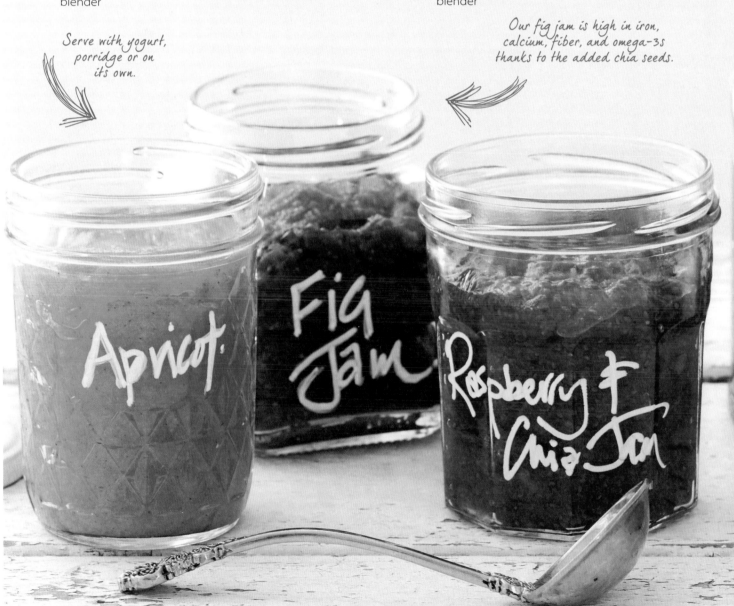

Chia Raspberry Jam

INGREDIENTS

2 cups (11¼ oz) frozen raspberries (or berries of choice)

2 tbs chia seeds

2 tbs maple syrup or raw honey (optional)

2 tbs filtered water

1 tbs coconut oil

1 vanilla pod, insides scraped out or ½ tsp vanilla extract

INSTRUCTIONS

In a small saucepan combine all ingredients, place over medium heat, and bring to a boil.

Turn heat down and simmer for around 10 mins, stirring occasionally.

Serve with yogurt, porridge, as a layer in Parfait (see page 249) or use as a pastry filling.

Rhubarb Compote

INGREDIENTS

1¼ cups (5⅓ oz) rhubarb, cubed

1 medium-sized red apple, peeled, cubed

10 dried apricots (sulphur-free), finely diced

1 vanilla pod, insides scraped out or ½ tsp vanilla extract

2 to 3 cups filtered water

2 tbs maple syrup or raw honey

INSTRUCTIONS

Place all the ingredients except the honey in a medium-sized pot and cover with filtered water.

Place over a medium heat, bring to a boil, reduce heat and cover with a lid. Simmer until water is evaporated. Add more water if necessary. The more you reduce the compote the more intense the flavor and thicker the consistency.

Sweeten with honey if it's too sour for your child's liking.

Blueberry Vanilla Compote

INGREDIENTS

2 medium-sized red apples, peeled, cored and cubed

1 cup (5 2/3 oz) frozen blueberries

1 vanilla pod, insides scraped out or ½ tsp vanilla extract

½ cup filtered water

EQUIPMENT

blender

INSTRUCTIONS

Place all ingredients in a medium-sized pot and bring to a boil.

Turn heat down and simmer for 25 mins or until all water has evaporated.

Put into a blender and blend until smooth and creamy.

Serve on it own, add to Bircher Muesli (see page 257) or porridge or as a topping for Pancakes (see page 51).

 Vegan
 Nut Free
 Gluten Free

Serving and storing leftovers: Serve immediately, store in a jar or in an airtight container in the fridge for up to 2 weeks or freeze for up to 4 months.

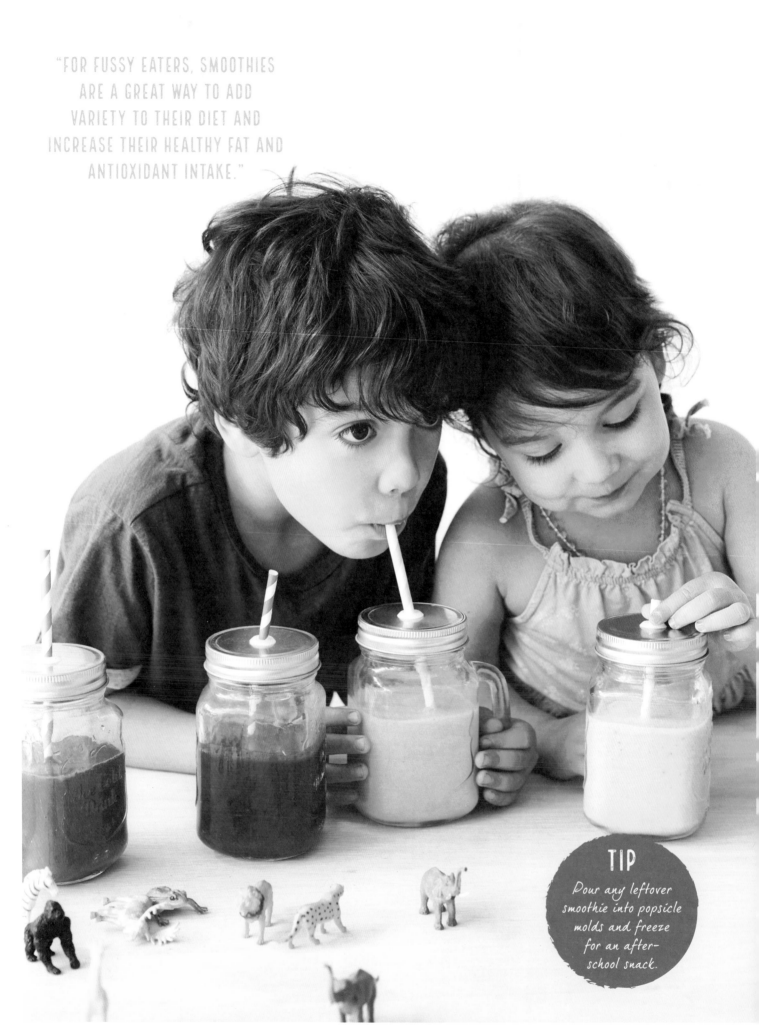

"FOR FUSSY EATERS, SMOOTHIES ARE A GREAT WAY TO ADD VARIETY TO THEIR DIET AND INCREASE THEIR HEALTHY FAT AND ANTIOXIDANT INTAKE."

TIP
Pour any leftover smoothie into popsicle molds and freeze for an after-school snack.

Vegan Gluten Free

Prep time: 5 mins
Serves: 4

Avocado Chocolate Smoothie

INGREDIENTS

1 ripe banana, frozen

½ ripe avocado

2 handfuls kale, rinsed

2 tbs cacao powder

2 tbs carob powder

4 Medjool dates, pitted

1½ cups almond milk

½ cup filtered water

EQUIPMENT
blender

INSTRUCTIONS

Place all ingredients in a blender and blend until smooth and creamy.

Serving and storing leftovers: Serve immediately, store in the fridge for up to 24 hours or freeze for up to 4 months.

Vegan Gluten Free

Prep time: 10 mins
(+ 2–4 hours soaking time)
Serves: 4

Strawberry & Banana Milkshake

INGREDIENTS

2 cups coconut or almond milk

½ cup (2⁴/₅ oz) cashews, soaked for 2–4 hours, rinsed, drained

1 cup (5 2/3 oz) strawberries, frozen

1 ripe banana, frozen

1 tsp chia seeds

1 cup cucumber, peeled and finely sliced

½ tsp pure vanilla extract

EQUIPMENT
blender

INSTRUCTIONS

Place all ingredients into a blender and blend until smooth and creamy.

Serving and storing leftovers: Serve immediately, store in the fridge for up to 24 hours or freeze for up to 4 months.

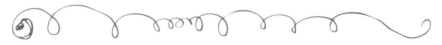

Vegan Gluten Free Nut Free

Prep time: 10 mins
Serves: 4

Beetroot Berry Smoothie

INGREDIENTS

½ cup (2⁴/₅ oz) beetroot, peeled, diced and frozen overnight (optional)

½ cup (2⁴/₅ oz) blueberries, frozen

1 ripe avocado

½ cup coconut water

juice of 1 orange

2 tbs lemon juice

EQUIPMENT
blender

INSTRUCTIONS

Place all ingredients into a blender and blend until smooth and creamy.

Serving and storing leftovers: Serve immediately, store in the fridge for up to 24 hours or freeze for up to 4 months.

Vegan Gluten Free

Prep time: 10 mins
Serves: 4

Tropical Turmeric Smoothie

INGREDIENTS

½ cup (2⁴/₅ oz) pineapple, frozen

1 cup (5¹/₂ oz) mango, frozen

1 cup (3 oz) carrot, peeled and grated

¼ cup (1¹/₅ oz) macadamias or blanched almonds

¼ tsp turmeric, fresh or dried

pinch ginger (optional)

2 cups coconut milk

EQUIPMENT
blender

INSTRUCTIONS

Place all ingredients into a blender and blend until smooth and creamy.

Serving and storing leftovers: Serve immediately, store in the fridge for up to 24 hours or freeze for up to 4 months.

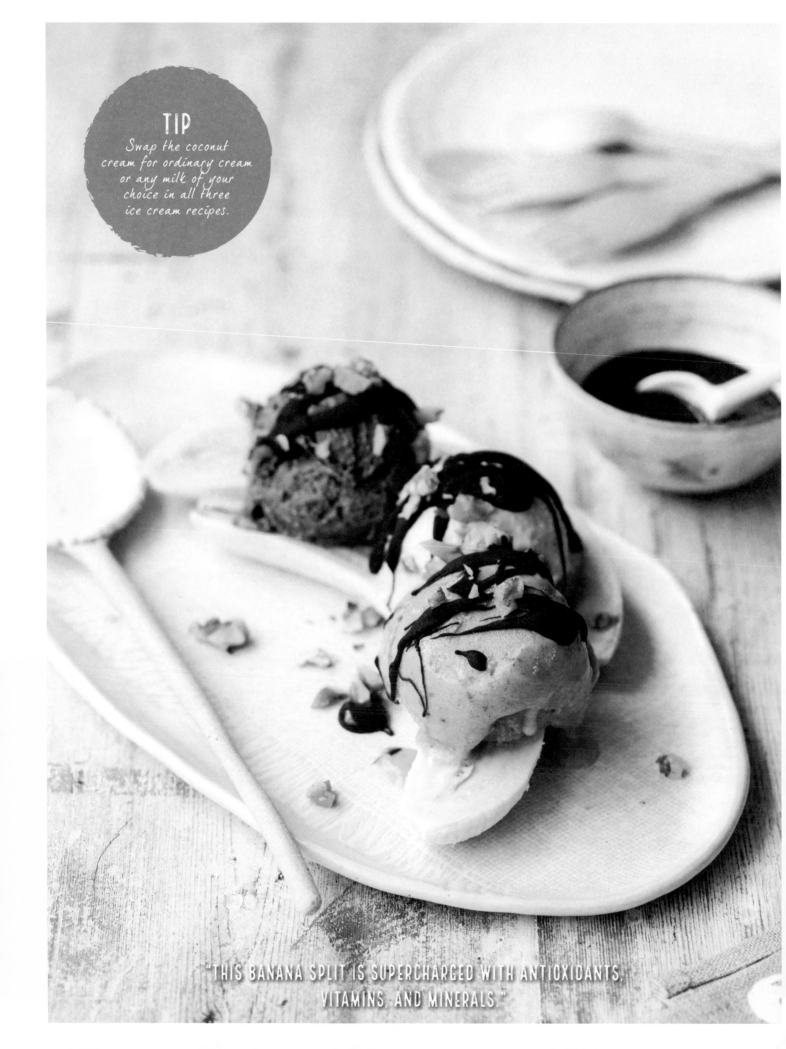

TIP
Swap the coconut cream for ordinary cream or any milk of your choice in all three ice cream recipes.

"THIS BANANA SPLIT IS SUPERCHARGED WITH ANTIOXIDANTS, VITAMINS, AND MINERALS."

Vegan Gluten Free

Prep time: 30 mins (+ 7 hours soaking time
and 4–5 hours freezing time)
Serves: 3

Banana Split Trio

Banana splits remind me of my childhood, so a version free of artificial colors and refined sugar was high on my list of desserts to share with my kids.

INGREDIENTS

3 ripe bananas, cut in half lengthways

MACADAMIA VANILLA ICE CREAM

1 cup (5 oz) macadamia nuts, soaked for 7 hours or overnight, rinsed and drained

1 cup coconut cream or milk

1 ripe banana, frozen

2 tbs maple syrup or raw honey

½ tsp pure vanilla extract

STRAWBERRY ICE CREAM

2 cups (11¼ oz) strawberries, frozen

1 cup coconut cream or milk

2 tbs maple syrup or raw honey

¼ tsp pure vanilla extract

AVOCADO CHOCOLATE ICE CREAM

1 ripe avocado

1 cup coconut cream or milk

1 tbs almond butter

generous 2–3 tbs maple syrup or raw honey

2 tbs cacao powder

¼ tsp pure vanilla extract

pinch Himalayan rock salt

OPTIONAL TOPPINGS:

melted dark chocolate

crushed walnuts

EQUIPMENT

high-powered blender such as Vitamix or Thermomix for smooth consistency

INSTRUCTIONS

For the macadamia vanilla ice cream place soaked macadamia nuts and coconut cream into a blender and blend until smooth.

Add banana, maple syrup, and vanilla and blend until smooth and creamy.

For the strawberry ice cream place all ingredients into a blender and blend until smooth.

Use the same method to make the avocado chocolate ice cream.

Pour the 3 mixtures into 3 separate airtight containers and freeze for at least 4–5 hours.

Thaw for 10 mins before serving. If you desire a creamier consistency, break ice cream apart and place back into your blender, then blend until smooth and creamy.

Place bananas on a serving plate and add a scoop of each ice cream to the centers. Drizzle with melted dark chocolate and sprinkle crushed walnuts on top.

Serving and storing leftovers: Serve immediately or store leftover ice cream in the freezer for up to 4 months.

VEG Gluten Free Dairy Free

Vegetarian

Prep time: 3–5 mins
Cooking time: 5 mins
Makes: 16 mini pancakes

Banana Pancakes

INGREDIENTS

2 eggs

1 ripe banana

1–2 tbs almond meal

1 tsp arrowroot

½ tsp ground cinnamon (optional)

pinch sea salt

coconut oil, for frying

EQUIPMENT

hand-held blender

INSTRUCTIONS

Using a hand-held blender, combine eggs and banana together until smooth consistency is reached.

Add almond meal, arrowroot, cinnamon, and salt and whisk to combine.

Heat coconut oil in a small frying pan over medium heat.
Place one tbs of mixture in pan and reduce heat.

Turn over when small bubbles appear or until golden brown on each side, approximately 1 min each side.

Serving and storing leftovers: Serve immediately or store in fridge for up to 4 days or freeze for up to 4 months.

Add 1 tsp of chia seeds, 1 tbs of almond meal, 1 tbs of coconut flour or 1 tbs of protein powder.

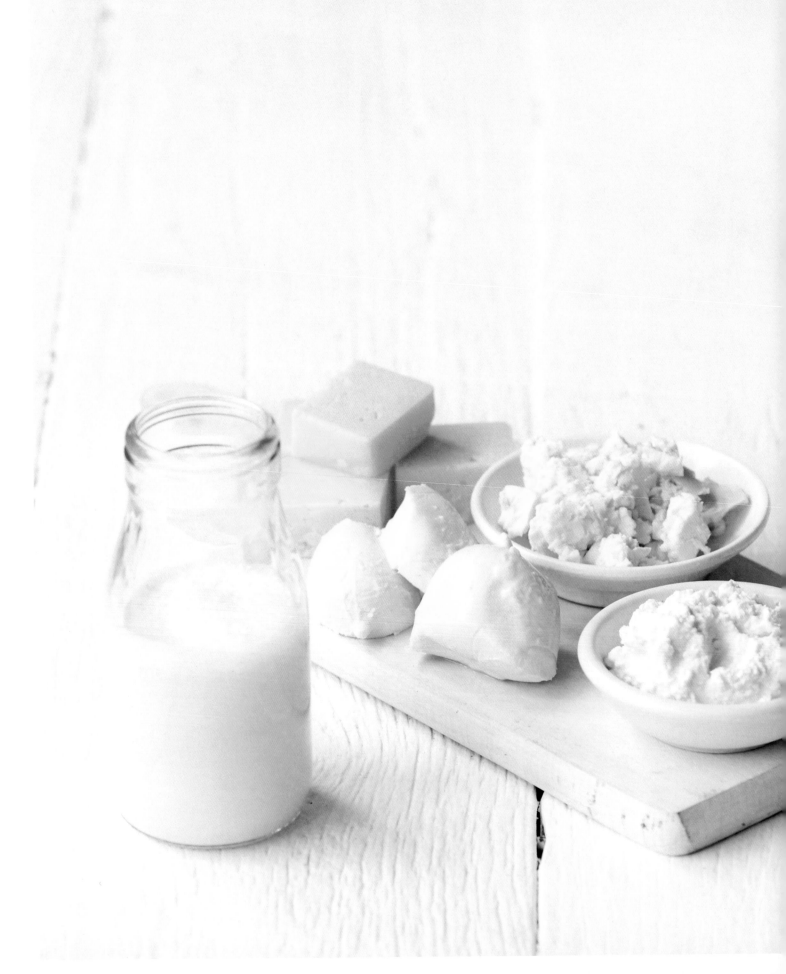

Rethink Dairy

MODERATE MILK CONSUMPTION AND FOCUS ON HIGH-CALCIUM FOODS

M ilk, yogurt, cheese, and ice cream are all firm favorites for many children, especially the fussy eaters. Milk products have long been touted as an essential part of a child's daily diet because they're considered an excellent source of calcium and contain potassium, vitamin D, magnesium, and protein. Dairy is not something I see most parents struggling to get their kids to eat, although of course there are exceptions.

Even so, speaking about dairy in my workshops always raises lots of questions: How much dairy should my child be eating or drinking? Is low fat or full fat/whole milk best? Why is it best to choose organic milk? These days our supermarket shelves are laden with so many options, it can be tricky for parents to pick out the best quality dairy products for their children. But more and more we are learning that the closer food is to its pure, natural form the better, and dairy products are no exception.

WHY SO MUCH FOCUS ON DAIRY?

It's no wonder that calcium-rich milk has been seen as a hero for growing children. Calcium is the most abundant mineral in the body, vital for the development of healthy bones and teeth in childhood. It is essential for building a healthy skeleton by the time we reach young adulthood. Along with strong bones, calcium helps muscles and nerves to work properly as well as aiding hormone and enzyme release. Rickets, a disease caused by calcium and/or vitamin D deficiency—thankfully now rare in Western societies—causes softening and even deformity of bones in babies and younger kids, as well as muscle pain and weakness.

It's easy to confuse the importance of calcium with the need for dairy in our diet. The reality is that it's not dairy per se that is so important but rather calcium which is crucial to the health of our children. The reason we focus on dairy is that although there are many non-dairy food sources of calcium, gram for gram dairy products rank high. However, it's growing increasingly common to see children on dairy-free diets due to food sensitivities, allergies, cultural or dietary preferences. A child

following a dairy-free diet should always be supervised by a qualified health practitioner, as calcium supplementation may become necessary.

CALCIUM-RICH FOODS ARE IMPORTANT FOR:

✓ Bone health
✓ Building strong teeth
✓ Aiding in proper muscle contraction
✓ Secreting and regulating hormones
✓ Transmitting messages through the nerves (transmitting nerve impulses)
✓ Proper clotting of the blood

HOW MUCH DAIRY (OR CALCIUM) DOES MY CHILD REQUIRE?

Ages two to three: 2 servings per day (700mg calcium)

Ages four to eight: 2½ servings per day (1000mg calcium)

BEST NON-DAIRY SOURCES OF CALCIUM:

3 oz of sardines with bones = 325mg

2⁴⁄₅ oz salmon canned with bones = 240mg

¼ cup almonds = 95mg

1 tbs of unhulled tahini = 50mg

3 oz tofu = 55mg–300mg

½ cup cooked broccoli = 35mg

SO WHAT'S THE PROBLEM WITH DAIRY?

The main issue I see in my practice with regard to dairy is that it takes up too much space in a child's diet. I often see young children who have five servings or more of dairy per day. A typical diet might look like this: milk and cereal for breakfast, a yogurt for a mid-morning snack, a cheese sandwich or string cheese in the lunch box, a flavored milk or ice cream after school, pasta with cheese for dinner plus a glass of milk before bed.

So often I see children who are eating too much dairy suffering from anemia. Too much

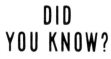

DID YOU KNOW?

99% of the body's calcium is stored in the bones and teeth.

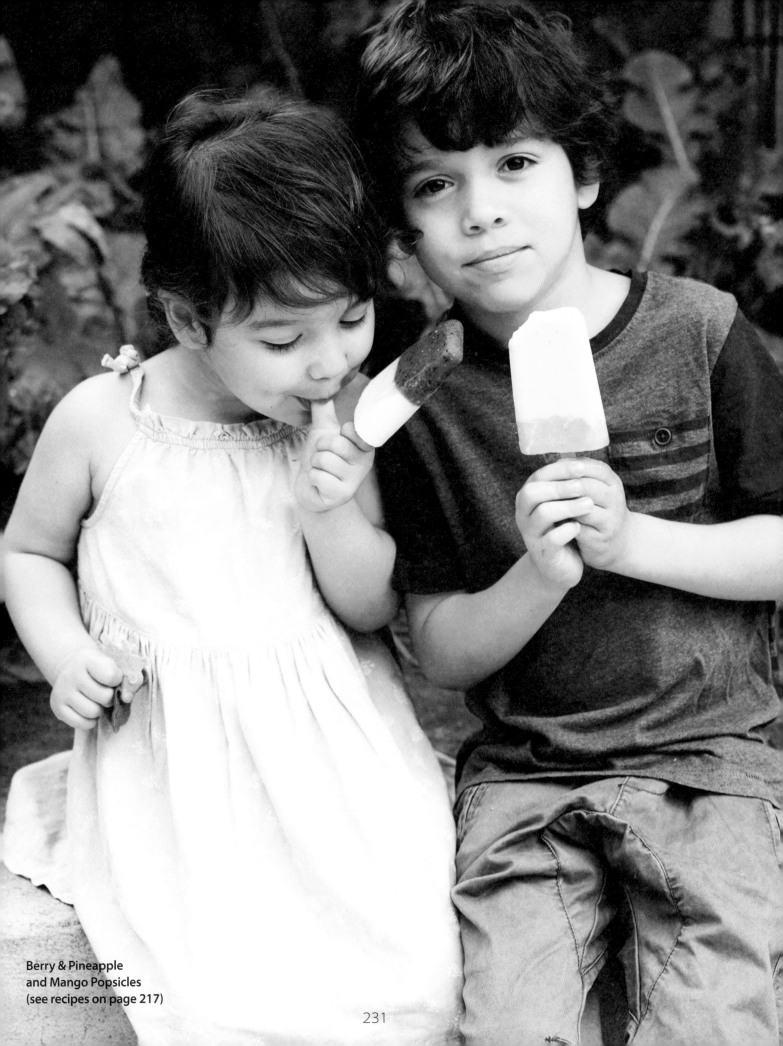

Berry & Pineapple
and Mango Popsicles
(see recipes on page 217)

231

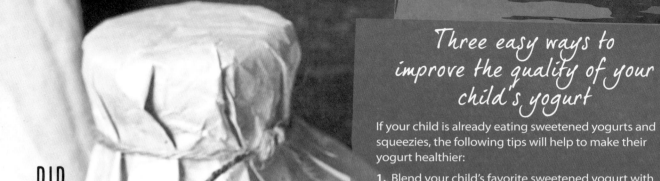

Three easy ways to improve the quality of your child's yogurt

If your child is already eating sweetened yogurts and squeezies, the following tips will help to make their yogurt healthier:

1. Blend your child's favorite sweetened yogurt with natural yogurt. Start at a ratio of 3:1 and slowly decrease the sweetened yogurt and increase the natural yogurt. This simple step will reduce sugar by up to 50 percent.

2. Let your child choose reusable yogurt pouches and fill with natural yogurt blended with a small amount of honey or pureed fruit (or try one of our fruit compotes or jams on pages 222–223).

3. Buy a small container and let your child decorate it with stickers. Blend natural yogurt and their favorite fruit together, place in the container, and freeze overnight. Remove from the freezer in the morning and by mid-morning it should be nice and slushy.

WHAT DOES ONE SERVING OF DAIRY LOOK LIKE?

DAIRY	SERVING	CALCIUM
milk	1 cup	300mg
whole milk yogurt	6 oz container	205mg
yellow cheese such as gouda, swiss or cheddar	1½ oz	300mg
white cheese such as ricotta or quark or goat cheese	½ cup	255mg

calcium in a child's diet can interfere with iron absorption and often takes the place of important iron-rich foods in their diet.

Another important lesson I learned when working on the MEND program, was that children over the age of one, unless breastfeeding or under pediatric supervision, should drink water over milk and save their calories for calcium-rich food instead.

Although milk is a good source of calcium, magnesium and vitamin D, there's no evidence that drinking it reduces bone fractures as we age. Additionally, these nutrients are available from many other food sources like yogurt, cheese, and leafy green vegetables. Milk is also filling for little tummies and may prevent your child from eating meals. Some studies show milk to be estrogenic, meaning it promotes the production of estrogen, and so possibly linked to hormonal issues.

While further research is needed, some experts believe drinking too much milk can contribute to obesity. And then there are concerns about pasteurized and homogenized milk losing good bacteria and enzymes that aid in digestion as well as questions over dairy from cows fed with grain that may be highly processed. My advice is to offer children no more than two servings of dairy a day and ensure they come from an organic source wherever possible. It's always best to offer cheese and yogurt over cow's milk as they are easier to digest. This does not apply to babies under one year of age on a cow's milk formula.

LOOK OUT FOR AND AVOID:

- Hormones
- Bovine growth promoters
- Preservatives
- Additives
- Sweeteners
- Vegetable oils (unless organic, cold-pressed)

LOW-FAT VS FULL FAT

This topic is causing heated debate. The Dietitians Association of Australia and the American Academy of Pediatrics continue to advise that children over the age of two move onto low-fat dairy products. There are many nutritionists like myself who disagree. Let's look at it from an empirical point of view: When fat is taken out of dairy products they become watery and unappetizing, so manufacturers cleverly add sugar, flavors and coloring to make them more appealing again. If you offer a young child a serving of whole natural yogurt like our

grandparents enjoyed, they will often happily eat it as is, or you may have to add a teaspoon of honey to sweeten it. You would never add 4–5 teaspoons of honey to 1 cup of yogurt, but that's often how much sugar is in flavored low-fat yogurts marketed to young children.

Consider the vitamins and minerals in dairy. These are fat-soluble vitamins A, D, E and K. Meaning without fat they are not as efficiently absorbed. Vitamin K, found naturally in butterfat, gets taken out of fat-free versions altogether. Certainly, if your child is overweight or obese and they are drinking more than one cup of milk per day, then I would recommend offering low-fat milk or preferably water instead. In my clinical experience, however, when I swap children over to full-fat dairy products they tend to eat less of it and stay fuller for longer. If your child is at a healthy weight and has no other medical conditions, my recommendation is that they continue to consume full cream milk products after age two, but in moderation (no more than two servings a day). It's best to buy organic whole milk from grass-fed cows and choose non-homogenized milk if possible (homogenization prevents liquid and fat from separating).

WHY ORGANIC MATTERS

We all know organic/biodynamic farming is better for the environment and better for cows, but it's also healthier for us too. Organic/biodynamic farming where cows are fed mostly pasture, produce superior milk free of pesticides, antibiotics and growth hormones and higher in omega-3s than conventional milk.

WHAT IS A2 MILK?

A2 milk is starting to gain popularity in places like Australia, New Zealand, UK, China and some parts of the US. A1 and A2 beta-casein are two types of milk protein. A long time ago, prior to domestication, there was only A2. However, after domestication some cows started to produce the A1 protein too. Some studies are suggesting that A2 is less likely to cause inflammation (which can lead to a raft of diseases) and is more easily tolerated by those who find ordinary milk hard to digest.

A connection has also been made between A1 milk and type 1 diabetes, heart disease, and autism. Human breast milk is A2, which also points to A2 being better for us—though it may be possible for a mother drinking A1 milk to pass this on in her own milk. Supermarket milk usually contains more A1 than A2 and pure-A2 cow's milk is now being marketed

DID YOU KNOW?

Calcium on its own is not enough. We need vitamin D to absorb the calcium. We can make our own vitamin D when our bare skin is exposed to sunlight, or get it from eating oily fish, cod liver oil, egg yolks, and fortified foods such as cereals and yogurt.

How to choose yogurt

Most yogurts aimed at children are high in added sugars. One squeezie yogurt can contain up to five teaspoons of sugar, and in my practice I see children who consume two to three squeezie yogurts a day.

Plain natural yogurt, if introduced early, can be one of the best ways to stretch your child's flavor range to include sour foods. Even if your child already prefers sweetened yogurt, encourage them to try natural yogurt with a drizzle of raw honey or pureed fresh fruit, or add natural yogurt to smoothies in place of milk.

- Choose organic natural, full cream yogurts or natural preservative-free yogurts..
- Choose yogurts with added probiotics to promote gut health.
- Try natural yogurts made with different milks and also vegan versions like coconut yogurt without any additives.

SHEEP'S MILK YOGURT. This is a rich and creamy full-flavored yogurt. I often recommend weaning babies onto this yogurt due to the fact it's easier on the digestive system, and high in fats which babies need.

GOAT'S MILK YOGURT. This is a full-flavored yogurt with a slightly more pronounced gamey flavor.

High in calcium, it may be easier to digest for some children. The best way to ensure your child likes this yogurt is to introduce it from when they are babies, or for older children add it to homemade smoothies or frozen popsicles.

WHOLE MILK YOGURT. The richest of the plain yogurts, whole-milk yogurt contains $1/5$ oz to $1/4$ oz of fat per cup. Some brands of whole-milk yogurt, called farm-style, come with a layer of yogurt cream on top.

GREEK YOGURT. A thicker, creamier type of yogurt, which has had the liquid removed so will have higher concentrations of fat and protein. Greek yogurt is traditionally strained and has the whey removed, resulting in a thicker yogurt. Always choose natural versions over ones with added sugar or fruit preserves.

NATURAL YOGURT. No added flavors, sweeteners, or preservatives.

FLAVORED YOGURTS. Added flavors, sugar, fruit, fruit concentrates (fructose)—it's best to avoid starting your children on these from a young age. Rather add a teaspoon of raw honey and pureed or chopped fresh fruit to natural yogurt.

POT SET. The ingredients used to make the yogurt (milk and cultures) are added directly to the pot where it sets, removing the need for added thickeners or stabilizers.

LABNEH (LABNE). This thick Middle Eastern yogurt 'cheese' is smooth and creamy like sour cream. It is often eaten with a drizzle of olive oil and chopped mint, and served with pita bread.

SOY YOGURT. Made from soy milk, this product has the texture and consistency of dairy yogurt. It's rare, however, to find a commercially available soy yogurt free from added sugars and flavors. This is my least favorite alternative.

COCONUT YOGURT. Made from coconut milk, it's fast gaining popularity. It's an excellent choice for children with dairy allergies or intolerances, however many of the quality brands available in health food stores come with a hefty price tag. If you want to make your own coconut yogurt see our recipe on www.wholesomechild.com.au. Due to the coconut flavor, it is most often sweetened. My sweetener of choice is stevia, monkfruit or other fruits.

KEFIR. Kefir is my number one go-to dairy product for kids, although it can also be dairy free. This cultured yogurt-like drink is naturally lower in lactose and provides greater natural probiotic properties for re-establishing healthy gut flora than yogurt, and can help improve digestion in kids. It is a great choice for anyone with lactose intolerance, as lactic acid bacteria have already got to work digesting the lactose for you. As it ferments, it develops a complex matrix of beneficial microorganisms including yeast. It's also rich in protein, calcium, and B-vitamins. Look for it in health food stores or make your own using kefir grains.

as a healthier choice for families. Goat, sheep, buffalo and camel milk is pure A2 too. Still, while many debate the healthiest choice for families with any history of dairy intolerance, my first choice for families with no-dairy sensitivities is to go for organic, grass-fed milk.

IS SHEEP'S OR GOAT'S MILK BETTER THAN COW'S MILK?

Along with being pure A2, often goat's milk and sheep's milk are lower in lactose than cow's milk. Another benefit is that both sheep and goats are able to produce good milk on a grass-fed diet and often do not have to be supplemented with grains—though of course one can't take it for granted that all sheep and goat milk have been produced this way. If you have trouble finding sheep's or goat's milk in your regular supermarket, try your local health foods store or online.

GOAT'S MILK

Pros: Goat's milk contains smaller molecules —more like breast milk, which may make it easier to digest—and goat cheese even more so. High in medium-chain fats and low in short-chain fats, goat milk has the healthiest fat content.

Cons: The flavor can be off-putting for some children. Many goat cheeses on the market contain preservative 202 (see page 266 for more information).

SHEEP'S MILK

Pros: The highest in minerals like calcium and iron, protein and vitamin C. Creamy yet still very low in lactose.

Cons: Higher fat content than cow's or goat's milk, plus the flavor can be off-putting for some children and it's not as easy to find.

WHY ARE CHEESE AND YOGURT EASIER TO DIGEST THAN MILK?

To digest lactose, the natural sugar in milk, we need lactase. Most people don't produce much lactase after infancy which can make them intolerant to lactose. Hard cheeses and yogurt lose lactose during the production process, and some quality branded yogurt has live cultures added which can help facilitate digestion, so children with mild sensitivities or intolerances may be able to handle these in small quantities a lot better than straight milk. However, if a child is suffering from an allergy to milk protein, rather than lactose, this won't help. A true milk allergy is an immune response to one or both of the milk proteins and can be severe.

WHAT ABOUT STRING CHEESE

String cheese are highly processed, high in sodium and more likely to be made with milk from grain-fed cows. I also think it's best to get children out of the habit of expecting everything to come in wrapping. It's harmful to the environment and also sets children up to expect that food should be individually wrapped and come from a supermarket. If your child likes string cheese, start to work on transitioning him to cheese shapes instead. Often when transitioning from string cheese I tell parents to buy a block of cheese which is often cheaper, lower in sodium and more environmentally friendly. Either grate cheese into a small container that fits into a lunch box or let your child cut it into fun shapes using cookie cutters.

WHAT IF MY CHILD WON'T EAT DAIRY?

Don't worry. Children can quite happily thrive without dairy as long as they are receiving adequate amounts of calcium from other sources. Try meat and vegetable stew, a sardine sandwich (don't knock it till you try it—I grew up eating these and they taste even better toasted), a rice paper wrap with organic tofu, hummus and shredded bok choy, a handful of almonds, a bliss ball that contains dried figs, sesame seeds and almonds, a Rich Chocolate Black Bean Brownie (see recipe on page 119). However, if your child has a limited diet due to fussy eating and adequate calcium sources are in short supply, working to get them to eat dairy will be a great way to ensure their calcium needs are met. Recipes for the following tips can be found throughout the book:

- Add yogurt to fruit smoothies.
- Make homemade ice cream using milk, cream or yogurt.
- Make mini-pizzas and top with cheese.
- Add grated cheese into omelettes.
- Serve scrolls or bread made with yogurt in the batter.
- Offer savory muffins or rice balls with cheese blended through.
- Offer pasta sauce with cheese or cream blended in.

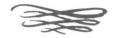

DID YOU KNOW?

Full-fat milk products contain less lactose, more vitamins, and will have less of an effect on blood glucose levels than low-fat milk products.

Consider this...

A healthy calcium intake for a child can be achieved by excluding cow's milk and including good-quality dairy products, like natural yogurt and goat cheese in moderation, and an abundance of non-dairy calcium-rich foods.

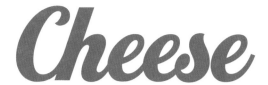

Cheese

While most cheese is high in calcium, it can also be high in sodium. As a general rule, look for low-sodium cheeses such as soft and semi-soft white cheeses.

HIGH SODIUM

GOUDA	CHEDDAR	FETA	PARMESAN	COTTAGE CHEESE
What is it? Children like its mild and smooth consistency, plus it's milder than cheddar. High in calcium but high in sodium too.	**What is it?** Stronger flavor than Gouda and available in different strengths, the strongest can be grainy, also high in calcium and sodium.	**What is it?** Although it's a white cheese, feta is extremely high in salt and contains moderate amounts of calcium compared to other cheeses. Many kids love feta and, if you are going to use it, it's best to soak in water overnight to reduce the sodium content.	**What is it?** A hard cheese with a distinct strong flavor, it is extremely high in calcium but also in sodium. Should be used sparingly—one tbs contains more than 25 percent of a toddler's daily recommended salt intake.	**What is it?** Though a firm favorite among health-conscious moms, most low-fat cottage cheeses are high in sodium and have more preservatives than the full fat versions. If your child likes cottage cheese, look for full cream, preservative free options.
How to use it Serve on its own, with fruit or added to sandwiches, as a pizza topping, or use in quiches or frittatas.	**How to use it** As with Gouda, a versatile cheese and good for cooking and melting.	**How to use it** Crumble over salad or vegetables, add to quiches, or toss with pasta.	**How to use it** Sprinkle sparingly over pasta or tarts, add to pesto sauce.	**How to use it** Add to salads, as a dip for veggies, on sandwiches, on top of baked potatoes or to lasagne. Cottage cheese is not the best choice for cooking or baking.

MODERATE SODIUM

MOZZARELLA	SHEEP'S MILK CHEVRE
What is it? A semi-soft white cheese with a sweet, mild flavor, it has a high calcium and moderate sodium content. It is a great option for children who do not like the strong flavor of yellow cheeses. For authentic mozzarella look for ones made from buffalo milk. Bocconcini (little bites or mouthfuls in Italian) are small mozzarella-style balls often made from cow's milk.	**What is it?** For children who are sensitive to cow's milk, I prefer to put them onto a sheep's milk chevre which has a similar consistency to cream cheese and is a good substitute. Sheep's milk chevre is high in fat, but has a good amount of calcium and moderate sodium.
How to use it Add to tomato salads with basil, add into pasta sauces or risotto, use in croquettes, frittatas, and to make rich and creamy sauces.	**How to use it** Spread on crackers or sandwiches, add to sauces, pizza, pasta, and salads.

LOW SODIUM

GOAT CURD	QUARK	CREAM CHEESE
What is it? Easier on the stomach than cow's milk, a good quality goat curd is naturally lower in sodium and calories than yellow cheese and still contains enough calcium.	**What is it?** A healthy white cheese alternative with a similar texture to yogurt, quark is used like a cottage cheese, but unlike other commercial cottage cheeses generally does not contain animal rennet, added sodium or preservatives.	**What is it?** Low in sodium but high in fat and low in calcium compared to other white cheeses. Avoid low-fat versions as they tend to have more additives.
How to use it Spread on crackers or wholegrain bread, add to quiches, frittatas, rice balls, and other savory dishes to replace yellow cheese.	**How to use it** Eat it sweetened with a drizzle of maple syrup, add to quiches or tarts, use as a topping for baked potato or sweet potato, use to create dips, in baked goods or spread onto crackers and sandwiches.	**How to use it** Spread on crackers and bagels, use for dips and pâtés in cheesecake and to make frosting.

Wholesome Child

- Let your child make shapes out of cheese using cookie cutters.
- Milk can be disguised in your child's favorite foods too. Try mixing it in oatmeal or add cream or blocks of cheese to tomato soup.

WHAT ABOUT DAIRY ALLERGIES?

There is a longstanding debate over the place of dairy, especially milk, in any mammal's diet once they have been weaned because dairy allergy or intolerance is extremely common in children. While some children have the constitution to handle cow's milk, others can react severely with eczema or gut irritation.

Growing evidence also suggests that children on the autism spectrum may benefit from a casein (milk protein) and gluten-free diet. Mainstream medical practitioners refute the link but clinical and anecdotal evidence has started to show more and more that for certain children a dairy-free diet can improve behavior and symptoms all round.

If there is a history of dairy allergy in the family look out for any of the following signs of sensitivity:

- Eczema flare-ups
- Loose stools
- Ear infections
- Constantly runny nose
- Bloating
- Cramps
- Rhinitis

If you notice any of these symptoms after your child has eaten dairy then consider decreasing or eliminating dairy for a period of three to six weeks under the supervision of a qualified healthcare practitioner to see if it will reduce their symptoms. Then slowly reintroduce dairy products in small amounts, one by one, and keep an eye out for any reactions.

By the same token, if your child shows no ill effects from consuming dairy products then there is no need for you to cut them out.

WHAT ARE THE BEST SOURCES OF CALCIUM?

Dairy products like milk, cheese, and yogurt contain calcium but there are many other non-dairy food sources such as sardines and tinned salmon plus good vegetarian options including almonds, basil, kale, bok choy, poppy, sesame, and chia seeds.

OTHER NON-DAIRY SOURCES OF CALCIUM

Wholegrain bread, soy milk, chicken, fish and meat broths, dried apricots, oranges, limes, kumquats, watercress, green beans, spring onions, parsley, watercress, nori seaweed, and leeks.

TOP FIVE HIGH-CALCIUM FRUITS

1. Rhubarb
2. Blackcurrants
3. Oranges
4. Kiwi fruit
5. Dried figs

TOP FIVE HIGH-CALCIUM VEGGIES

1. Okra
2. Broccoli
3. Kale
4. Leeks
5. Chinese cabbage (pak choi)

ARE NON-DAIRY ALTERNATIVES A SUITABLE REPLACEMENT FOR MILK?

Non-dairy alternatives (see page 240), should not be used for infants, but you can start introducing them between the ages of one and two. However, they do not offer the same nutritional benefits as whole milk, as they are low in protein and low in fat. And even if they are fortified with calcium, it's often in the form of calcium carbonate, which is not easily absorbed and has been proven to reduce the acidity of the gut harming the absorption of other nutrients too.

The simple truth is that nature cannot be easily replicated by synthetic additives like those found in fortified milks. Calcium needs fat and vitamin D to be absorbed and dairy alternatives are often lacking in both. Offering a child a glass of almond milk after school is not sufficient in itself; however, an almond milk smoothie, blended with whole almonds as well as banana, kale and chia seeds, would be an optimal choice as it contains a higher percentage of nutrients from other calcium rich sources.

Many children's diets include these milk replacements as they may have lactose intolerance, or for a variety of reasons, may be following a dairy-free diet. I don't urge everyone to go dairy-free, but I do believe in mixing up the diet, and rotating the milks you are using.

As discussed earlier, many children are suffering

DID YOU KNOW?

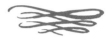

Drinking milk from grass-fed cows can help our balance of omega-3 to omega-6 fatty acids.

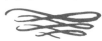

In general, white cheeses are naturally lower in sodium and fat and are a good addition to your child's diet. Feta is an exception, as it is high in sodium.

from what I perceive to be a dairy overload. If your child is drinking two to three glasses of milk daily, there is no need to use additional cow's milk in your cooking or smoothies. By introducing alternatives like almond or coconut milk to replace the milk in smoothies, cereal, porridge or baking, you can actually reduce your family's overall consumption of whole milk and introduce alternative sources of nutrition (especially if you are using homemade nut milks).

If you choose to use these dairy alternatives as a straight-up replacement for cow's milk, it's better to make your own. Store-bought almond milk can have as little as 2 percent almonds, while better brands may only be as high as 10 percent. Homemade almond milk is often prepared with a higher percentage of almonds than supermarket varieties and therefore has higher levels of naturally occurring vitamin E and calcium.

Ultimately, my advice is don't rely on non-dairy milk replacements as a suitable alternative source of calcium.

If your child is unable to consume whole milk, make sure to include calcium-rich foods in their diet, such as almonds, sesame seeds, canned sardines, and salmon.

It is definitely worth keeping store-bought non-dairy milks in your pantry, however, as they are very handy for cooking and baking. If you are time-poor and need to rely on commercially available milk alternatives, become a label-reader and try to avoid those that contain preservatives, additives, added sugars, vegetable oils, flavorings, and colorings.

THREE ADDITIVES TO AVOID IN NON-DAIRY MILKS

Just because a carton of almond or rice milk claims to be "organic" and "heart healthy," does not mean it should be a part of your child's diet. Always read the ingredients label carefully and look out for:

❶ **Carrageenan.** This red seaweed extract is natural but it's also extremely inflammatory and can cause digestive distress and gut irritation. The World Health Organization classifies one type of carrageenan as a "possible human carcinogen."

❷ **Added sugars.** Many milk alternatives are loaded with sugar in the form of cane sugar and agave syrup. Always choose unsweetened options.

❸ **Added vegetable oils.** Canola and sunflower oil are usually extracted with toxic solvents as well as high heat and pressure. Corn and soybean oils are most likely extracted from heavily sprayed GMO crops. Unless you're buying organic, avoid them.

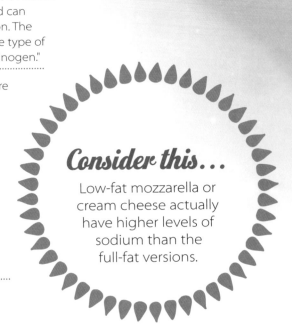

Consider this...
Low-fat mozzarella or cream cheese actually have higher levels of sodium than the full-fat versions.

Five ways to boost your child's calcium intake without milk

1. Substitute canned salmon for tuna in sandwiches at lunch.

2. Blend kale with frozen fruit in a smoothie—they won't notice the difference!

3. Offer dark leafy greens as a side dish or mixed in casseroles.

4. Include bliss balls and trail mixes filled with almonds and calcium-rich seeds.

5. Add a layer of tahini to a peanut butter sandwich or use as a dip for apples and celery sticks.

LACTOSE INTOLERANCE VS COW'S MILK ALLERGY

	LACTOSE INTOLERANCE	COW'S MILK ALLERGY
CAUSE	Not enough lactase to digest lactose.	An immune response to one or both milk proteins.
SYMPTOMS	Uncomfortable but not dangerous: stomach pain, bloating, gas, diarrhea.	Potentially severe: Vomiting, hives, diarrhea, wheezing. Can also trigger life-threatening anaphylaxis.
TREATMENT	Remove or restrict lactose intake. In some cases lactase can be taken.	See your doctor and go to the emergency room if there are any signs of anaphylaxis.
PROGNOSIS	This may not mean an end to dairy. Try lactose-free milk or lower lactose dairy food like Greek yogurt and hard cheeses.	Most children should grow out of it. Be very careful about reintroduction if the reaction was severe. This may need to be done in a hospital setting.

Milk Replacements

RICE MILK	ALMOND MILK	COCONUT MILK	OAT MILK	SOY MILK	HEMP MILK
WHAT IS IT? Generally made from brown rice and water.	**WHAT IS IT?** Generally made from almonds and water.	**WHAT IS IT?** Generally made from the flesh of the coconut and water. Coconut milk contains lauric acid, a medium-chain fatty acid that is easily absorbed and used by the body for energy. It's also completely free from dairy, soy, nuts or grains making it an excellent option for anyone allergic to dairy, nuts or grain-based milks.	**WHAT IS IT?** Made from oats, water and oat flour. (You can make your own by soaking steel-cut oats or whole groats in water overnight, blending the mixture, and then straining it).	**WHAT IS IT?** Made from soybeans and water.	**WHAT IS IT?** Made from hemp seeds and water.
Pros: Nut free. Rice milk is popular as it's naturally sweet and also has a neutral taste.	**Pros:** It has a subtle nuttiness and light texture. If you are on a budget then homemade almond milk is definitely the way to go. See our recipe on page 245.	**Pros:** Coconut milk is my first choice for cooking or baking. I make my own (see recipe on page 249) or buy unsweetened 100% pure coconut milk blended with almond milk. If choosing coconut milk or cream from a can, always choose organic and ensure that it's a BPA free can.	**Pros:** Oat milk is slightly higher in protein than almond and rice milk and much lower in sugars. Oat milk has the added benefit of dietary fiber, which may help to lower blood cholesterol levels. Even unsweetened varieties are naturally sweet and creamy.	**Pros:** One of the highest sources of plant protein (5–10g per 250ml serve) making it similar to dairy milk, very versatile.	**Pros:** Higher in protein than other dairy-free milk except for soy and high in omega 3s—you'll get half of the RDI in a single 250ml serve.
Cons: Can be very low in protein and calcium and high in sugars and calories. The UK Food Standards Agency advises against offering rice milk to children aged between one and four and a half as an alternative to breast milk or cow's milk due to unacceptable levels of arsenic in relation to a young child's body weight.	**Cons:** Store-bought options can be expensive, low in protein and calcium and only contain small amounts of real almonds. Can contain sugar and nasty additives.	**Cons:** Coconut flavor can be strong and as a milk replacement some children don't enjoy the texture. It contains little protein and calcium.	**Cons:** Not suitable for children on a gluten-free diet unless you make your own using gluten-free oats.	**Cons:** With so much controversy surrounding soy, this is my least preferred alternative for children. Even vegans and vegetarians may be better off eating their soy in fermented forms rather than commercial, non-organic GMO brands. There is a 15–20 percent chance that children with dairy allergies or intolerances will react to soy, so do not offer to sensitive children.	**Cons:** Becoming more commercially available but still not as easy to find as other milks. Also, there is some evidence to suggest that vegetarian sources of omega 3 may not have these same health benefits as those in oily fish.
How to use Great for using in small quantities in cakes, muffins, pancakes or waffle recipes.	*How to use* Extremely versatile in smoothies, ice pops, porridge, cooking and baking. Just remember that if you use almond milk in your cooking or baking then whatever you create is no longer school friendly.	*How to use* Most of the recipes in the sugar chapter use coconut milk, as it adds a sweetness to homemade dishes. For dairy-free baking and cooking, coconut cream is the best replacement for cream. You can also blend coconut milk and coconut water for a delicious and light smoothie.	*How to use* Replace normal milk in baked goods, puddings, or heat it over the stove with a dash of cinnamon.	*How to use* Add to porridge, cereal, sauces, baking and cooking.	*How to use* It's thick and creamy with a strong taste. Use in savory dishes or as an alternative to soy milk when baking.

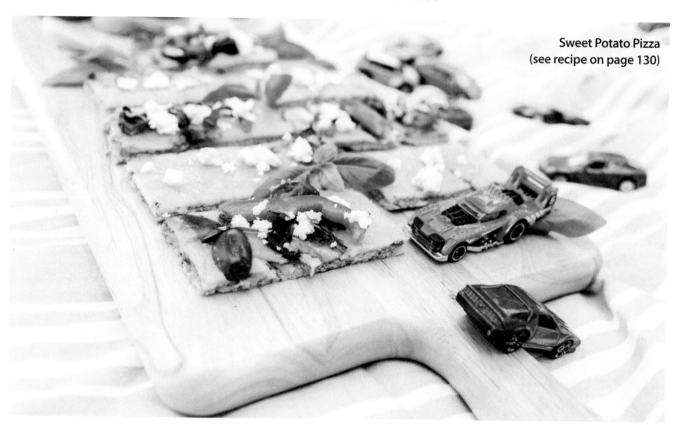

Sweet Potato Pizza
(see recipe on page 130)

GOAL 7: AVOID REPETITIVE EATING

What is a repetitive eater?

One of the most common signs of a fussy eater is a child who wants to eat the same foods, prepared in the same manner, for the same meals day in and day out. My eyes were really opened to this phenomenon during my training with the brilliant Dr. Kay Toomey, PhD, a pediatric psychologist who developed the Sequential Oral Sensory (S.O.S.) approach to feeding workshop, a trans-disciplinary program for assessing and treating children from birth to eighteen years with feeding difficulties and weight or growth problems. Dr. Toomey calls repetitive eating "food jagging," a term I've come to use too. Often I ask parents to keep food diaries for a couple of days, and when I take a look, I see three days where the exact same foods have been eaten at the exact same meals. These parents are usually desperate to make changes to their child's diet but their kid refuses to try anything new. (Remember that great Dr. Seuss book, *Green Eggs and Ham*?).

Aside from a lack of variety and high quality nutrition, the main issue when we give in to a child's food jag, is that eventually after eating their favorite foods for long enough they become bored, tire of them, and refuse to eat them too.

Consider this...

Reactions to dairy are not always what they seem. One of my clients was concerned about a recurring rash around her son's mouth. Studying his diet, I realized he was eating flavored yogurt at daycare. When this was changed to natural, unflavored yogurt sweetened with honey, the rash did not reappear. So if children are reacting to products like flavored yogurts, chocolate milk or dairy products with additives, it may be the additives and not the milk that is causing the problem. By improving the quality of the dairy foods the symptoms may subside.

HOW TO PREVENT REPETITIVE EATING

1. Introduce a wide variety of foods as early as possible and remember to exercise enormous amounts of patience in the face of rejection. It can take a young baby ten to sixteen tries to accept a new food.

2. When offering a new food, start with small portions even if this means only one taste or teaspoon at a time.

3. Set realistic expectations. Getting your child to move from white bread to a white preservative-free sourdough is a small step but can make a big change at a nutrition level.

4. As your child gets older, continue to offer variety. Even if your child has fifteen things on their food list, introduce more. If your child loves a bagel with cream cheese, for example, and typically eats it every day for school, start offering it every other day.

5. Rotate your meals so that your child becomes familiar with a wider range of different foods (see our menu planners on page 284).

6. Don't be afraid to use herbs and spices. Work with your child to identify herbs and spices they may like to try. Start, for example, with a sprinkle of oregano on a pizza.

7. Choose a new vegetable and spark your child's interest by letting them get involved with preparing it in various ways. For example, zucchini can be eaten steamed, roasted, cut into strips and cooked like pasta or blended into chocolate muffins (see recipe on page 127).

8. If you are stuck for ideas take into consideration the eating preferences of the fussiest member of your family and choose meals and recipes based on the foods they love to eat. For example, if your child loves pizza, try a cauliflower or sweet potato pizza base (see recipes on page 131).

9. Stretch their food choices focusing on the foods they love to eat. If they are an avid cheese sandwich eater, then offer them a wrap with cheese instead of a sandwich. Then move on to cheese melted over a baked potato, then add tuna to the melt. Or if they love chicken nuggets, offer homemade turkey schnitzel.

10. Most importantly, seek help early. Obviously every child is different, but if you find that meal times are way more stressful for you than they are for your peers, it's time to speak to a nutritionist or feeding therapist. Remember, the final goal is to bring the joy back into meal times.

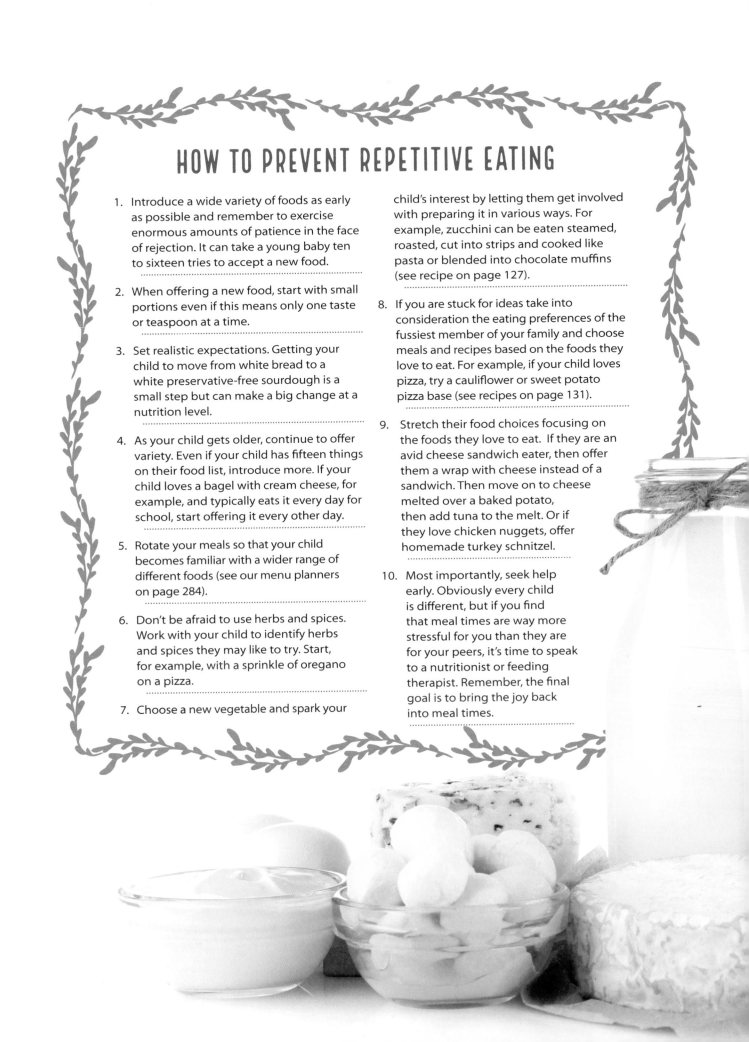

👍 DO ...	👎 DON'T ...
offer children new foods ten to sixteen times before giving up.	feel guilty if your child is a repetitive eater. It's very common and things can improve.
offer one new food with one snack and/or one meal a day.	give in to your child's demands for the same food day in and day out.
offer a new food with an accepted or favorite food.	offer "easy" foods over and over again.
use transitional foods between bites of new foods (i.e., a piece of accepted food, or drink of accepted fluid).	forget to praise your child, even just for a small taste.
take notice of your child's favorite foods and offer new foods with similar properties—may look the same, be the same color, same texture.	insist your child finishes what's on his plate.
be a role model by enjoying a wide and varied diet yourself.	forget to challenge yourself by stretching your own food choices.
ask for help if mealtimes become too stressful.	allow mealtimes to turn into battlefields.

If your child eats a wide range of foods—more than thirty—but loves avocado, for example, and wants to eat it daily, it won't matter too much when they become bored and refuse it, as they have twenty-nine other foods to choose from. However, if your child eats a limited range of foods (less than ten), losing one favoured food is a big deal, especially if it's the only food in a particular food group. Also, kids prone to food jagging are typically obsessed with salt laden, carbohydrate-rich foods such as sandwiches on white bread, potato chips, or sweetened dairy products such as squeezie yogurts or ice cream.

Most kids will go through stages where they prefer certain foods, then tire of these foods, and then resume eating them again. For serious repetitive eaters, though, once their favorite food is no longer desirable it's unlikely they will go back to it.

The most common issue I see in my practice is children who are stuck in a rut, hooked on chicken nuggets, fries, pizza or pasta. These are the same kids who demand the same brand of bread with the same amount of butter. Some children who display fussy eating behaviors have underlying medical conditions such as sensory processing disorders. However, more than 50 percent of the children I see simply started out as typical picky eaters. Their parents just needed the tools to avoid giving in to repeated demands for their favorite foods. Over time, if children eat the same foods daily, their food choices dwindle down so much that their diets become nutritionally lacking and can cause lethargy, poor concentration and nutritional deficiencies, which demand attention.

As discussed in the fussy eating section (see page 20), children with limited diets are often low in iron, zinc, and B12 and this can suppress the appetite and cause further fussiness due to lack of interest. I had one three-year-old client who would only eat five foods. This was a nutritional nightmare, and put a huge amount of pressure on her parents, as they had to prepare all her meals ahead of going anywhere or find restaurants that could cater to her limited repertoire. Identifying repetitive eating behaviors early on, and using positive strategies to deal with it, is highly recommended.

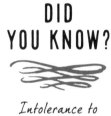

DID YOU KNOW?

Intolerance to dairy affects three-quarters of the population.

243

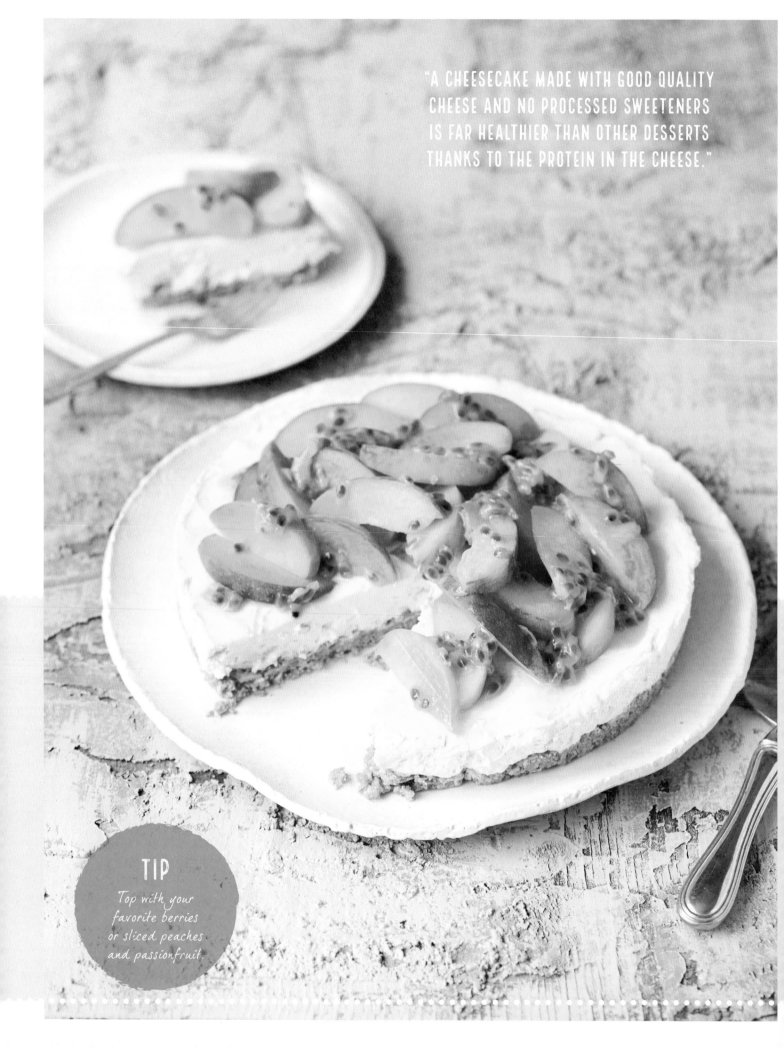

"A CHEESECAKE MADE WITH GOOD QUALITY CHEESE AND NO PROCESSED SWEETENERS IS FAR HEALTHIER THAN OTHER DESSERTS THANKS TO THE PROTEIN IN THE CHEESE."

TIP

Top with your favorite berries or sliced peaches and passionfruit.

"A CHEESECAKE MADE WITH GOOD QUALITY CHEESE AND NO PROCESSED SWEETENERS

Vegetarian · **Gluten Free** · **Egg Free** · **Nut Free**

Prep time: 20 mins (+ 4 hours chilling time)
Serves: 10

No-Bake Cheesecake

I grew up eating my mom's classic cheesecake. I created this healthier but equally delicious version for my family to enjoy.

INGREDIENTS

BASE:

2 cups (6²/₅ oz) Quick Homemade Granola (see page 275)

3 tbs coconut oil, melted

1–2 tbs maple syrup

FILLING:

2 cups (1¹/₈ lbs) cream cheese or mascarpone, at room temperature

2 tbs thick Greek yogurt, unsweetened

1 tsp pure vanilla extract

1 tbs lemon juice

¹/₄ cup raw or Manuka honey

pinch stevia (optional)

EQUIPMENT

high-speed food processor

INSTRUCTIONS

Line a 9" round cake pan with baking paper.

For the base, place all ingredients in a blender and blend until you reach a fine crumble.

Put the mixture into the cake pan and press it down evenly. Place in the freezer to firm up while preparing the filling.

Meanwhile, place the cheese in the food processor and process until smooth and creamy.

Slowly add all other ingredients and process until smooth and creamy.

Pour the cheese mixture on top of the base and spread evenly.

Refrigerate for at least 4 hours before serving.

Serving and storing leftovers: Serve immediately, store in the fridge for up to 4 days or freeze for up to 4 months.

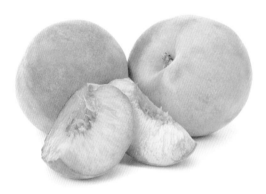

Vegan · **Gluten Free**

Prep time: 10 mins (+12–14 hours soaking time)
Makes: 3 cups to 4 cups

Almond Milk

INGREDIENTS

1 cup (5²/₃ oz) raw almonds

3 cups to 4¹/₄ cups (750ml-1L) filtered water (less water makes it thicker)

EQUIPMENT

High-powered blender (such as Vitamix or Thermomix)

INSTRUCTIONS

Soak almonds in a bowl covered with filtered water for 12–14 hours.

Rinse and drain almonds then place into a blender along with the filtered water.

Blend for 3–5 mins until smooth and creamy

Place a nut milk bag or a thin tea towel over a large bowl and slowly pour the almond milk mixture into the bag. Gently squeeze the bottom of the bag to release the milk. If using a tea towel, carefully gather the corners and lift up. Then squeeze until all of the liquid is extracted.

Transfer milk to a jar or covered bottle and refrigerate. Shake well before drinking as it tends to separate.

Serving and storing leftovers: Serve immediately, store in the fridge in a very cold spot for 4 days or freeze for up to 4 months.

To sweeten, add 2 pitted Medjool dates to blender and 1 tsp of vanilla. before straining. Alternatively, add a pinch of stevia.

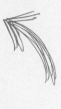

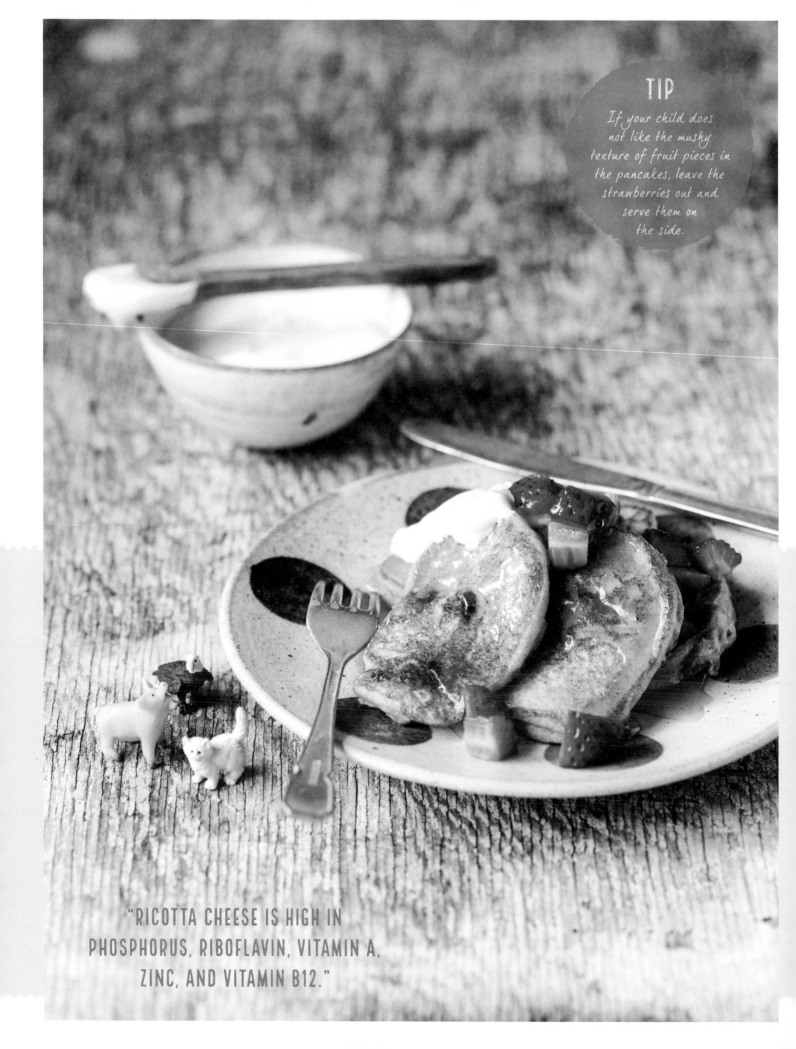

TIP

If your child does not like the mushy texture of fruit pieces in the pancakes, leave the strawberries out and serve them on the side.

"RICOTTA CHEESE IS HIGH IN PHOSPHORUS, RIBOFLAVIN, VITAMIN A, ZINC, AND VITAMIN B12."

Nut Free   Vegetarian

Prep time: 5–7 mins
Cooking time: 10 mins
Makes: 20

Ricotta Pancakes

I always need to make a double batch of these pancakes. My husband demolishes them before the kids even get to try them.

INGREDIENTS

2 eggs, separated

1 cup (8³⁄₄ oz) ricotta

¹⁄₂ cup milk of choice

1–2 tbs maple syrup (optional)

³⁄₄ cup (3²⁄₃ oz) whole spelt flour or buckwheat flour

1 tsp baking powder

¹⁄₂ tsp ground cinnamon

pinch sea salt

1¹⁄₂ cups (8¹⁄₂ oz) strawberries, cubed

coconut oil, butter or ghee for frying

EQUIPMENT
electric handmixer

INSTRUCTIONS

In a small bowl, beat egg whites until stiff. Set aside.

In another bowl, add egg yolks, ricotta cheese, milk, and maple syrup and beat until well combined. Add flour, baking powder, cinnamon, and salt and beat until well incorporated.

Gently fold egg whites into the batter. Do not over-mix the batter.

Add strawberries and gently stir to combine.

Heat a teaspoon of coconut oil in a large frying pan over medium heat. Drop in heaped tablespoons of batter and cook for a minute on each side. Continue with remaining batter.

Serving and storing leftovers: Serve immediately, store in a container in the fridge for up to 4 days or freeze for up to 4 months.

Vegetarian   Gluten Free

Prep time: 1 hour
Cooking time: 10 mins
Makes: 12

Strawberry Coconut Dumplings

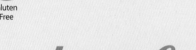

INGREDIENTS

DOUGH:

¹⁄₂ cup (2⁷⁄₈ oz) buckwheat flour

¹⁄₂ cup (2³⁄₄ oz) polenta or semolina

4 tbs coconut oil, melted

1 cup (8³⁄₄ oz) ricotta cheese

1 egg

FILLING:
12 strawberries

COATING:
1 tbs coconut oil

¹⁄₄ cup (1 oz) almond meal

¹⁄₄ cup (²⁄₃ oz) rice bread crumbs

¹⁄₄ cup (1¹⁄₅ oz) coconut sugar

EQUIPMENT
blender

INSTRUCTIONS

Mix all dough ingredients together to a smooth consistency. Place in the fridge for 45 mins.

Take some of the dough and wrap it around a strawberry to form a little ball. Continue with the rest of the dough.

Bring lightly salted water to boil in a saucepan and reduce to simmer. Cook the balls for 10 mins. They are ready when they float on the surface and flip in the water.

In a large frying pan, melt 1 tbs coconut oil and add almond meal, rice crumbs and coconut sugar. Stir through until everything is well combined then take off the heat.

Roll strawberry dumplings in the almond mixture until they are covered in crumbs.

Serve with pureed strawberries.

Serving and storing leftovers: Serve immediately, store in the fridge for up to 4 days or freeze for up to 4 months. You can also freeze them uncooked.

 For a chocolate version, swap the strawberries for a tablespoon of our Healthy Chocolate Spread (see page 275).

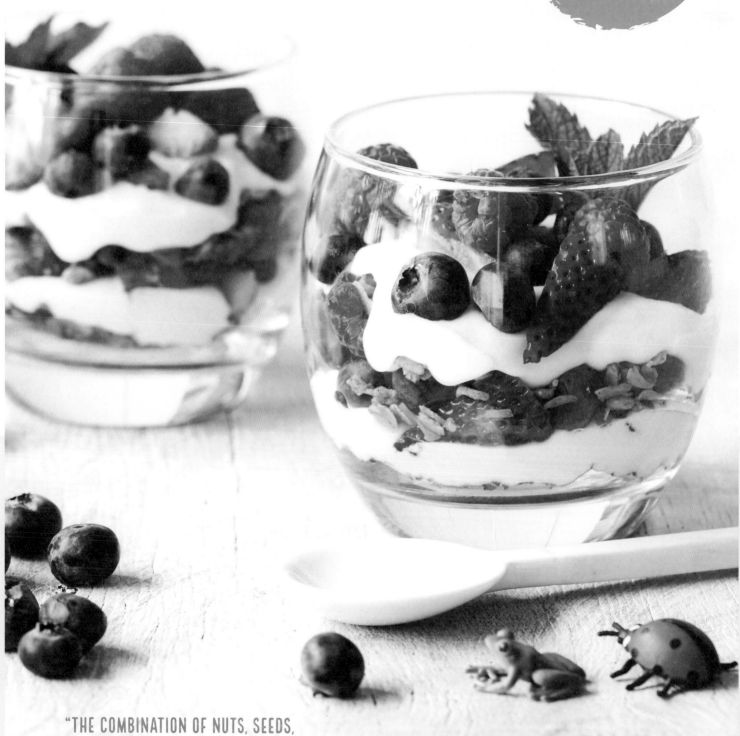

TIP

Replace the coconut cream with coconut yogurt or natural yogurt. Use fruit of choice to replace berries.

"THE COMBINATION OF NUTS, SEEDS, OATS, BERRIES, AND COCONUT GIVES AN ANTIOXIDANT HIT FOR THE WHOLE FAMILY."

V
Vegan

Wheat Free

Prep time: 45 mins (+ 7 hours refrigeration time)
Cooking time: 30 mins
Serves: 4

Berry & Granola Parfait

My three-year-old loves layering her own parfait cup. Some days she's in a berry mood and other days she asks for mango layers. It's so good to see her involved and creating her own meals.

INGREDIENTS

GRANOLA:
2 cups (8½ oz) whole rolled oats

1 cup (5 oz) almonds and pecans, slivered

⅓ cup (⅞ oz) shredded coconut

⅓ cup (1⅞ oz) seeds (sunflower seeds, pepitas)

¼ cup (1⅘ oz) flaxseeds

½ tsp ground cinnamon

pinch Himalayan rock salt

¼ cup maple syrup or raw honey

¼ cup coconut oil, melted

1 tsp pure vanilla extract

PARFAIT:
1 can (13½ fl oz) coconut cream, refrigerated upside down for 7 hours or overnight

1½ cups (8½ oz) fresh strawberries or blueberries

INSTRUCTIONS

Preheat oven to 300°F and line a baking tray with baking paper.

To make the granola, place oats, nuts, coconut, seeds, cinnamon, and salt in a big bowl and stir to combine.

In another bowl, combine maple syrup, coconut oil, and vanilla extract.

Pour maple syrup mixture over oat mixture and use clean hands to mix well and toss to coat.

Spread mixture onto the baking tray and roast in the oven for 30 mins, stirring halfway through cooking.

Allow granola to cool completely to obtain a crunchy texture.

To make the whipped coconut cream, turn the chilled coconut cream can upside down, and pour off the clear liquid at the top until all that is left is the solidified cream. If the cream hasn't solidified, then pour off as much clear liquid as possible.

Transfer coconut cream to a mixing bowl and beat with a standing or hand mixer until it's whipped, approximately 5 mins.

Spoon granola into the bottom of four serving bowls or glasses. Then add a layer of strawberries. Spoon coconut whipped cream on top of the strawberries. Repeat the layers using the strawberries and cream mixture.

Serving and storing leftovers:
Serve immediately. Store leftover granola in an airtight container at room temperature for up to 4 weeks or freeze for up to 4 months. Store leftover whipped coconut cream in an airtight container in the fridge for up to 4 days.

V
Vegan

Gluten Free

Nut Free

Prep time: 10 mins
Makes: 4 cups

Coconut Milk

INGREDIENTS

2 cups (5⅓ oz) unsweetened shredded coconut or the flesh and water from two fresh coconuts

2 cups filtered water

EQUIPMENT

high-powered blender (Vitamix or Thermomix)

INSTRUCTIONS

Place flesh and water of fresh coconut in blender and add 2 cups of water. If using shredded coconut add 4 cups of water.

Blend on highest setting for 3–5 mins minutes until thick and creamy. If you prefer a thinner consistency add more water to your blender before rinsing and add to milk.

Add another ½ cup of water to blender and give it a quick spin to get every last bit.

Place a nut milk bag or a thin tea towel over a large bowl and slowly pour the milk into the bag. Gently squeeze the bottom of the bag to release the milk. If using a tea towel, gather the corners and lift up. Squeeze until all of the liquid is extracted.

Transfer milk to a jar or covered bottle and refrigerate. Shake before drinking.

Serving and storing leftovers: Serve immediately, store in the fridge for 4 days or freeze for up to 4 months.

To sweeten, add 2 pitted Medjool dates to blender and 1 tsp of vanilla before straining. Alternatively, add a pinch of stevia.

Vegetarian · Gluten Free · Nut Free

Prep time: 10 mins
Cooking time: 15 mins
Serves: 4

Leftover Vegetable Omelette

INGREDIENTS

4 eggs

1 tbs milk or cream of choice

1/2 cup (1²/₅ oz) yellow cheese, low sodium or sheep milk cheese

1 tsp chia seeds

1 tbs fresh parsley, finely chopped

sea salt and pepper, to taste

1 tbs extra virgin olive oil or coconut oil

1/2 yellow onion, finely diced

1 garlic clove, finely diced

1 cup (8³/₄ oz) leftover vegetables, finely diced (cauliflower, carrot, broccoli, sweet potato, peas, green beans)

INSTRUCTIONS

In a bowl, combine eggs, milk, cheese, chia seeds, parsley, and salt and pepper. Whisk until well combined.

Heat oil in a large frying pan over medium heat.

Add onion and sauté for 2–3 mins or until soft.

Add garlic and sauté for another 1–2 mins.

Add vegetables and cook for 2–3 mins.

Pour egg mixture in pan with vegetables, swirling the egg around the pan.

Reduce the heat to low and cook, without stirring for 1–2 mins.

Turn off the heat, cover with a lid and leave for 3–5 mins, or until egg is cooked through.

Cut into 4 triangles and serve with homemade bread (see page 283).

Serving and storing leftovers: Serve immediately or store in the fridge for up to 4 days. Does not freeze well.

Vegetarian · Gluten Free · Egg Free

Prep time: 5 mins
Cooking time: 5–10 mins
Makes: 2½ cups

Béchamel Sauce

INGREDIENTS

2 tbs organic, unsalted butter

1/4 cup (1 oz) arrowroot

2 cups almond milk or milk of choice

1/2 cup–1 cup (1²/₅ oz to 2⁴/₅ oz) cheddar cheese, grated

sea salt, to taste

INSTRUCTIONS

In a saucepan, melt the butter over medium heat.

Add arrowroot and whisk to combine quickly, then add milk, one cup at a time, and cook until it thickens, whisking regularly.

Stir in grated cheese, season with sea salt, and set aside.

Use for any kind of bakes or our Tuna, Vegetables & Chia Lasagne (see page 63).

Serving and storing leftovers: Serve immediately or store in the fridge for up to 3 days.

For a dairy-free option, use 2 tbs of coconut oil and omit cheese. Use for non-dairy dishes that require béchamel sauce.

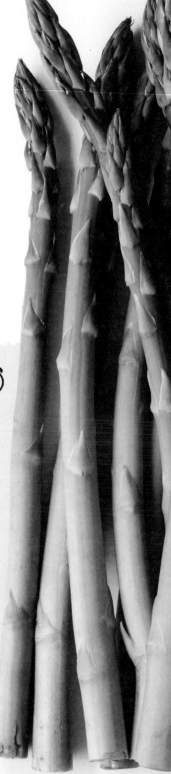

Egg
Free

Prep time: 15 mins
Cooking time: 20–25 mins
Makes: 10 scrolls

Savory Scrolls 4 Ways

These scrolls are a big hit in the lunch box or at birthday parties.

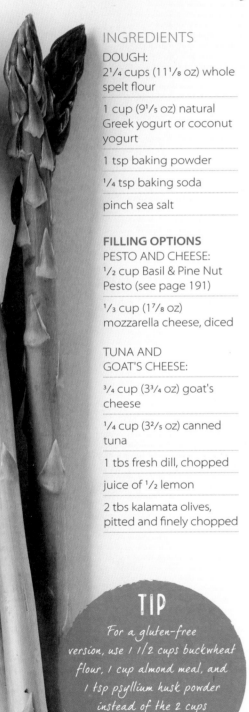

INGREDIENTS

DOUGH:

2¼ cups (11⅛ oz) whole spelt flour

1 cup (9⅕ oz) natural Greek yogurt or coconut yogurt

1 tsp baking powder

¼ tsp baking soda

pinch sea salt

FILLING OPTIONS

PESTO AND CHEESE:
½ cup Basil & Pine Nut Pesto (see page 191)

⅓ cup (1⅞ oz) mozzarella cheese, diced

TUNA AND GOAT'S CHEESE:

¾ cup (3¾ oz) goat's cheese

¼ cup (3⅖ oz) canned tuna

1 tbs fresh dill, chopped

juice of ½ lemon

2 tbs kalamata olives, pitted and finely chopped

sea salt and pepper, to taste

PIZZA:
½ cup Homemade Ketchup (see page 283)

⅓ cup (1 oz) grated cheese (mozzarella/ gouda/cheddar)

¼ cup (1¾ oz) kalamata olives, pitted and diced

1 tbs fresh basil, finely chopped

PROVENCALE:
½ cup (2¾ oz) sundried tomatoes, diced

½ cup (2¾ oz) sheep or goat feta, crumbled

1 garlic clove, crushed

¼ cup (1¾ oz) kalamata olives, pitted and diced

½ tsp dried oregano

EQUIPMENT
high-speed food processor

INSTRUCTIONS

Preheat oven to 355°F and line a baking tray with baking paper.

Place all dough ingredients into a food processor and process until smooth.

Remove the dough, shape it into a ball and place between two sheets of baking paper and roll it into a rectangle shape about ⅛" to ⅓" thick. If dough seems too sticky, lightly flour the baking paper and sprinkle some flour on top of the dough before rolling out. Remove the top sheet.

For the pesto filling, simply spread pesto onto the dough, leaving out 1cm on the longer sides and sprinkle with cheese.

For the tuna filling, place all ingredients in a blender and blend until desired consistency (you can also just mix the ingredients together without a blender if you prefer more texture). Then spread onto dough, leaving ⅓" on the longer sides.

For the pizza filling, spread dough with ketchup and sprinkle with cheese, olives, and basil. Be careful to leave ⅓" on the longer sides.

For the provencale filling, place all ingredients in a small bowl and mix to combine. Spread mixture onto the dough, leaving ⅓" on the longer sides.

Roll dough into a log shape and cut into even slices to make scrolls. Brush or drizzle with olive oil or coconut oil.

Place on the lined baking tray and bake for 20–25 mins.

Leave to cool on a wire rack before serving.

Serving and storing leftovers: Serve immediately, store in an airtight container in the fridge for up to 3 days or freeze for up to 4 months.

TIP

For a gluten-free version, use 1 1/2 cups buckwheat flour, 1 cup almond meal, and 1 tsp psyllium husk powder instead of the 2 cups of spelt flour.

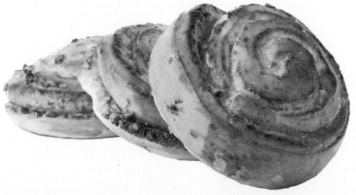

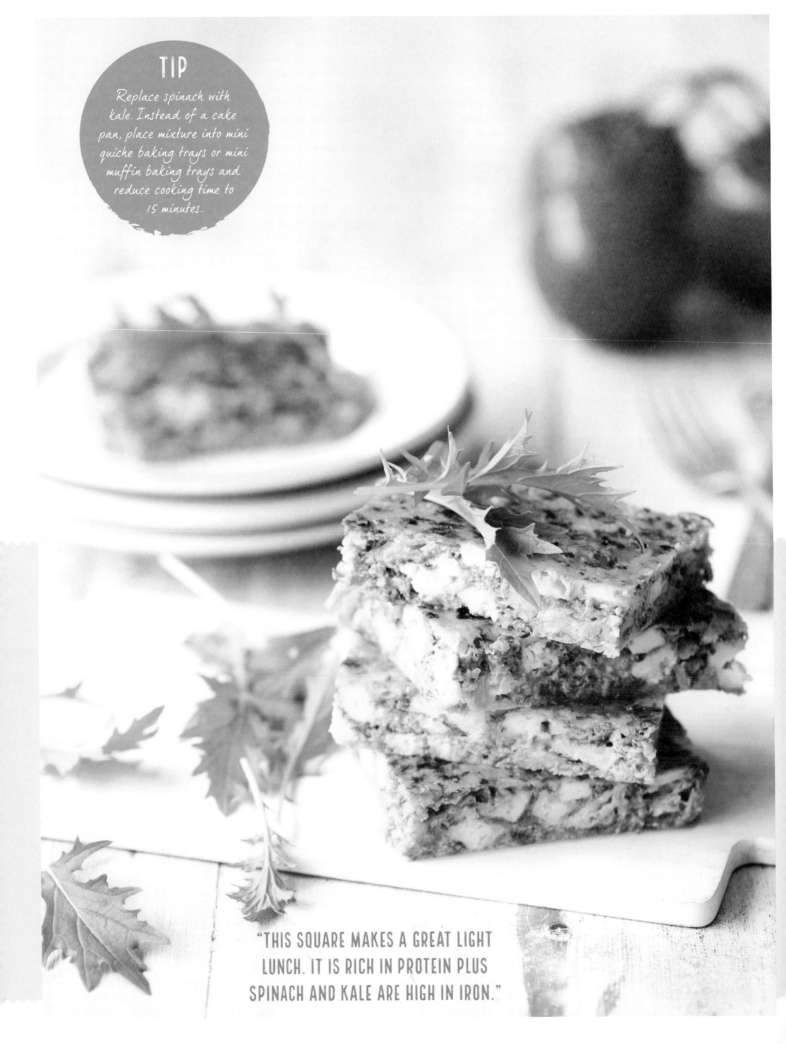

TIP
Replace spinach with kale. Instead of a cake pan, place mixture into mini quiche baking trays or mini muffin baking trays and reduce cooking time to 15 minutes.

"THIS SQUARE MAKES A GREAT LIGHT LUNCH. IT IS RICH IN PROTEIN PLUS SPINACH AND KALE ARE HIGH IN IRON."

VEG
Vegetarian   Gluten Free   Nut Free

Prep time: 15 mins
Cooking time: 30–40 mins
Makes: 12–15 squares

Spinach & Feta Squares

This tasty square is one of my son's favorite lunch box meals. I soak the feta overnight in water to reduce the sodium content.

INGREDIENTS

1 tsp extra virgin olive oil

4 eggs

1¹⁄₃ cups (7 oz) feta cheese, crumbled

1 cup (⁷⁄₈ oz) spinach or kale, finely chopped

1 medium-sized carrot, peeled and finely grated

1 cup (2⁴⁄₅ oz) gouda, mozzarella or Swiss cheese, grated

EQUIPMENT

electric hand mixer

INSTRUCTIONS

Preheat oven to 390°F and grease a tart tin (10") with olive oil.

In a large bowl, beat eggs and remaining ingredients.

Pour into prepared tart tin.

Bake for approximately 30–40 mins.

Serving and storing leftovers: Serve immediately, store in an airtight container in the fridge for 4 days or freeze for up to 4 months.

Nut Free   Gluten Free

Prep time: 30 mins
Cooking time: 25–30 mins
Makes: 24 small or 12 large quiches

Mini Salmon Quiches

INGREDIENTS

1 tbs coconut or olive oil, plus extra for greasing tray

½ yellow onion, chopped

¼ cup (¹⁄₆ oz) spinach or kale, steamed and finely sliced

7 oz salmon fillet, grilled and flaked, or canned salmon, rinsed and drained

½ cup (4½ oz) ricotta cheese or coconut cream

½ cup (4½ oz) pumpkin, peeled and steamed

2 tbs coconut flour or almond meal

4 eggs

1 cup milk of choice

sea salt, to taste

½ tsp mixed herbs or dill

EQUIPMENT

high-speed food processor

INSTRUCTIONS

Preheat oven to 355°F. Grease a mini muffin tray or a quiche mold with coconut oil or butter.

Heat 1 tbs olive oil in a frying pan and sauté the onion and spinach for 2 mins or until soft. Remove the vegetables and set aside. Add the salmon and pan fry until lightly cooked.

In a processor, add onion mixture, flaked salmon, ricotta, pumpkin and flour and process until smooth.

In a large bowl, beat eggs lightly; add milk, salt and herbs.

Combine egg mixture with salmon mixture and stir thoroughly.

Pour mixture into prepared muffin tray and bake for 25 mins.

Serve with Tzatziki Dip or Homemade Ketchup (see recipes on page 283).

Serving and storing leftovers: Serve immediately, store in the fridge for up to 3 days or freeze for up to 4 months.

TIP

For a dairy-free version swap the ricotta cheese for 1/2 cup coconut cream.

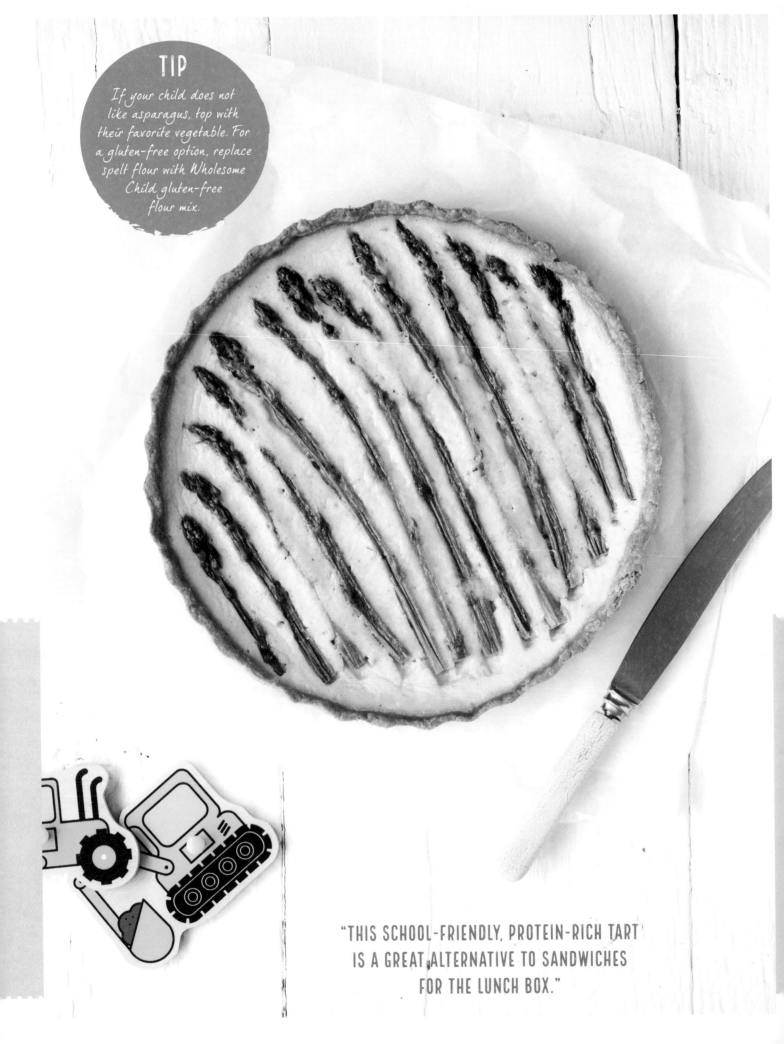

TIP

If your child does not like asparagus, top with their favorite vegetable. For a gluten-free option, replace spelt flour with Wholesome Child gluten-free flour mix.

"THIS SCHOOL-FRIENDLY, PROTEIN-RICH TART IS A GREAT ALTERNATIVE TO SANDWICHES FOR THE LUNCH BOX."

VEG
Vegetarian

Nut
Free

Prep time: 35 mins
Cooking time: 50–60 mins
Makes: 16 tarts

Asparagus & Cheese Tart

This easy-to-make crust is free of the nasties that you'll find in store-bought versions.

INGREDIENTS

CRUST:

½ cup (2⅞ oz) whole spelt flour

½ cup (2⅞ oz) buckwheat flour

½ cup (2¾ oz) butter, cubed (plus additional for greasing tin)

¾ cup (2⅙ oz) cheddar cheese, finely grated

1–2 tbs cold filtered water

FILLING:

3 eggs

½ cup milk of choice

¾ cup (6⅞ oz) quark or ricotta cheese

½ cup (1⅖ oz) cheddar cheese, finely grated

sea salt and pepper, to taste

10½ oz asparagus, trimmed and cut in half lengthwise

INSTRUCTIONS

Preheat oven to 355°F and grease a 10" tart tin with butter.

To make the crust, place both flours into a bowl, add the butter to the flour and rub in with your fingertips until it resembles bread crumbs.

Add the grated cheddar into the pastry and mix. Add 2 tbs cold water and mix until the pastry forms a ball. Wrap in cling film and chill for 5 mins in fridge. Remove and lightly knead.

Lightly dust the work surface with flour, roll out the pastry and line the tin. Chill in the freezer for 20 mins, then line the pastry tin with baking paper, To prevent pastry from rising, fill with uncooked beans and rice or a suitable baking weight, and cook for 15 mins. Remove the beans or rice and paper, then return the pastry tin to the oven for 10 mins.

To make the filling, combine eggs, milk, quark, ¼ cup of cheese, and salt and pepper and whisk to combine. Pour batter into pastry shell and top with asparagus and remaining cheddar cheese.

Bake for 30–35 mins or until the egg mixture is set.

Serving and storing leftovers: Serve immediately, store in an airtight container in the fridge for up to 4 days or freeze for up to 4 months.

VEG
Vegetarian

Gluten
Free

Dairy
Free

Prep time: 10 mins
Cooking time: 25 mins
Serves: 4

Beetroot & Coconut Frittata

INGREDIENTS

1 tbs coconut oil

1¼ cups (7 oz) beetroot, peeled and roasted (make sure it's a sweet one)

½ cup coconut cream or ricotta cheese

4 eggs

2–4 tbs almond meal

EQUIPMENT

high-speed food processor

INSTRUCTIONS

Preheat oven to 355°F and grease a baking dish/quiche tin with the coconut oil.

Place all ingredients in a processor and process until smooth.

Pour batter into prepared baking dish.

Bake for approximately 25 mins or until it sets.

Allow to cool, then cut into little squares.

Serving and storing leftovers: Serve immediately, store in an airtight container in the fridge for up to 4 days or freeze for up to 4 months.

Substitute the beetroot with sweet potato, pumpkin, carrot, broccoli or cauliflower.

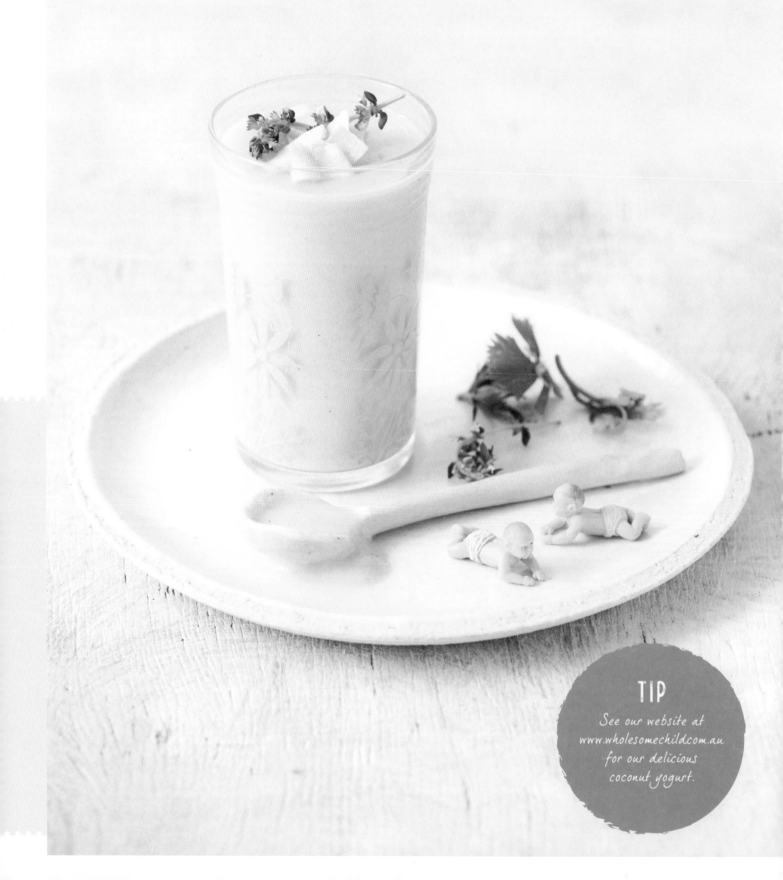

Vegetarian Gluten Free Nut Free

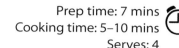

Prep time: 7 mins
Cooking time: 5–10 mins
Serves: 4

Coconut Custard

Custard is a comfort food for many of us. I really love this recipe because it contains added protein from eggs and has no artificial colorings or preservatives.

INGREDIENTS

2 cups coconut milk

2 tsp pure vanilla extract

2 tbs maple syrup

2 eggs

1 tbs arrowroot

zest of ¹/₂ lemon

INSTRUCTIONS

In a medium-sized saucepan, add coconut milk, vanilla extract, and maple syrup, whisk and bring to a boil. Take off the heat immediately and set aside.

In a small bowl combine eggs and arrowroot until smooth (avoid any lumps). Add to the milk mixture with the lemon zest, whisking continuously, and gently bring back to a boil over medium heat.

Let simmer for about 3-5 mins, until it thickens up, whisking occasionally.

Transfer into 4 small glasses or bowls and serve warm or refrigerate for an hour before serving. Top with fresh fruits or homemade Chia Raspberry Jam (see recipe on page 223).

Serving and storing leftovers: Serve immediately, store in the fridge for up to 4 days or freeze for up to 4 months.

Vegetarian Wheat Free Egg Free

Prep time: 10 mins (+7 hours refrigeration time)
Serves: 4

Bircher Muesli

INGREDIENTS

1 cup (4¹/₄ oz) rolled oats

¹/₂ cup almond milk

¹/₂ cup filtered water

³/₄ cup (4¹/₄ oz) mixed nuts and seeds of choice, crushed in a blender

1 tbs goji berries

1 tbs shredded coconut (optional)

1 medium-sized pear, peeled and grated

¹/₂ cup (4³/₅ oz) natural yogurt

¹/₂ tsp ground cinnamon

1 tbs maple syrup or raw honey

¹/₂ cup (2⁴/₅ oz) frozen berries

EQUIPMENT
blender

INSTRUCTIONS

Place oats, almond milk, water, nuts and seeds, goji berries, shredded coconut, and pear in a bowl and mix to combine with a wooden spoon.

Cover and refrigerate for 7 hours or overnight.

Add yogurt, cinnamon, and maple syrup and mix to combine.

Transfer to 4 small bowls and top with frozen berries.

Serving and storing leftovers: Serve immediately or store in the fridge for up to 4 days.

TIP
Replace almond milk with any milk of choice and natural yogurt with coconut yogurt for a dairy-free option.

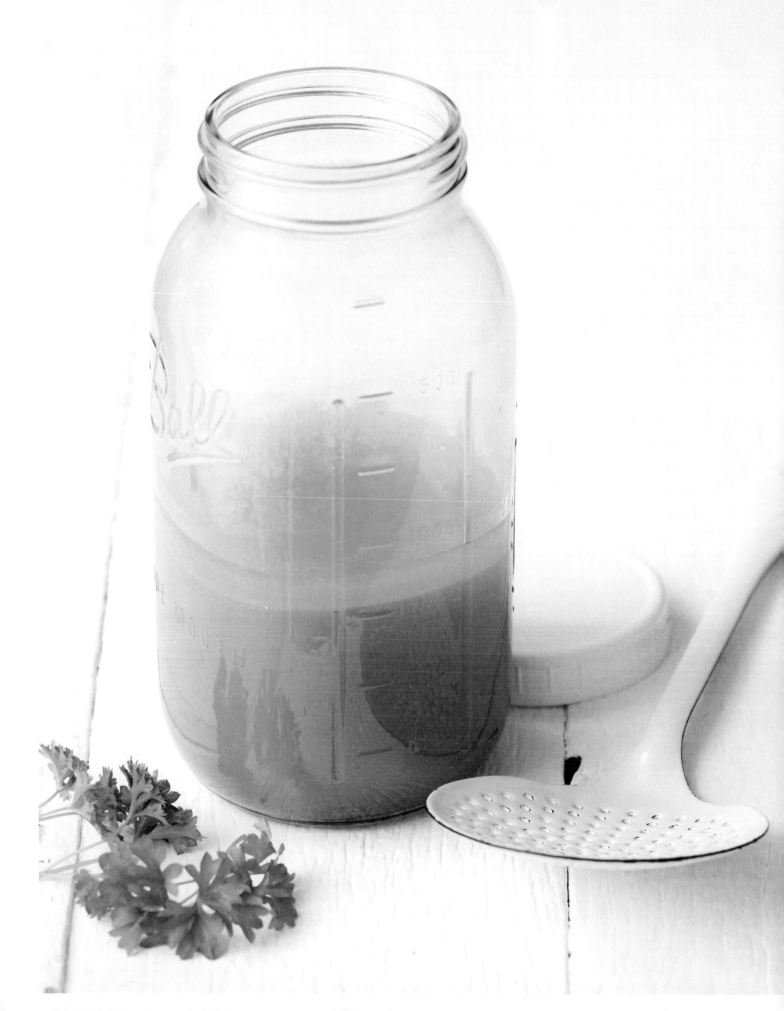

Avoid Nasties

EAT REAL FOOD THAT IS FREE OF PRESERVATIVES, ADDITIVES, ARTIFICIAL COLORS, GM INGREDIENTS, AND EXCESSIVE SODIUM

*W*hen I think about what motivated me to start *Wholesome Child* and what continues to drive me to keep making changes in my own family's diet, the diets of my clients and those that I reach through my website, it's that I believe we all deserve to eat real food.

To do this, we need to be informed so we can make the right decisions for our families when faced with multiple options. Many of us don't have the time to cook every meal from scratch and we have to rely on a certain amount of packaged food. My ultimate aim is to help you navigate the supermarket shelves to ensure you choose the most wholesome options available, free of the nasties that are present in many foods.

I believe a child's diet should contain a variety of different foods (of course the less healthy items deserve far less of a place), but my main concerns are the preservatives, additives, artificial colors, GM ingredients, and excessive sodium in many of our foods.

If your child ate seven tablespoons of sugar in the form of a few slices of homemade chocolate cake or brownies, it would still be far healthier for him than if he ate five tablespoons of food coloring or three tablespoons of an artificial sweetener like aspartame—substances that can be really detrimental to our children's behavior, moods, and general health. Some food additives are even listed as possible carcinogens by the World Health Organization, yet manufacturers continue to use them.

WHAT IS A FOOD ADDITIVE?

Additives are substances allowed in food because they perform a technical function like reducing the tendency of food particles to clump or stick together, restoring color or enhancing the texture or taste, without contributing significantly to its calories. Many food additives are listed by their class name followed by the number—for example, beta-carotene (160a)—but some are only listed as numbers, which means you need to play detective if you want to know exactly what is in your food.

ADDITIVES TO AVOID

Look out for these potentially harmful nasties:

1 FOOD COLORING Artificial food colorings have been controversial since the 1970s, when pediatrician Benjamin Feingold published findings suggesting a link between food dyes and hyperactive behavior. However, scientists have yet to reach a consensus on the extent of this risk.

While the 2007 Southampton study in the UK found a link between food coloring and hyperactivity in children, there is ongoing debate around the validity of this finding and the Food and Drug Administration (FDA) in the US believes more research is needed to warrant a warning.

Norway first banned the use of synthetic colorings in food back in 1978 and other EU countries now require products containing the worst offenders to carry the warning: "May have an adverse effect on activity and attention in children." A 2010 report by the US Center for Science in the Public Interest called for artificial colors to be replaced by natural colors. And in possibly the biggest stand taken to date, global supermarket chain Aldi has removed all artificial food coloring from its products.

However, in Australia, the US, and many other countries, additives and artificial colorings are still widespread in food products, especially baked goods marketed to children.

What to look out for:

Amaranth (123)	Quinoline yellow (104)
Brown (154)	Azorubine (122)
Ponceau (124)	Brilliant black (151)
Patent Blue V (131)	

Found in:
Processed colored foods such as cakes, cookies, chocolate, ice cream, soda, and baked goods.

Potential effects on children:
• Hyperactivity
• Irritability
• Loss of concentration
• Allergic response (rash, hives, asthma)

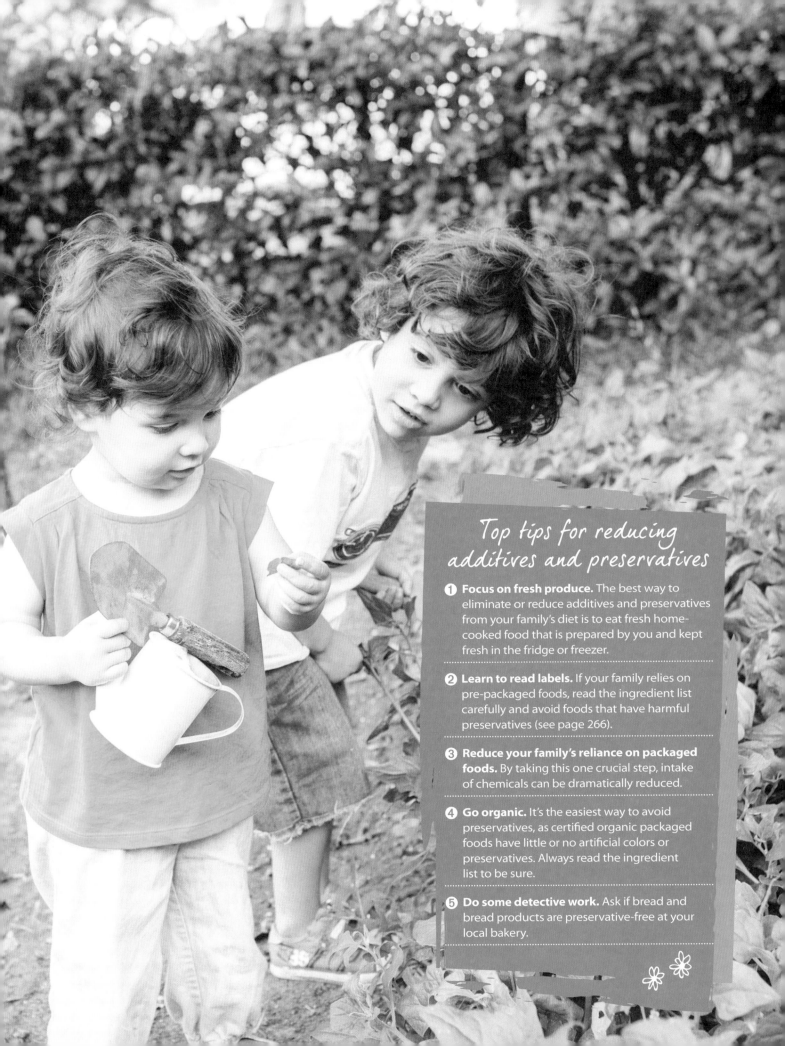

Top tips for reducing additives and preservatives

1 **Focus on fresh produce.** The best way to eliminate or reduce additives and preservatives from your family's diet is to eat fresh home-cooked food that is prepared by you and kept fresh in the fridge or freezer.

2 **Learn to read labels.** If your family relies on pre-packaged foods, read the ingredient list carefully and avoid foods that have harmful preservatives (see page 266).

3 **Reduce your family's reliance on packaged foods.** By taking this one crucial step, intake of chemicals can be dramatically reduced.

4 **Go organic.** It's the easiest way to avoid preservatives, as certified organic packaged foods have little or no artificial colors or preservatives. Always read the ingredient list to be sure.

5 **Do some detective work.** Ask if bread and bread products are preservative-free at your local bakery.

DID YOU KNOW?

Strawberry artificial flavor can contain up to 50 chemical ingredients.

Better choices:

Choose foods that use natural food coloring, which is indicated by ingredients such as betacarotene, beet powder, paprika, saffron, turmeric, and vegetable juice. However, take care with the following three "natural" food colors that are often marketed to unsuspecting shoppers with the label "No artificial coloring," but are not necessarily safer than synthetic ones:

- **Cochineal (120)**, derived from the dried pregnant bodies of scale insects—important information for people following a diet based on a philosophy (e.g., vegetarians) or on a religious belief (e.g., Kosher or Halal).

- **Annatto (160b)**, an orange-yellow coloring almost always found in children's food products such as yogurts, etc. Safe alternatives include beta-carotene (160a).

- **Caramels (150a to150d)**, often described as "natural colors" but produced synthetically.
  Caramel I (150a)—plain
  Caramel II (150b)—caustic sulphite process
  Caramel III (150c)—ammonia process
  Caramel IV (150d)—ammonia sulphite process

❷ FLAVOR ENHANCERS Contrary to what you may think, children don't only go for sweet and salty foods. There are many who like sour and bitter tastes too—as well as the fifth taste, known as umami.

A twenty-first century buzzword, umami combines the Japanese characters for "delicious" and "taste" to describe the strong, savory flavor associated with foods. Glutamic acid, or glutamate, is a naturally abundant amino acid that creates the savory umami flavor in many foods such as tomatoes and cheese.

It's little wonder then that food manufacturers created monosodium glutamate (MSG). This commercially produced sodium salt of glutamic acid gives many processed foods their palatable, savory flavor.

While some people can safely eat food that contains MSG, many experience symptoms if they eat a large amount of MSG in a single meal. "No added flavors" does not necessarily mean there is no MSG in a food product—it is often listed as a "flavor enhancer" instead and can have up to 129 different names.

Found in:

Ready-made soup, stocks, seaweed snacks, flavored crackers, seasonings, flavored chips, dips, sauces, processed meat like sausages, and fast foods.

Potential effect on children:

- headaches
- numbness
- tingling
- digestive disturbances
- drowsiness
- difficulty breathing for asthmatics

What to look out for:

Glutamic acid (620)

Monopotassium L glutamate (622)

Monosodium glutamate (621) (MSG)

Six ways to reduce MSG in your family's diet

❶ Cook with fresh ingredients wherever possible.

❷ Avoid instant soups and store-bought marinades. Try our quick, easy marinades on pages 278–9.

❸ Wean your kids off yeast extract spreads such as Vegemite or Marmite. If they are eating them five days a week, reduce to four, then three, and so on. Start to introduce healthier spreads such as almond butter, tahini, avocado, raw honey, low-sodium cheese, hummus or try our Fig or Chia Raspberry Jam on page 222–3.

❹ Choose plain crackers over flavored ones. Make them more interesting by offering dips and healthy toppings. Check the ingredients even if you know a brand.

Many well known brands offer natural wholegrain crackers which are free from preservatives but also a full range of flavored crackers (rice crackers, corn cakes etc) which contain hidden MSG.

❺ Snack-size seaweed packs often contain plenty of unwanted additives and flavorings. A better bet? Purchase plain, unflavored Nori sheets and cut them into small strips. You can also use them as wraps.

❻ Many packaged herb mixes contain yeast extract and other flavor enhancers. It's best to introduce your child to a variety of fresh herbs from a young age. If you're dealing with an older "fussy" child blend herbs into their food.

Hydrolyzed soy/vegetable protein (HVT)

Textured vegetable protein (TVP)

Yeast extract

Other flavor enhancers to avoid:

Calcium glutamate (623)

Monoammonium L-glutamate (624)

Magnesium glutamate (625)

Disodium 5/inosinate (631)

Disodium 5/Guanylate (627)

Disodium 5/ ribonucleotides (635)

Better choices:

If your child loves savory yeast extract spreads then their tastebuds are craving the umami flavor sensation. Here are some alternatives you can try:

✓ Spread a small amount of organic miso paste on wholegrain bread or crackers to replace savory spreads that contain yeast extract.

✓ Roasting, stewing or searing can enhance the natural flavor of chicken and meat without the need for marinades.

✓ Pan-roast or caramelize tomatoes and mushrooms as they both contain naturally occurring glutamates. Add a touch of tamari and herbs. (Note: there are many individuals who will react to naturally occurring glutamates too. If this is the case, avoid both synthetic and natural forms).

✓ Often soy is used to create the umami flavor. I prefer wheat-free tamari to soy sauce; however, if you are using soy sauce look for an organic, wheat-free version.

❸ **ARTIFICIAL SWEETENERS** Often hidden in non sugar-free items to add sweetness without adding further calories, these are best avoided in young growing bodies. They have been linked to digestive disorders, hormonal disruption, and even neurological disorders. And studies have found they can actually contribute to weight gain as they create a desire for more sweet foods.

Found in:

Chewing gum, fizzy drinks, yogurts, low-fat desserts and milk, chocolate, and hard candies.

Potential effect on children:

• While there is ongoing debate as to the detrimental effects of these sweeteners on adults, there is no doubt that children remain vulnerable. One or two low-fat yogurts, a low-sugar jelly on toast or a low-calorie fruit drink can contain enough aspartame, for example, to put a young child over the FDA's recommended intake limit of 50mg/kg of body weight. The European Food Safety Authority (EFSA), which regulates food additives in the European Union, recommends a slightly lower acceptable daily intake (ADI) for aspartame, at 40mg/kg.

• Some studies in rats have found aspartame to be carcinogenic, but the findings have been questioned and the jury remains out on aspartame's safety for human consumption. However, when it comes to children, it's best to err on the side of caution and not offer them products containing artificial sweeteners, especially aspartame (for more on the safety of aspartame and other artifical sweeteners, see page 79).

What to look out for:

Acesulphame-K (950)

Aspartame (951)—Nutrasweet and Equal

Cyclamates (952)

Sucralose (955)

Saccharin (954)

Aspartame Acesulfame Salt (962)—Twinsweet

Better choices:

The best option is to avoid artificially sweetened foods and drinks altogether.

✓ Avoid foods labelled "low fat," "diet," "low sugar," "lite," or "low calorie."

✓ If a member of your family is overweight or has a medical condition such as diabetes or candidiasis, choose products sweetened with natural stevia or monk fruit extract, both calorie-free sweeteners that do not carry the same side effects.

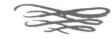

DID YOU KNOW?

Even the term "natural food"— once used to describe whole fruits, vegetables and unrefined grains—has now been expanded to include packaged, processed foods, many of which contain a wide array of chemicals.

Consider this…

A survey by Kalsec, a natural spice and flavor company, found that 80% of respondents worry about the mental health and behavioral effects of food chemicals on children.

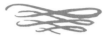

DID YOU KNOW?

Sensitive babies with a susceptibility to food intolerances, can have reactions even while still exclusively breastfed. This is because chemicals from the mother's diet may get into the breast milk and cause colicky, irritable behavior, loose stools, eczema and nappy (diaper) rashes. If the mother goes onto an elimination diet, baby's symptoms are likely to settle rapidly.

What about sugar alcohols?

Many reduced-calorie foods contain sugar alcohols that, although not as potentially harmful as artificial sweeteners, can cause extreme stomach upset in kids. Products containing these ingredients carry the warning: "Excessive consumption may have a laxative effect." Xylitol (967) is the only sugar alcohol that is vaguely beneficial as it can help reduce the risk of dental cavities.

What to look out for:

Sorbitol (420)

Erythritol (968)

Isomalt (953)

Maltitol or hydrogenated glucose syrup (965)

Mannitol (421)

❹ STABILIZERS Carrageenan (170), an indigestible polysaccharide that is extracted from edible red algae, is most commonly used in food as a thickener or stabilizer. In 2016, the National Organic Standards Board, an independent body that advises the US Department of Agriculture, announced it would no longer permit carrageenan as an additive in organic food. Current research remains inconclusive but has shown a link to digestive disorders and inflammation in lab animals. Although the evidence may be inconclusive, the fact that it is related to digestive issues means I recommend avoiding carrageenan for young children.

Found in:

Shelf-stable dairy beverages, milk alternatives such as almond milk, coconut milk, flavored chocolate milks, ice cream, yogurt and yogurt alternatives, cottage cheese, whipped cream, fruit jellies, ready-to-eat infant formula.

Potential effect on children:

Inconclusive, though animal studies have shown that carrageenan can cause inflammation and intestinal damage in some animals.

What to look out for:

- **Carrageenan (170).** Carrageenan may be found in a final product but not listed on the ingredients list when it is used as a "processing aid"—for example, in cream. Contact the manufacturer directly to ask whether carrageenan is in the final product. The website www.cornucopia.org has a shopping guide to help consumers avoid organic foods containing carrageenan.

WHAT IS A PRESERVATIVE?

Preservatives are food additives that have been around since humans began preparing food. Perhaps the best-known preservative is salt. They are certainly useful to keep food safe by preventing mold from forming, however some modern-day chemical preservatives can have unintended side effects on our health.

Today, our children consume food differently to the way we once did. When I was a child, a cake was always a homemade treat and if we were having guests for Sunday afternoon tea, my mother would spend the whole morning baking. We loved these occasions and did not expect the leftover treats to last more than a few days, but these days a supermarket cake can last a week or more thanks to preservatives. In one infamous experiment, a McDonald's burger kept in a jar was able to last for thirty days without growing any mold!

Of course some preservatives are necessary, but unfortunately many companies are more concerned with taste and shelf life than with what's healthy for the consumer. With their lower body weights, young children are far more vulnerable to preservatives than we are.

As a new mother I remember being advised by a well-meaning nurse to feed my infant the same food as the rest of the family when I started giving him solids. Fortunately for my son the food we ate was mostly homemade, but it is not uncommon to see some babies being fed French fries dipped in additive-filled mayonnaise—and then suffering from colic or wind.

There are also some preservatives that must be avoided to attain optimal health, especially for young children. Australian food intolerance expert Sue Dengate and her husband Dr. Howard Dengate provide independent information about the effects of food on behavior, health and learning in children. They also offer support for families following low-chemical elimination diets. Some of the information that follows is based on their research.

NATURAL CHEMICALS

Natural chemicals like salicylates, amines, and glutamates found in many healthy foods can create the same problems for sensitive people as artificial food additives. Small amounts of natural chemicals present in a particular food may not be enough to cause a reaction the first few times that food is eaten. However, because these chemicals are common to many different regularly eaten foods they accumulate in the body eventually causing a reaction when a child's threshold is exceeded. Therefore it can be quite easy to blame the last food eaten prior to the reaction, instead of looking at the many foods that contain natural chemicals.

Note: Always consult your GP, pediatrician, dietician, or nutritionist before following an elimination diet for your child.

The following natural chemicals may be problematic for sensitive children:

SALICYLATES Plant-based chemicals found naturally in certain fruits, vegetables, nuts, herbs, and spices, jellies, honey, yeast extracts, tea, coffee, juices and flavor additives used in foods, drinks and liquid medications, including herbal.

Potential effects on children:
• Headaches
• Rashes
• Gastric disturbances
• Asthma
• Rhinitis
• Behavioral issues
• Insomnia
• Night terrors
• Bed wetting
• Anxiety and depression

AMINES These come from the breakdown of protein. Foods such as cheese, fish, and meat increase their amine content as they age. They are also present in fruits such as bananas, avocado, and olives and, as these fruits ripen, the amine levels increase. Plus you'll also find them naturally occurring in sauces, fruit juices, chocolate, flavored spreads, nut and seed pastes, jellies, and fermented products such as pickles and yeast extract.

Potential effects on children:
• Behavioral issues
• Migraines and headaches
• Rashes
• Digestive disorders

GLUTAMATE Glutamate is an amino acid building block of all proteins and is found naturally in most foods. In its free form, (not linked to protein) it enhances the flavor of food. This is why foods rich in natural glutamate such as cheese, tomato, mushrooms, soy sauce, meat extracts and yeast extracts are used to add flavor to meals. For the same reason, MSG (pure monosodium glutamate) is used as an additive in savory snack foods, soups, sauces, and Asian cooking.

Potential effects on children:
• Behavioral issues
• Migraines and headaches
• Rashes
• Digestive disorders

DID YOU KNOW?

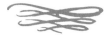

Infants and young children are more vulnerable to toxins than adults.

How to find out if a member of your family is sensitive to sulphites

1 Familiarize yourself with the sulphite numbers and names listed in the table on the following page and look through your pantry to see which products contain sulphites.

2 Keep a food diary for one week and record any symptoms that are triggered from eating a particular food—check to see if it contains sulphites.

3 Eliminate all sulphite-containing products from your pantry and avoid when eating out. It most likely won't be possible to eliminate them entirely as they occur naturally in some food, but you can drastically reduce them. Try to follow a wholefood diet and choose organic, preservative-free products wherever possible.

4 After four to six weeks, check in to see if your child's symptoms have reduced. Are they less wheezy, having fewer asthma attacks? Has their rash reduced, are migraines less frequent, or has behavior improved?

5 If you find there is an improvement in any of the symptoms, continue following a low-sulphite diet and replace favorite foods with preservative-free alternatives where possible.

Preservatives to Avoid

BHA AND BHT

Found in
Vegetable oils, margarine, spreadable butter, cookies, cakes, cereal, pastries, sweets, chewing gum, milk powder, frozen dinners, bread, wraps, frozen French fries.

There is ongoing debate about the safety of BHA (Butylated hydroxyanisole) and BHT (Butylated hydroxytoluene), both petroleum-derived antioxidants commonly used to prevent rancidity in fats and oils. Although BHA, which is a heat stable additive used in baked products, is a suspected carcinogen and banned in the UK (in instant foods), in parts of Europe and in Japan, the US Food and Drug administration categorizes it as GRAS (generally regarded as safe).

Potential effects on children
Suspected carcinogen, gastrointestinal disturbances, aggression, hyperactivity, mood disturbances (depression, insomnia), asthma, eczema, dermatitis, hives, rashes.

What to avoid
Along with BHA (320) and BHT (321) avoid: Propyl gallate (310); Octyl gallate (311); Dodecyl gallate (312); tert-Butylhydroquinone (319), tertiary butylhydroquinone (tBHQ)

Suggestions
- Avoid products that contain vegetable oils.
- Choose foods that say "preservative free" on the pack or organic packaged foods as they contain little or no synthetic colors or preservatives.
- Look for products containing ascorbic acid (300). Infant products use ascorbic acid or vitamin C, a far safer antioxidant than the above mentioned ones and you'll also find it in other products lining the supermarket shelves too.
- Another safer antioxidant option is citric acid although it may provoke mild symptoms in sensitive individuals.

Note: Unless a product is certified organic, both ascorbic acid and citric acid may be derived from GM sources.

SORBATES

Found in
Orange juice, cheese, pickles, yogurt, dips, dried meats, soft drinks, ice cream, baked goods.

Sorbic acid and its calcium, sodium, and potassium salts (collectively referred to as sorbates) are another group of preservatives used to inhibit the growth of mold. Derived from petroleum, they can provoke an allergic reaction in sensitive children and are often included in pediatric elimination diet's "to avoid" lists. Sorbates are banned in foods for infants and two studies have found them to have the potential to disrupt our DNA.

Potential effects on children
Headaches and migraines, asthma, allergic reactions (rhinitis, skin irritation), hyperactivity; gastrointestinal upset.

What to avoid
Preservatives 200–203; 200 is also known as sorbic acid while 202 can be called potassium sorbate

Suggestions
- Ascorbic acid (300); Sodium ascorbate (301); Calcium ascorbate (302); Potassium ascorbate (303); Ascorbyl palmitate (304).
- Prepare home-made fruit sorbets and ice creams (see recipe on page 227).
- Make your own fresh squeezed orange juice (diluted with water is always best).
- Choose natural yogurts which contain no additives.

PROPIONATES

Found in
Pre-packaged breads and wraps, cheese, pasta, bakery products, bread crumbs.

Derived from propionic acid, calcium propionate (282) is most commonly known as the "bread preservative." It's often added to supermarket breads and other commercially baked goods to prevent mildew and bacterial growth (now you know why some loaves can last for up to ten days outside the fridge). Studies have found that although calcium propionate may have little to no side effects for the average person, irritability, restlessness, inattention, and sleep disturbance in some children can be attributed to this preservative being consumed daily in their diet.

Potential effects on children
As food intolerance expert Sue Dengate states, "If you wanted to create a nation of underperforming children, you could hardly do better than to add a preservative known to cause learning difficulties to an everyday staple food."

What to avoid
Propionic acid (280), Sodium propionate (281), Calcium propionate (282), Potassium propionate (283), Cultured whey, Cultured wheat, Cultured dextrose

Suggestions
- Follow our guidelines for choosing supermarket bread on page 42.
- Visit an organic bakery or local bakery and ask if they use any form of propionic acid (including cultured whey, wheat or dextrose in their bread).
- Choose freshly baked bread at your local supermarket as it's more likely to not contain propionates (always ask before purchasing).
- Beware of wraps. In my Lunch Box Solutions workshop I show many examples of wraps that have nearly as many preservatives as ingredients. Most contain 280 or 282.

A quick-glance guide to avoiding nasties

BENZOATES	SULPHITES	NITRATES AND NITRITES
Found in	*Found in*	*Found in*
Fruit-based syrups, orange juice, vegetable juice, soft drinks, cheese, yogurt, ice cream, sauces, toppings, baked goods, cough medicines, ointments.	Dried fruit (especially dried apricots and raisins), cordials, sausages, hamburger patties, rissoles, fruit juice, soft drinks, grapes, processed dried vegetables, deli meats, baked goods, glucose syrup, molasses, pickles, garlic powder.	Processed meats like ham, salami, roast beef, chicken, turkey, bacon, sausages, frankfurters, smoked fish, pickled vegetables.
Benzoates, also known as flowers of benzoin, phenlycarboxylic acid, benzene carboxylic acid or carboxybenzene, are one of the oldest preservatives. They are prohibited in foods for infants. Benzoates (especially sodium benzoate 211) are another asthma-causing preservative. Sodium benzoate, when combined with vitamin C, forms benzene. Benzene is a carcinogen and is known to contribute to the formation of many different types of cancer. However, the FDA states that food products containing both vitamin C and sodium benzoate express benzene levels that are below the dangerous limit.	Sulphites are the most common preservatives in foods. Sulphur dioxide, the synthetic form, is used to extend shelf life and protect food from bacteria. They are used to preserve color and moisture in dried fruit. They've been banned in the US in meat since 1959 but can still be found in other foods like frozen french fries. In 1999 the World Health Organization estimated that 20–30 percent of asthmatic children react to sulphites. Sensitivity is dependent on how much a child is exposed to sulphur dioxide or sulphites from all sources over a short period of time.	Smoked and cured foods like ham and sausages are many a parent's answer to protein hits for their kids. Most, however, contain nitrates and nitrites to extend shelf life, preserve color, and prevent bacterial growth. These preservatives have been proven to convert into carcinogenic nitrosamines in the body. According to the American Cancer Society, an increased risk of stomach cancer is seen in people with diets that contain large amounts of smoked foods, salted fish and meat, and pickled vegetables. Nitrates and nitrites can be converted by certain bacteria, such as H pylori, into compounds that have been shown to cause stomach cancer in lab animals. There is also a reported increased risk of bowel cancer.
Potential effects on children	*Potential effects on children*	*Potential effects on children*
Asthma, headaches, hyperactivity, skin irritation, stomach upsets.	Asthma, eczema, skin rashes, headaches, behavior disturbances.	Recurrent infections, headaches, irritable bowel symptoms, stomach cancer, bowel cancer.
What to avoid	*What to avoid*	*What to avoid*
Benzoic acid (210), Sodium benzoate (211), Potassium benzoate (212), Calcium benzoate (213), and the less commonly used 214–219	Sulphur dioxide (220), Sodium sulphite (221), Sodium bisulphite (222), Sodium metabisulphite (223), Potassium metabisulphite (224), Potassium sulphite (225), Potassium bisulphite (228)	Potassium nitrite (249), Sodium nitrite (250), Sodium nitrate (251), Potassium nitrate (252)

Suggestions (Benzoates)

- Avoid soft drinks, cordials and commercial orange juices that contain preservatives.
- Offer ¼ cup freshly squeezed orange juice mixed with ¾ cup water.
- If your child is used to sodas, offer ¼ cup fruit juice of choice with ¾ sparkling water.
- Replace soft drinks and cordials with an occasional smoothie. See recipes on page 225.

Suggestions (Sulphites)

- Make sure dried apricots, other dried fruits, and any other common sulphite-containing foods are labelled "sulphite free."
- Dried apricots, cordial, sausages and hamburger patties are the greatest source of sulphites for children and should be avoided as much as possible.

Suggestions (Nitrates and Nitrites)

- Minimize your consumption of processed and cured meat products such as hot dogs, sausages and cold cuts.
- Visit a reputable organic butcher and ask for preservative-free sausages, meatball patties, and other deli meats.
- Choose organic salmon or other forms of smoked fish which say "nitrite or nitrate free."
- Read labels. It's not uncommon for nitrates and nitrites to be found in canned or frozen vegetables or quiches that contain bacon or packaged seafood.

DID YOU KNOW?

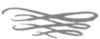

Babies and small children with reduced-salt diets have lower blood pressure, eat healthier foods overall and are likely to have fewer health problems and better eating patterns into adulthood.

THE BOTTOM LINE

The continuing debate around the safety of additives and preservatives highlights the need for regulatory bodies to ensure that food additives, when being approved for use in our food, are initially tested for safety and continue to undergo long-term monitoring for their effects on chronic health conditions—especially in young children.

If the harm from these substances could potentially have on your family's health (especially babies and children under six) concerns you, then the best option is to avoid or minimize processed foods, use fresh ingredients when possible, read food ingredient labels and become more aware of what is in the products your family is eating.

THE TRUTH ABOUT SALT

While we are warned to reduce our salt intake, it is actually essential for health, helping to maintain and regulate fluid levels, balance blood sugar and transport nutrients around the body. But too much can increase blood pressure and lead to heart and kidney disease.

Table salt is 40 percent sodium (the other 60 percent is chloride) and this mineral is important for nerves, muscles and the cardiovascular system. Salt can help your child's body to absorb other important nutrients more effectively, too.

Celtic sea salt, Himalayan rock salt and natural sea salts are far better than white table salt as they contain beneficial trace elements and minerals. However, only use sparingly in your children's diets. Too much salt can be harmful, especially for growing bodies, as it can produce a serious rise in blood pressure. For children, this will get progressively worse with age.

Tiny tastebuds are impressionable too, so a salty childhood sets up cravings for salty food—a difficult habit to break and a potential route to illnesses including kidney stones and stroke.

SO HOW MUCH SODIUM IS SAFE FOR CHILDREN?

Children's diets can contain as much as 75 percent more salt per day than they need. Most salt is hidden in processed foods such as bread, deli meats, cookies, cheese, chips, sausages, canned soups, ready-prepared meals, chicken patties or nuggets, take-out food, or pasta with sauce. And don't be fooled—one cheese sandwich can contain 1000mg of sodium or more. That's already the entire daily allowance for an under three-year-old in a single sandwich.

Tolerable Upper Intake Levels (UL)

1 to 3 years: 1500mg sodium/day
(1000 -1500mg/day)

4 to 8 years: 1900 mg sodium/day
(1200-1900mg/day)

9 to 13 years: 2200mg sodium/day
(1500-2200mg/day)

DO CHILDREN NEED IODINE?

Humans require trace amounts of iodine, a non-metallic mineral, for proper development and growth. It is true that iodine deficiency is on the rise, because of the lack of iodine-rich soil.

Most white table salts have been iodized, meaning iodine has been added to them, but table salt is usually stripped of its naturally occurring minerals first and then potassium iodide is added back in along with anti-caking agents and other additives.

If your child is eating a healthy, balanced, varied diet, he's probably getting enough iodine (iodine can be found in dairy from cattle who graze on iodine-rich grass as well as veggies grown in iodine-rich soil). Instead of using iodized salt, offer your child a range of iodine-rich foods such as saltwater fish and nori seaweed.

SHOULD YOU AVOID GMOS?

A genetically modified organism (GMO) has had its DNA altered in a laboratory in order to exhibit different characteristics. Crops like soy, corn, and wheat have been changed in this way to make

How to reduce salt intake

1 Cut out processed foods wherever possible. This immediately lowers sodium intake.

2 Reduce salt slowly in cooking so your family's taste buds can adapt.

3 Don't put salt or salty condiments on the table (table salt, ketchup, soy sauce etc).

4 Choose low-sodium, preservative-free stocks, sauces, and salad dressings or make your own.

5 Rinse canned foods like beans or chickpeas.

DID YOU KNOW?

Low salt does not mean low flavor if you experiment with herbs and spices instead.

The sodium content of packaged foods is part of the Nutrition Facts panel. The label gives the sodium in milligrams in one serving of the food. It also gives the Percent Daily Value (%DV), which is the percent of sodium in one serving compared to the daily recommended amount for a 2,000 calorie diet. If a food has 140mg sodium or less per serving, or 5% DV or less, it is low in sodium; if it has 20% DV or more, it is high in sodium.

HOW MUCH SODIUM IS YOUR CHILD EATING?

1. To determine whether a food is high in sodium, check the Nutrition Facts, which is usually found on the side or back of the product package. The label gives the sodium in milligrams in one serving of the food. It also gives the Percent Daily Value (%DV) of sodium, which is the percent of sodium in one serving compared to the daily recommended amount for a 2,000 calorie diet. If a food has 140mg sodium or less per serving, or 5% DV or less, it is low in sodium; if it has 20% DV or more, it is high in sodium.

2. To quickly identify foods that contain less sodium, check if there is a nutrient claim on the front of the product package. If it says the product is reduced in sodium, that means it has at least 25% less sodium than the regular product. If it says the product is low sodium, that means it has 140mg or less sodium per serving; if it says it is very low sodium, it has 35mg or less sodium per serving.

3. An overall guide is:
   140mg or less per serving is low (the healthiest choice)
   Over 140mg to 460mg is moderate.
   460 mg or more per serving is high (limit or avoid these foods)

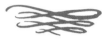
them toxic to bugs or immune to weed-killers and so easier to cultivate.

The entire GM crop can be blanket sprayed with a herbicide, like Roundup, without harming the cash crop. The American conglomerate Monsanto is a driving force behind GM crops and also the producer of Roundup. Monsanto has also produced an artificial hormone to increase milk yields in cows, something the Organic Consumer's Association has campaigned against since the mid-1990s.

WHY I DON'T BUY GM FOODS

One of my greatest dietary concerns is the inclusion of GM ingredients in young children's food. A child's digestive system is immature; their cells and organs are still growing. While GM advocates will tell you that there are no long-term trials proving GMOs are harmful, equally there are no long-term clinical trials proving them safe, so is it really worth taking the chance?

With no scientific consensus on safety, it can take decades for the true effects of a new product containing GMOs to be known. Trans fats are an example of an ingredient initially thought to be potentially healthy turning out to be hazardous to our health.

The World Health Organization (WHO) has termed glyphosate, a primary ingredient of Monsanto's Roundup, "probably carcinogenic to humans" and genetic modification has allowed a much greater use of this herbicide.

Lobby group Moms Across America has found worrying levels of glyphosate in tests on breast milk, suggesting there may be a risk of bioaccumulation (a build-up of a substance in

the body). I believe natural is best and changing the genetic makeup of food could set up a chain reaction that affects important gut-flora and lead to illness in the long term.

Most important is our right to know if a food contains GM ingredients so that parents can choose whether or not to use that particular product or food.

HOW TO AVOID GMOS

This is not as easy as you might think. Many foods can often contain ingredients like GM vegetable oils, soy lecithin, and corn syrup. If a product does not clearly state that it is GMO-free, then it probably isn't.

1. **Cook from scratch.** Processed foods, especially anything made using vegetable oil, is a prime source of GMOs. Be aware of this when buying bread, dips, margarine, chips, crackers, cereals, dairy-free milk replacements and baked goods like cakes and muffins.

2. **Buy seasonal, local vegetables and fruits.** Eat them fresh or freeze them.

3. **Consider what your food has been fed.** There is no way to recognize animal products from animals fed GM feed, so going for 100% grass-fed meat (remember grass-fed labeling may be grain-finished, so look for grass-fed and grass-finished where possible) and organic dairy and poultry is the only way to be sure.

4. **Buy certified organic or Non-GMO Project verified food.** Look for the butterfly icon

FOOD ALLERGY VS FOOD INTOLERANCE: WHAT'S THE DIFFERENCE?

FOOD ALLERGY	FOOD INTOLERANCE
Involves the immune system (IGE antibodies). Usually begins in the first twelve months.	Doesn't involve the immune system at all. Triggered by various natural food chemicals and/or artificial additives which cause reactions by irritating nerve endings in different parts of the body. Occurs at any age.
Symptoms appear within minutes or in one to two hours, usually atopic eczema—an intensely itchy chronic skin rash. Some children experience potentially life-threatening anaphylaxis.	Symptoms can appear within hours or take days, making it difficult to investigate cause. They include irritable behavior (colic/screaming, disturbed sleep, leg aches and pains, ADHD). Reflux from birth, eczema/itchy rashes and nappy rash.
Needs to be supervised by a medical allergy specialist.	Can be diagnosed by an elimination diet, food challenges or blood test (not as reliable as elimination diet).

or download the free Non-GMO Project Shopping Guide app.

5. **Beware of corn and soy.** Most corn and soy products are GM-derived.

FOOD ALLERGIES, FOOD INTOLERANCES, AND SENSITIVITIES

If you suspect your child has a food allergy or intolerance, see your GP or pediatrician straight away. It also helps to do the following:

- Keep a food diary and record food eaten and any reactions. Include what food was eaten, how much, what symptoms, how long they lasted and if any medication was given.

- If a reaction occurs in a restaurant or at a friend's home, find out exactly what was in the food given to your child.

- If a symptom arises, such as a rash, take a photograph to show to your doctor.

- If a symptom occurs after eating a particular packaged food, save the packaging with the nutrition label or take a photo to show your GP or pediatrician.

- Remove suspected foods from the diet for a period of two to six weeks or until symptom fades (discuss first with GP or pediatrician).

- Slowly reintroduce the foods, in a controlled manner, one at a time, recording any symptoms if they should appear.

- Have a detailed record of any allergy history on both sides of the family.

GOAL 8: SET GOALS & REWARDS

One of the points of difference in my approach as a clinical nutritionist is that I combine nutritional advice with behavioral change techniques. From my own experience as a child, and as a qualified practitioner and mother-of-two, I know kids do not eat new food just because we want them to. Often they need encouragement and parents need to be guided on how best to motivate their child to display positive eating behaviors and to let go of negative ones.

Encouraging children to try new foods can be daunting for them (and frustrating for you) at the best of times. Setting goals and offering rewards can be a very powerful tool to encourage children to broaden their repertoire, as long as it is age appropriate and achievable.

Don't set your child up for failure by setting goals that are too advanced or too far out of their comfort zone.

USE THE SMART APPROACH

When I worked on the MEND program I spent time with Dr. Paul Chadwick, an expert in behavior change for children. Dr. Chadwick, who works as Professional Lead for Psychology Services at Camden Integrated Practice Unit for Diabetes in the UK, developed the behavioral aspect of the MEND program using a reward system based on SMART goals.

The SMART goal approach can be applied to help break unhealthy food and inactivity behaviors and to establish new ones. Setting goals with kids from a young age can reinforce their internal motivation to do something new—and when applied to new eating behaviors, can be very effective.

WHAT SMART STANDS FOR

S = Specific The goals you set for your child need to be specific (e.g., eat one new vegetable each week, eat half the amount of chocolate on the weekend, eat breakfast before school).

M = Measurable You need to be able to measure if your child has achieved their goal. Did they eat a carrot this week? Did they eat two less chocolate bars on the weekend? How many mornings included breakfast before school?

A = Achievable Does your child have the ability or skills to achieve this goal? Is it age appropriate? An example of a non-achievable goal for a fussy child who hates vegetables would be eating a new vegetable at every meal for a week. An achievable goal is trying a new vegetable at one meal each day for the week.

R = Relevant Try to choose a goal that will have most benefit for your child. There's no point setting a goal to reduce chocolate cake in their diet if they are low in iron and only have cake at their grandmother's house once a week. Start with something they can work on in their day-to-day life. Example: Try to eat iron-rich meatballs at two meals this week.

T = Time-limited Young children are more inclined to work towards a goal if there is immediate gain. Stretching a goal over too long a timeframe is not as productive as working towards a goal with a clear end in sight. So instead of making the goal "eat carrots more often," make it "eat carrots three times before Monday."

DID YOU KNOW?

Cow's milk, egg, peanuts, tree nuts, fish, shellfish, soy and wheat are most likely to cause an allergic reaction in children. Most kids will grow out of milk and egg allergies.

DID YOU KNOW?

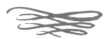

The most effective rewards are daily praise, affection, and giving children time and attention. For these to have the most effect give them as close to the positive behavior as possible. For example, if your child tries a new food, praise them for trying, even if they stop at a lick.

NEVER USE FOOD AS A REWARD

Romy Kunitz, a Sydney-based child psychologist, endorses my belief that we should try as much as possible to not use food as a reward or punishment, however tempting this may be. I am often disappointed by the amount of candies used to reward or incentivise children at school and even at some doctor's offices.

Using food as a reward teaches children to value sweet treats over other foods, to eat when they are not hungry and to develop lifelong habits of rewarding or comforting themselves with unhealthy foods. We are reinforcing from such a young age, that certain foods are more valuable than others, and as a result children learn to prefer unhealthy foods.

Nutrition principles, taught in a classroom or at home, are undermined if they are contradicted by sweet rewards. We are saying to children "you need to eat healthy foods to feel good and perform your best, however when you do well we will reward you with unhealthy food.'"

On the other hand, withholding food as a punishment may lead children to worry that they will not get enough food. For example, sending them to bed without any dinner may cause them to worry they will go hungry. As a result, they may feel deprived and eat whenever they get the chance. Note: This is different to not offering your child a second choice when they refuse the food you've offered them at a meal.

GOOD NON-FOOD REWARDS

- A play date or sleepover with a special friend.
- A favorite outing—zoo, movie or aquarium.
- Child gets to choose a movie to watch.
- Child gets to stay up later than usual.
- Child gets to choose a weekend activity.

HOW TO SET GOALS AND REWARDS

1. **Agree on the goal together.** You cannot enforce a goal. Your child needs to feel comfortable and be motivated to reach it.

2. **Manage your disappointment.** If your child fails to achieve their goal, it may mean the goal was too difficult or that they are not ready for it. Don't give up. Eventually they will succeed and their confidence will be raised.

3. **Choose a reward system.** Sticker and reward charts are usually effective for children from the age of three onwards. The reward system that I use with my own children and with clients (starting from four and a half years) is what I call The Bead System, inspired by my son's preschool teacher. One day when I went to pick up my son, I found him counting what looked like golden rocks. The educator explained she was rewarding the children with "golden nuggets" for things like listening, sharing and taking turns. At the end of each week she had what she called a 'market day'. The children could exchange their nuggets for rewards such as stickers, pencils and erasers. I decided to use a version of this system in my home. I was struggling to get my son to sit in his chair during mealtimes, so we agreed that for every meal where he sat in his seat to eat, he would receive a bead, which we placed in a glass jar. At the end of the week we counted his beads and I put out a few items for "market day" and he exchanged his beads for a set of stickers. Over time this system has changed and often we exchange beads for an adventure or movie. Now my daughter also participates and they love counting their beads.

Reward Do's and Don'ts

👍 DO...	👎 DON'T...
ensure the goal set is agreed upon with your child.	use food as a reward or punishment.
reward small goals with small rewards and larger goals with larger rewards. If you start out with big rewards for small goals, you can run into trouble.	punish your child for not achieving their goal—even the anger in your voice could be experienced as punishment.
ensure that rewards are not given in the distant future. Children want instant gratification.	make your child feel like a failure for not achieving their goal. Encourage them to try again.
make sure that the goal set is achievable.	set them up for failure with unachievable goals.

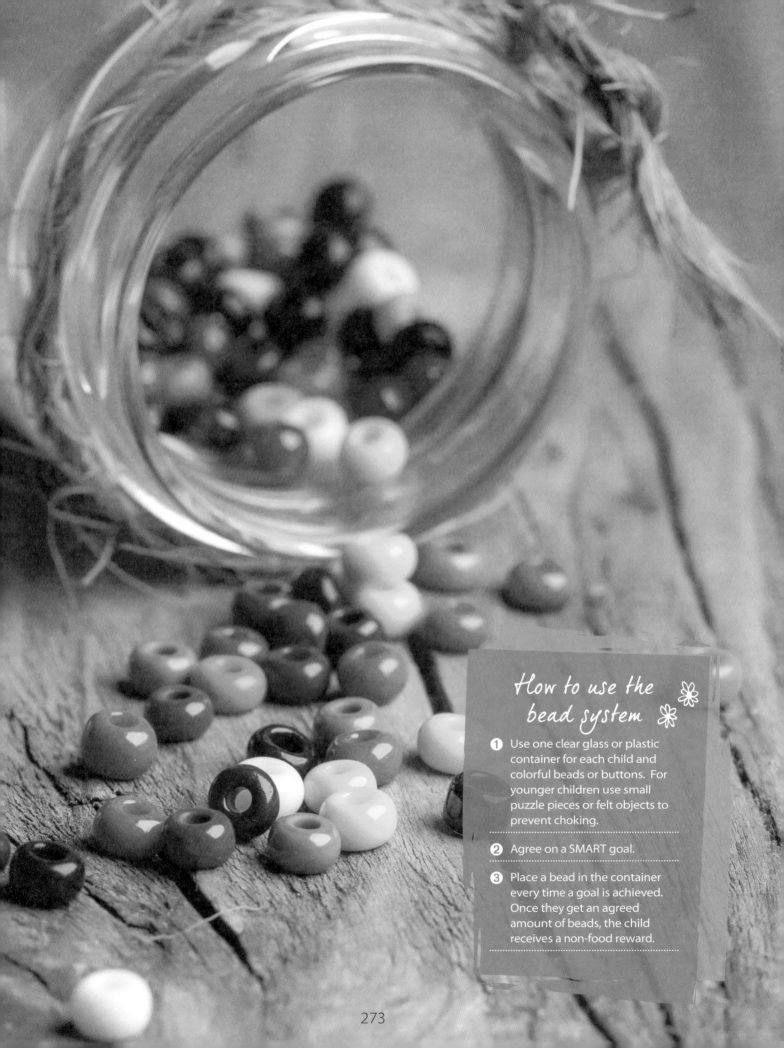

How to use the bead system ❀ ❀

1 Use one clear glass or plastic container for each child and colorful beads or buttons. For younger children use small puzzle pieces or felt objects to prevent choking.

2 Agree on a SMART goal.

3 Place a bead in the container every time a goal is achieved. Once they get an agreed amount of beads, the child receives a non-food reward.

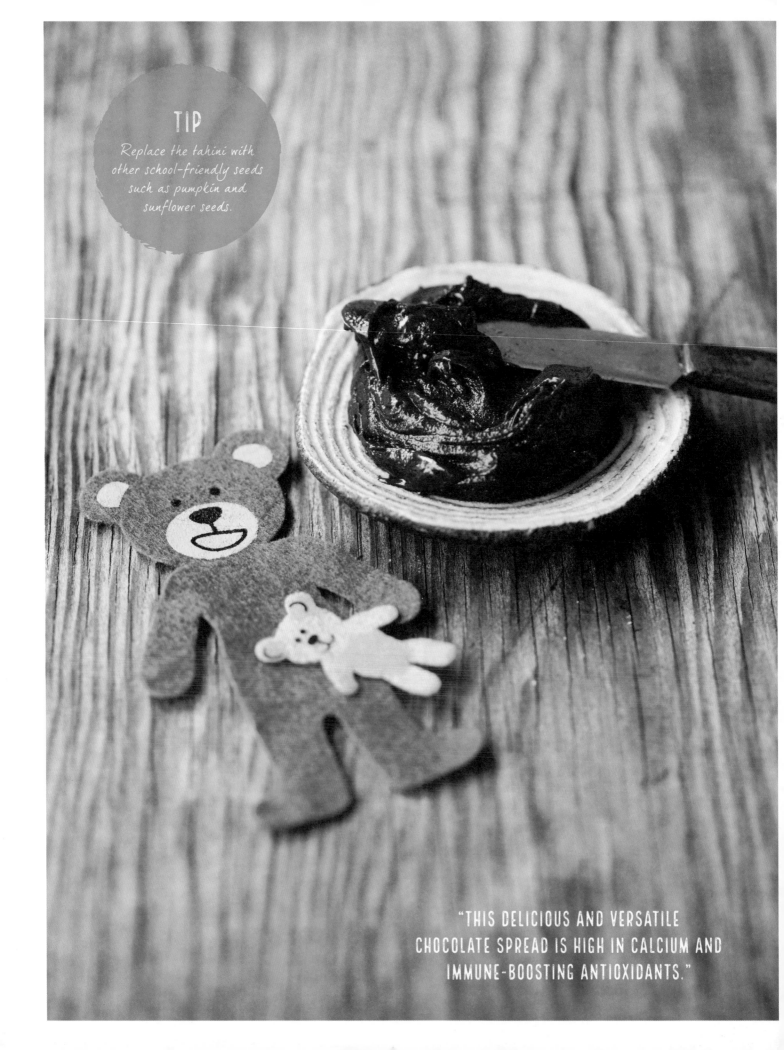

TIP

Replace the tahini with other school-friendly seeds such as pumpkin and sunflower seeds.

"THIS DELICIOUS AND VERSATILE CHOCOLATE SPREAD IS HIGH IN CALCIUM AND IMMUNE-BOOSTING ANTIOXIDANTS."

Vegan Gluten Free Nut Free

Prep time: 5 mins
Makes: 1 cup

Healthy Chocolate Spread

I came up with this healthy substitute during my first pregnancy when the chocolate cravings hit hard. The bonus is that my kids love it!

INGREDIENTS

¼ cup (⅞ oz) carob powder

¼ cup (⅞ oz) cacao powder

½ cup maple syrup or raw honey

¼ cup (2⅞ oz) hulled tahini

1 tbs coconut oil, melted

1 tbs filtered water

EQUIPMENT
hand-held blender

INSTRUCTIONS

Place all ingredients in a medium-sized bowl, and using a hand-held blender, blend until a smooth consistency is reached.

If it is too thick, add an additional tablespoon of water and keep adding until desired consistency is reached.

Serving and storing leftovers:
Serve immediately, store in an airtight container in the fridge for up to two weeks or freeze for up to 4 months.

Vegan Gluten Free

Prep time: 5 mins
Makes: 2 cups

Malted Chocolate Drink

INGREDIENTS

1 cup (5⅔ oz) mixed nuts (almonds/cashews/macadamias/pecans/Brazils)

¼ cup (1⅖ oz) mixed seeds (sunflower/pumpkin)

2 tbs black chia seeds

½ cup (2¾ oz) coconut sugar

¼ cup (⅞ oz) cacao powder

½ cup (1¾ oz) carob powder

1 tsp pure vanilla extract

1 glass non-dairy milk

EQUIPMENT
high-speed food processor or high-powered blender

INSTRUCTIONS

Place all the nuts and seeds in a high-speed food processor and process until it resembles a fine powder, not a paste.

Transfer to a bowl, add coconut sugar, cacao, carob, and vanilla and mix thoroughly until well combined.

To use, add 1–1½ tbs of the mixture to a glass of non-dairy milk and stir until well combined. It

won't dissolve completely because of the nuts and seeds.

Serving and storing leftovers: Store in an airtight container in the fridge for up to 2 months or freeze for up to 4 months.

Can also be used as a chocolatey topping on sweet treats like our homemade ice creams (see page 227).

Vegan Wheat Free Nut Free

Prep time: 5 min
Cooking Time: 15 min
Makes: 4 cups

Quick Homemade Granola

INGREDIENTS

4 cups (1 lbs) whole rolled oats

2 tsp pure vanilla extract

¼ cup maple syrup or raw honey

⅓ cup coconut oil, melted

INSTRUCTIONS

Preheat oven to 340°F and line a baking tray with baking paper.

In a large bowl, combine all ingredients and stir until all oats are coated with honey oil mixture.

Spread mixture onto the baking tray and bake in the oven for 15 mins, stirring occasionally.

Allow to cool on the tray before transferring into a glass jar or an airtight container.

Serving and storing leftovers: Serve immediately with some non-dairy milk or store in a glass jar or airtight container in a cool, dry spot for up to 1 month or freeze in an airtight container for up to 6 months.

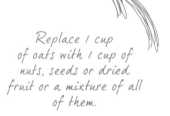

Replace 1 cup of oats with 1 cup of nuts, seeds or dried fruit or a mixture of all of them.

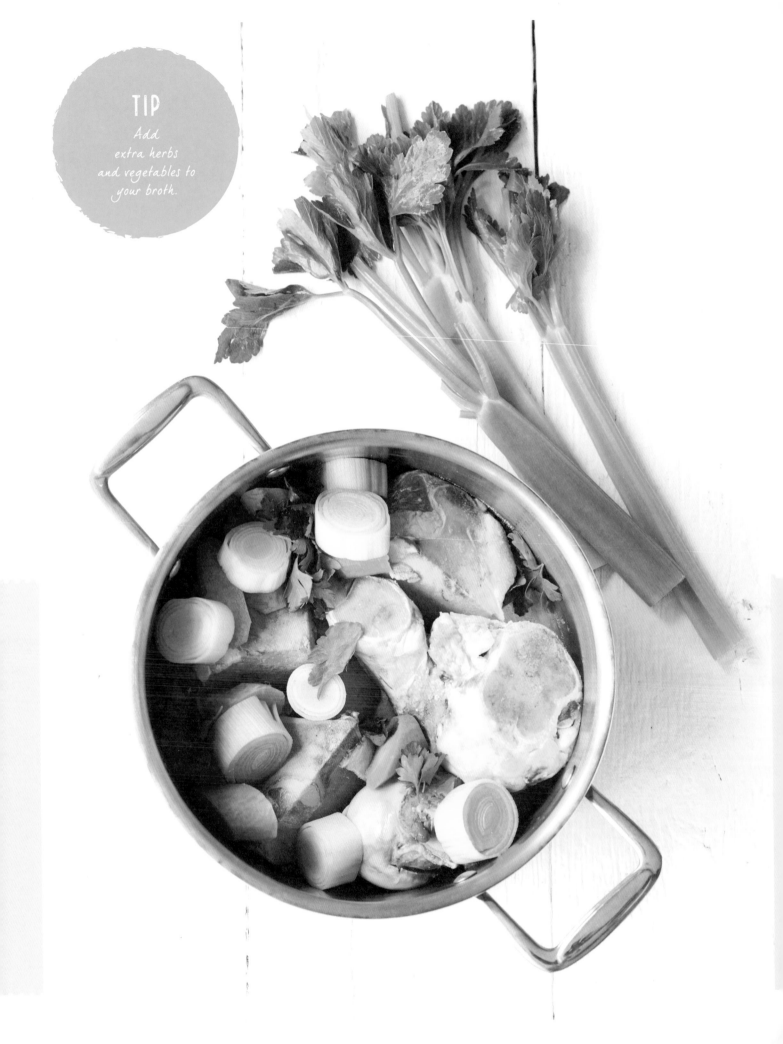

TIP
Add
extra herbs
and vegetables to
your broth.

Egg Free
 Gluten Free
 Nut Free
 Dairy Free

Prep time: 5–30 mins
Cooking time: 4–18 hours
Makes: 3½ to 4 quarts

Bone Broth

This is my go-to broth when my kids don't feel well. It's an excellent source of bio-available nutrients in an easy-to-digest form, is healing for the gut, boosts the immune system, and soothes sore tummies.

INGREDIENTS

3¼ lbs beef or chicken bones, grass fed and organic

1 leek, finely sliced

2 large carrots, chopped

2 stalks of celery, roughly chopped

2 tbs apple cider vinegar

1 tsp Himalayan rock salt

filtered water

1 bunch flat-leaf parsley

INSTRUCTIONS

Preheat your oven to 355°F and roast the bones for approximately 30 mins. (This step is optional).

Place bones in a large pot or a slow cooker, add vegetables, vinegar and salt and cover with filtered water. If using a slow cooker, it should be ¾ full.

Cook uncovered for at least 4 hours. Add more water if necessary. If using a slow cooker set on low and allow to cook for approximately 12–18 hrs.

Add parsley in the last 15 mins of cooking.

Allow to cool, remove bones and store the liquid in small freezer containers.

Add to purees, meat dishes, sauces, roast veggies.

Serving and storing leftovers: Serve immediately, store in fridge for up to 3 days or freeze for up to 4 months.

 Vegan
 Gluten Free
 Nut Free

Prep time: 10 mins
Cooking time: 2 hours
Makes: 2 quarts

Vegetable Stock

INGREDIENTS

1 large yellow onion, unpeeled and cut in half

2 garlic cloves, unpeeled and crushed

½ celery root (7 oz), roughly peeled and chopped

2 large carrots, chopped

1 leek, chopped

½ fennel (4¼ oz), roughly chopped

1 medium-sized parsnip, chopped

1 tomato, quartered

10 cups (2¾ quarts) filtered water

1 small bunch of parsley

3 bay leaves

½ tbs peppercorns

½ tbs cilantro seeds

1 sprig thyme

3 cloves

sea salt, to taste

INSTRUCTIONS

Heat a large pot over medium heat. Place onions in pot and let brown underneath.

Add water, herbs, and spices and allow to cook, uncovered, for at least 2 hours. Add more water if necessary.

Pour the stock through a sieve. Discard the vegetable pieces or reserve for another use.

Store in the fridge or freeze in portions.

Serving and storing leftovers: Serve immediately, store in an airtight container in the fridge for up to 4 days or freeze for up to 4 months.

Dairy
Free

Gluten
Free

Egg
Free

Nut
Free

Prep time: 10
Cooking time: 1 hour (+15 mins resting time)
Serves: 4

Roast Chicken in Marinade

This delicious marinade was inspired by my wonderful mother who often has us over for a roast chicken dinner. Thanks Mom!

INGREDIENTS

1 whole organic chicken (3¼ lbs)

½ cup extra virgin olive oil

1 tbs mild paprika powder

4–6 garlic cloves, crushed

2–3 tbs fresh sage, finely chopped

2–3 tbs fresh parsley, finely chopped

2–3 tbs fresh rosemary, finely chopped

sea salt and pepper, to taste

1 organic lemon

2–3 extra rosemary sprigs

INSTRUCTIONS

Pre-heat the oven to 390°F.

Rinse the chicken, pat dry with paper towel, and place in a roasting tin.

Whisk the olive oil in a small bowl along with the paprika, garlic, sage, parsley, rosemary, salt and pepper.

Pour the mixture over the top of the chicken and rub all over. Make sure the chicken is coated evenly.

Place the lemon inside the chicken's cavity along with a few extra rosemary sprigs.

Tuck the chicken wings behind the back to keep them from burning in the oven and tie the legs together with a piece of kitchen twine (optional).

Roast the chicken for about an hour, (turning half way) or until cooked through.

Remove from oven and allow to rest for 15 mins before slicing and serving.

Serving and storing leftovers: Serve immediately, store in the fridge for up to 3 days or freeze for up to 4 months

Add potatoes or sweet potatoes and vegetables such as carrots, celery, parsnips and onions, drizzle with extra virgin olive oil and 1/2 cup of water, and roast with the chicken.

Dairy
Free

Gluten
Free

Egg
Free

Nut
Free

Prep time: 5 mins
Makes: ¾ cup
(enough for 1 lb meat)

Red Meat Marinade

INGREDIENTS

10 thyme stalks, stems removed and leaves chopped

¼ cup fresh lemon juice

juice of half an orange

1 tbs capers

2 garlic cloves, crushed

¼ cup extra virgin olive oil

pinch sea salt and pepper

INSTRUCTIONS

Mix all ingredients together in a small bowl until well combined.

Marinate meat (beef, lamb or pork) with the mixture and let sit for at least 1–2 hours before cooking.

Serving and storing leftovers: Serve immediately, store in an

airtight container in the fridge for up to 2 weeks or freeze for up to 4 months.

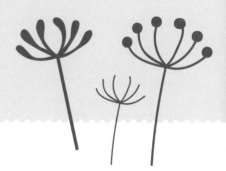

Egg Free   Gluten Free   Dairy Free

Prep time: 10 mins
Cooking time: 10 mins
Serves: 4

Beef Stir Fry

A delicious and fragrant stir-fry that is not too spicy for tiny tastebuds.

INGREDIENTS

2 tbs coconut oil

3 cloves garlic, finely minced

1 tsp ginger, finely minced

1 bunch broccolini, roughly chopped

1 medium-sized red pepper, cut into thin strips

1¹⁄₈ lbs to 1¹⁄₃ lbs beef fillet, thinly sliced

¹⁄₄ cup (¹⁄₆ oz) fresh basil, roughly chopped

¹⁄₄ cup (¹⁄₆ oz) fresh cilantro, roughly chopped

¹⁄₂ cup (2⁴⁄₅) activated or roasted cashew nuts, chopped

SAUCE:

3 tbs tamari

juice of 1 lime

¹⁄₃ cup beef stock or filtered water

¹⁄₂ tsp cold pressed sesame oil (optional)

1 tsp arrowroot

INSTRUCTIONS

Heat oil in a wok or a large frying pan over medium heat.

Add garlic and ginger and sauté for a minute.

Add broccolini and pepper and cook for 2–3 mins or until just cooked through. Transfer to a bowl and set aside.

Add beef strips to the wok or frying pan and cook for 2–3 mins or until browned. Transfer to the bowl with the veggies and set aside.

Combine all sauce ingredients in a small bowl, then add to the wok/pan and simmer for a minute or until thickened.

Return veggies and meat to the wok/pan along with the herbs and nuts (if using) and cook for another minute, stirring through until well combined.

Serve with coconut rice.

Serving and storing leftovers: Serve immediately, store in fridge for up to 3 days or freeze for up to 4 months.

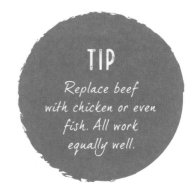

TIP

Replace beef with chicken or even fish. All work equally well.

Dairy Free   Gluten Free   Egg Free   Nut Free

Prep time: 5 mins
Makes: ¾ cup
(enough for 1 lb fish)

Easy Fish Marinade

INGREDIENTS

¹⁄₃ cup extra virgin olive oil

¹⁄₄ cup fresh lemon juice

4 sprigs thyme, stems removed and chopped

1–2 cloves of garlic, crushed

1 tbs fresh basil, finely chopped

¹⁄₄ tsp sea salt

pinch pepper

INSTRUCTIONS

In a small bowl combine all ingredients and mix well.

Use to marinate fish for at least an hour before cooking.

Serving and storing leftovers: Serve immediately, store in the fridge for up to 2 weeks or freeze for up to 4 months.

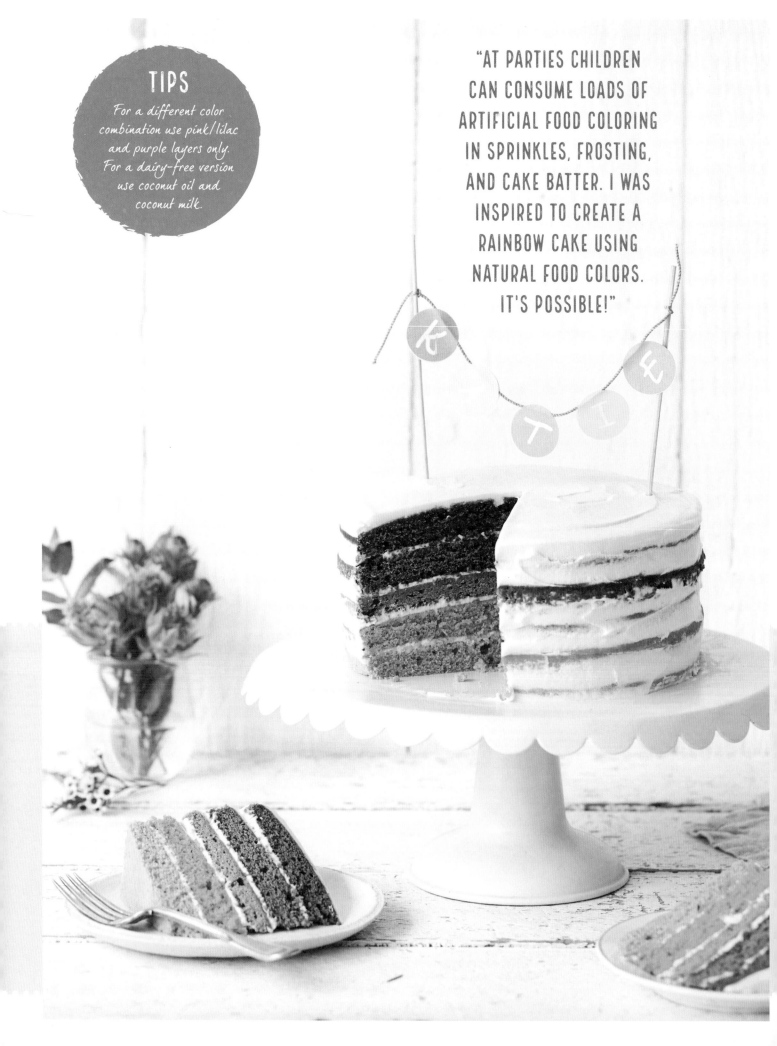

TIPS

For a different color combination use pink/lilac and purple layers only. For a dairy-free version use coconut oil and coconut milk.

"AT PARTIES CHILDREN CAN CONSUME LOADS OF ARTIFICIAL FOOD COLORING IN SPRINKLES, FROSTING, AND CAKE BATTER. I WAS INSPIRED TO CREATE A RAINBOW CAKE USING NATURAL FOOD COLORS. IT'S POSSIBLE!"

VEG
Vegetarian

Nut
Free

Prep time: 40 mins
Cooking time: 15–25 mins
Makes: 32 kid-sized pieces

Natural Rainbow Cake

INGREDIENTS

Cake

2 cups (9¹⁄₅ oz) spelt flour

1¹⁄₂ cups (7²⁄₅ oz) whole spelt flour

1 tbs baking powder

1 tsp baking soda

¹⁄₂ tsp sea salt

1 cup (8¹⁄₂ oz) organic butter, room temperature

1¹⁄₂ cups maple syrup

4 large eggs

2 tsp pure vanilla extract

¹⁄₄ cup coconut milk

1 tbs lemon juice

Natural food colors

Yellow: plain batter

without any coloring

Orange: 1–2 tsp turmeric powder mixed with 1–2 tsp filtered water + 2 tsp lemon juice

Lilac/pink: 4 tbs raspberry juice + 1 tbs lemon juice + 1 tbs spelt flour

Purple: 4 tbs blueberry juice + 1 tbs lemon juice + 1 tbs spelt flour

Green: ¹⁄₄–¹⁄₂ tbs Spirulina powder + 1 tbs lemon juice

EQUIPMENT
electric handmixer

INSTRUCTIONS

Juice for food colors:
For the raspberry and blueberry juice, heat 1 cup of frozen raspberries and 1 cup of frozen blueberries in 2 small saucepans over medium heat and simmer for 5 mins. Using a sieve, drain the juice out of the berries and set aside.

Cake:
Preheat oven to 340°F and grease and flour five 8" cake tins with a little butter and flour.

In a large bowl, add flour, baking soda, baking powder and salt. Stir to combine.

In a medium-sized bowl, beat butter and maple syrup with an electric handmixer. Add eggs, vanilla, milk, and lemon juice and mix for another minute.

Carefully fold dry ingredients into wet ingredients until well combined.

Divide the batter into 5 equal parts. Add one natural food color per part and mix well.

Pour batters into prepared pans and bake for 15–25 mins, or until a cake tester comes out clean.

Leave to cool on a wire rack before icing with your frosting of choice (see recipe below).

Serving and storing leftovers: Serve immediately, refrigerate in an airtight container for up to 4 days or freeze for up to 4 months.

Nut
Free

V
Vegan

Gluten
Free

Prep time: 15 mins (+7½ hours refrigeration)
Makes: Enough for one rainbow cake with five layers

Coconut Cream Frosting

INGREDIENTS

2 x 13¹⁄₂ fl oz cans coconut cream, refrigerated for 7 hours or overnight

2 scoops 100% natural stevia

½ tsp pure vanilla extract

EQUIPMENT
electric hand mixer

INSTRUCTIONS

Remove the coconut cream from the fridge and turn the can upside down. Using a can opener, open from the bottom and discard water that has separated from the cream.

Add the cream, stevia, and vanilla extract to a medium-sized bowl and whip with a hand mixer until light and fluffy.

Place in the fridge for half an hour before frosting the cake.

Serving and storing leftovers:
Use immediately, store in the fridge in an airtight container for up to 4 days or in the freezer for up to 4 months

For a thicker consistency, replace one can of coconut cream with one can of organic thick cream.

Vegan Gluten Free Nut Free

Prep time: 10 mins
Makes: 1½ cups

Egg Free Gluten Free Nut Free Dairy Free

Prep time: 5 mins
Cooking Time: 15–20 min
Makes: 1½ cups

Basic Hummus

INGREDIENTS

1½ cups (9½ oz) cooked chickpeas (See tips for preparing chickpeas on page 30) or 1 x 14 oz can chickpeas, rinsed and drained

½ tbs tahini, hulled

1 garlic clove

sea salt to taste

1 tbs lemon juice

½ tbs fresh cilantro

¼ tsp ground cumin

2 tbs filtered water

pinch pepper

EQUIPMENT
blender

INSTRUCTIONS

Place all ingredients in a blender and blend until smooth and creamy.

Use as a dip for veggie sticks or homemade crackers (see page 64).

Serving and storing leftovers: Serve immediately or store in the fridge for up to 4 days or freeze for up to 4 months.

BBQ Sauce

INGREDIENTS

1 cup tomato puree

1 tbs tomato paste

¼ cup balsamic vinegar

¼ cup (2⅞ oz) unsweetened apple sauce

1 tbs raw honey

1 tbs pomegranate molasses

1 tbs butter or ghee

1 garlic clove

1 tbs arrowroot

1 tsp smoked paprika

1 tsp tamari

sea salt and pepper, to taste

EQUIPMENT
hand-held blender

INSTRUCTIONS

Combine all ingredients in a medium-sized saucepan and bring to a boil.

Simmer on a low heat for 15–20 mins, or until thickened.

Blend with a hand-held blender until smooth.

Transfer to a sealed glass jar and use as a dip for grilled meat and vegetables or sweet sweet potato fries.

Serving and storing leftovers: Serve immediately or store in a glass jar or an airtight container in the fridge for up to 2 weeks.

You can also use dried fruits such as prunes, plums or dates (2-3) instead of honey.

Nut Free Dairy Free Vegetarian

Prep time: 10 mins
Cooking time: 20 mins
Makes: 4

Pita Bread

INGREDIENTS

1 egg

⅓ cup milk of choice

2 tbs filtered water

1 tbs extra virgin olive oil or coconut oil

1 cup (5 oz) whole spelt flour

¼ tsp baking soda

½ tsp sea salt

INSTRUCTIONS

Preheat oven to 355°F and line a baking tray with baking paper.

Add egg, milk, water, and oil to a bowl and whisk to combine.

Add remaining ingredients and stir well.

Divide the mixture and pour each half onto the baking sheet. Using a spatula, spread each mixture into a circle, about ¾" thick.

Bake for 20 mins.

Leave to cool, then cut in half and fill with favorite fillings.

Serving and storing leftovers: Serve immediately, store in an airtight container for up to 3 days or in the fridge for up to 5 days, or freeze for up to 3 months.

For a gluten-free version swap the spelt flour for 1 1/4 cup Wholesome Child gluten-free flour mix, 1 tbs coconut flour, and 1/2 tsp psyllium husk powder.

Gluten Free • Nut Free • Egg Free

Tzatziki Dip

INGREDIENTS

1 large cucumber (12¹/₃ oz to 14 oz)

1 cup (9¹/₅ oz) Greek yogurt

1 cup (8¹/₂ oz) sour cream

1–2 cloves garlic, crushed

¹/₂ tsp fresh dill, finely chopped

¹/₂ tsp fresh mint, finely chopped

sea salt and pepper, to taste

INSTRUCTIONS

Finely grate the cucumber and drain through a sieve or wrap in a cloth to remove excess water.

Place all ingredients in a medium-sized bowl and stir to combine.

Serve chilled with meat or vegetables.

Serving and storing leftovers:
Serve immediately or store in the fridge for up to 4 days.

Vegan • Gluten Free • Nut Free

Prep time: 5 mins
Cooking time: 15–20 mins
Makes: 3 cups

Homemade Ketchup

INGREDIENTS

1¹/₂ lbs ripe tomatoes or 2³/₄ cups bottled tomato puree

1–2 tbs extra virgin olive oil

1 large yellow onion, chopped

2 cloves garlic, crushed

4 tbs of tomato paste, no added salt

¹/₂ cup (1⁴/₅ oz) carrot, grated

¹/₂ cup (4³/₄ oz) unsweetened pear or apple puree

1–2 tbs maple syrup or coconut sugar (optional)

4 dried apricots (sulphite-free), finely diced

¹/₂ tsp Himalayan rock salt

1 tsp dried oregano

1 tbs arrowroot (optional)

INSTRUCTIONS

If using fresh tomatoes, place in a large bowl of boiling water for two mins then drain, allow to cool, and carefully remove skin. Finely chop the flesh before cooking.

Heat olive oil in a large saucepan. Add onion and sauté until soft for about 2–3 mins.

Add garlic and sauté for another 1–2 mins.

Add tomatoes, tomato paste, carrot, pear or apple puree, apricots, salt and oregano.

Bring to boil, reduce heat and allow to simmer uncovered for 15 mins.

Add 1 tbs of arrowroot flour if necessary to thicken and cook for a further 3 mins.

Serving and storing leftovers:
Serve immediately, store in the fridge for up to 4 days or freeze for up to 4 months.

Nut Free • Vegetarian

Prep time: 10 mins (+ 30 mins resting time)
Cooking time: 10–15 mins
Makes: 4

Naan Bread

INGREDIENTS

¹/₄ cup milk of choice

2 tbs butter or coconut oil

¹/₄ cup (2¹/₃ oz) natural yogurt or coconut yogurt

1¹/₄ cups (6¹/₅ oz) whole spelt flour

1 tsp baking powder

¹/₄ tsp coconut sugar

¹/₂ tsp sea salt

INSTRUCTIONS

Add milk and butter to a small saucepan and heat until butter is melted. Set aside to cool.

Add yogurt to the warm milk and butter mixture and whisk to combine.

Place all dry ingredients into a bowl and whisk to combine. Add wet mixture and, using your hands or a wooden spoon, form a smooth dough.

Let dough rest in the bowl, covered with a tea towel, for half an hour. Divide dough into 4 equal portions.

On a lightly floured surface, roll out each portion into a ¹/₃" thick circles or ovals.

Preheat pan to medium high heat, but don't add any oil. Put dough into the pan and cook for 1–2 mins on each side. Wrap the bread in a kitchen towel while baking the rest.

Cut in half and fill with chicken, tzatziki, lettuce, tomatoes, or hummus.

Serving and storing leftovers: Serve immediately, store in an airtight container for up to 3 days, in the fridge for up to 5 days or freeze for up to 3 months.

Menu Planners

GENERAL MENU PLANNER *Suits children and families without allergies or intolerances*

	MON	TUES	WED	THURS	FRI	SAT	SUN
BREAKFAST	Pumpkin Porridge with blueberries and chopped walnuts.	Leftover Vegetable Omelette. Orange slices.	Crunchy Chocolate Coconut Granola with milk of choice. Chopped strawberries.	Omega-3 Smoothie. Wholesome Kamut Tortilla Wraps with almond butter.	Quinoa Blueberry Porridge with crushed hazelnuts.	Shakshuka with Quinoa & Greens. Sliced nectarine.	Almond Coconut Waffles with Blueberry Vanilla Compote.
SNACK	Teff & Parmesan Crackers with Basic Hummus. Veggie sticks.	Mini Banana Cinnamon Scroll. Veggie sticks.	Mini Naan Bread with boiled egg. Veggie sticks.	Lunch Box-Friendly Muesli Bar. Veggie sticks.	Natural yogurt in reusable yogurt pouch or container with 1 tsp of Fig Jam and chia seeds. Veggie sticks.	Mini Pita Bread with peanut butter and Chia Raspberry Jam. Veggie sticks.	Beetroot Berry Smoothie. Veggie sticks with Watercress & Cashew Pesto.
LUNCH	Lamb Koftas with baked sweet potato wedges and assorted raw vegetables.	Cheesy Cauliflower Falafels and assorted vegetables.	Miso Chicken with Vegetables and quinoa.	Mini Salmon Quiches with Tzatziki Dip and assorted raw vegetables.	Lentil & Vegetable Soup served with Gluten-Free Yogurt Bread.	Fish Fingers with baked French fries and Homemade Ketchup. Raw vegetables.	Sticky Chicken Casserole served with baked vegetables.
SNACK	Natural yogurt tub with a sprinkle of Quick Homemade Granola, chopped almonds, and sliced banana. Veggie sticks.	Mango Chia Pudding. Veggie sticks.	Kiwi & Coconut Popsicle. A handful of sunflower seeds, pumpkin seeds or chopped cashew nuts. Veggie sticks.	Flaxseed Crackers with Roasted Garlic Guacamole or ricotta cheese. Veggie sticks or one piece of fruit.	Watermelon & Feta salad. Veggie sticks.	Vanilla Cupcake. Veggie sticks.	Banana Split Trio. Veggie sticks.
DINNER	Easy Fish Curry with brown rice and steamed vegetables (save leftover veggies for tomorrow's breakfast).	Coconut Lamb Meatloaf with baked pumpkin and sweet potato.	Tuna & Chia Lasagne with a side of steamed vegetables.	Adzuki Bean Stew with brown rice.	Chicken Drumstick Casserole with quinoa and a side of grilled vegetables.	Mac 'n' Cheese with a side of roast vegetables.	Hamburger Patties with Gluten-Free Hamburger Buns and optional extras such as avocado, tomato, cucumber slices, and grated beetroot.

NOTE All suggestions appear as recipes in this book. Wherever possible use homemade versions of sauces, marinades and milks. Recipes for vegetable side dishes are available on the website: www.wholesomechild.com.au

284

VEGETARIAN *including egg and dairy (no meat)*

	MON	TUES	WED	THURS	FRI	SAT	SUN
BREAKFAST	Choc Coconut Porridge with natural yogurt.	Strawberry & Ricotta Pancakes.	Apple Buckini Porridge with chopped cashew nuts.	Paleo Granola with Almond Milk or milk of choice. Mixed berries.	Pumpkin Porridge with chopped almonds.	Gluten-Free Yogurt Bread with sunflower butter and Chia Raspberry Jam.	Banana Pancakes.
SNACK	Beetroot Bliss Ball. Veggie sticks.	Superseed Bar. Veggie sticks.	Walnut Hummus, Watercress & Cashew Pesto and Tzatziki Dip. Veggie sticks.	Teff & Parmesan Crackers with Basil & Pine Nut Pesto Veggie sticks.	Naan Bread with Basic Hummus. Veggie sticks.	Choc Chia Pop. Veggie sticks.	Tropical Turmeric Smoothie plus a handful of chopped mixed nuts. Veggie sticks.
LUNCH	Cheesy Cauliflower Pizza Base with vegetable toppings.	Asian-style Rice Paper Rolls with tofu, egg or cheese. Assorted raw vegetables.	Asparagus & Cheese Tart with steamed vegetables.	Quinoa Fried Rice with Vegetables and egg.	Sweet Potato Pizza with vegetables and Basil & Pine Nut Pesto topping.	Shakshuka with Quinoa & Greens and roasted vegetables.	Mixed Bean Salad with mini Pita Bread and chopped vegetables.
SNACK	Flaxseed Crackers with Tzatziki Dip. Veggie sticks.	Strawberry & Banana Milkshake. Veggie sticks.	Carrot, Walnut & Apple Salad. Veggie sticks.	Pecan Quinoa Muesli Bar. Kiwi fruit.	Berry and Pineapple Popsicles. Veggie sticks	Avocado Chocolate Smoothie (frozen into popsicle). Veggie sticks.	Rich Chocolate Black Bean Brownie.
DINNER	Lentil & Vegetable Soup with quinoa.	Brazil & Cashew Nut Patties with steamed vegetables.	Asparagus & Cheese Tart with assorted grilled vegetables.	Cheesy Cauliflower Falafel Patties with steamed vegetables.	Black Bean Tortillas with Arrowroot Tortillas.	High-Protein Veggie Hamburger with Gluten-Free Buns. Raw vegetables.	Adzuki Bean Stew with brown rice and steamed vegetables.

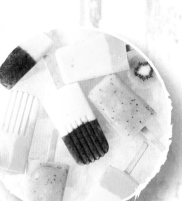

ASPARAGUS & CHEESE TART
page 255

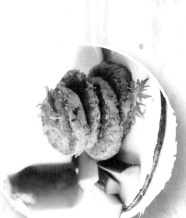

BERRY AND PINEAPPLE POPSICLES
page 217

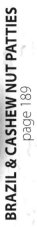

BRAZIL & CASHEW NUT PATTIES
page 189

BEETROOT BLISS BALLS
page 115

Menu Planners

GLUTEN-FREE AND DAIRY-FREE A guide for sensitive or allergy-prone family members

	MON	TUES	WED	THURS	FRI	SAT	SUN
BREAKFAST	Strawberry & Banana Milkshake with 1 slice of Gluten-Free Yogurt Bread (made with coconut yogurt) and almond butter.	Shakshuka with Quinoa & Greens. (replace feta with crumbled tofu) and avocado slices.	Apple Buckini Porridge with crushed walnuts.	Vegan Cashew Cheese with Pita Bread.	Chocolate Rice Puffs with Almond Milk, crushed almonds and chia seeds.	Mango Chia Pudding.	Almond & Buckwheat Pancakes with blueberries.
SNACK	Flaxseed Crackers and Roasted Garlic Guacamole. Veggie sticks.	Sweet Potato Pancakes. Veggie sticks.	Choc Chia Pop. Veggie sticks.	Beetroot & Coconut Frittatas. Veggie sticks.	Arrowroot Tortillas with Roast Garlic Guacamole. Veggie sticks.	Pecan Quinoa Muesli Bar. Veggie sticks.	Veggie sticks with Walnut Hummus.
LUNCH	Quinoa Fried Rice with Vegetables.	Asian-style Rice Paper Rolls with fish, tofu or chicken.	Vegetable Muffins (swap cheese for coconut cream) with assorted raw vegetables.	Salmon & Millet Rissoles with Cashew & Cauliflower Mayonnaise and assorted raw vegetables.	Mezze-style lunch: gluten-free Pita Bread with Chicken Liver Pâté, Basic Hummus, Olive Tapenade and roast vegetables.	Sliced roast chicken (leftover from dinner) on Gluten-Free Buns with lettuce and Homemade Ketchup.	Grilled cod (or similar) with Easy Fish Marinade and brown rice.
SNACK	Gluten-free Pita Bread with almond butter. Veggie sticks.	Omega-3 Smoothie. Veggie sticks.	Flaxseed Crackers with Watercress & Cashew Pesto and/ or Chicken Liver Pâté. Veggie sticks.	Berry & Pineapple Popsicle. Veggie sticks.	Mini Salmon Quiche (use coconut cream instead of cheese) Veggie sticks.	Raw Caramel Chocolate Square. Veggie sticks.	Apple and Cinnamon Doughnut with coconut cream/ Macadamia Vanilla Ice cream.
DINNER	Shepherd's Pie with steamed vegetables.	Orange Lamb Cutlets with baked sweet potato, broccoli and carrot.	Easy Fish Curry with quinoa and steamed vegetables.	Beef & Veggie Meatballs with Homemade Ketchup and mashed potato and cauliflower (use recipe from Shepherd's Pie).	Roast Chicken in Marinade and roasted pumpkin, potato and green beans.	Supercharged Spaghetti Bolognaise with gluten-free pasta and steamed vegetables.	Chicken Nuggets with baked sweet potato and parsnip chips.

NOTE
- 1–2 pieces of fruit can be added daily to these menu planners either in the lunch box or after dinner, for example.
- For children who are not hungry at snack time, swap suggestions with simple options such as a piece of fruit, a slice of cheese or a handful of nuts.
- Always offer veggie sticks at snack times with or without dips.
- Even if veggies are disguised in main meals, it's still advisable to offer a side of raw or cooked vegetables.
- Dessert is not essential. If your child is used to having dessert after their meal, then either offer a piece of fruit with natural yogurt or see dessert suggestions on page 291.

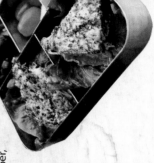

GUIDELINES

1. Choose two vegetables to include for mid-morning snack (for fussy eaters, this can be one they like paired with one they dislike).

2. If your child is eating the same lunch every day, then begin with including one of these choices for the first week. Then try to include two of these choices for the second week and slowly build up. Remember, change is a slow process and you need to work with what your child can tolerate.

3. Choose 2–3 extras (see below) to include with the lunch box.

OPTIONAL LUNCH BOX EXTRAS:

- Popcorn, lightly salted.
- Trail mix (sunflower seeds, pumpkin seeds, goji berries, s golden raisins).
- Wholegrain crackers—ensure they contain no additives.
- Chickpeas (roasted or plain) or beans.
- Low-sodium cheese, grated or sliced.
- Natural yogurt in reusable container and sweeten with pureed fruit, raw honey or chopped fresh fruit and a sprinkle of Quick Homemade Granola.
- Dips such as hummus, guacamole, tzatziki or pesto.
- Berries are low in sugar and great for lunch boxes: raspberries, strawberries, blueberries, mulberries, blackberries.
- Dried fruit is high in sugar so offer it in small quantities. If your child is used to the mini sultana boxes from supermarkets, pour half out, and fill with pumpkin seeds and sunflower seeds to create a school-friendly trail mix.
- Healthy fats: boiled egg, avocado slices, pitted and sliced olives (soak overnight to remove excess sodium), sunflower seeds, pumpkin seeds.
- Fresh vegetables: carrots, tomatoes, snow peas, pepper, carrot, kohlrabi, cucumber, celery.
- Cooked vegetables: sweet potato wedges, pumpkin, broccoli, cauliflower, green beans.

LUNCH BOX MENU PLANNER *for adventurous eaters*

	MON	TUES	WED	THURS	FRI
MID MORNING SNACK	Flaxseed Crackers with Basic Hummus. Veggie sticks.	Vegetable Muffins. Veggie sticks.	Sweet Potato Pancakes. Veggie sticks.	Mixed Bean Salad. Veggie sticks.	Teff & Parmesan Crackers with cheese. Veggie sticks.
LUNCH	Cheesy Cauliflower Falafel Patties in wraps. Assorted veggies.	Lamb Koftas with brown rice in thermos. Assorted veggies.	Quinoa & Brown Rice Chicken Balls. Assorted veggies.	Mini Salmon Quiches. Assorted veggies.	Beef & Veggie Meatballs with Homemade Ketchup in thermos.
MID AFTERNOON SNACK	Superseed bar. Veggie sticks.	Pita Bread with Basic Hummus and salad. Veggie sticks and sliced apple.	Beetroot Bliss Ball. Veggie sticks.	Gluten-Free Yogurt Bread with Roasted Garlic Guacamole. Veggie sticks.	Gluten-Free Chocolate Biscuit or Chocolate Spelt Biscuit. Veggie sticks.

LUNCH BOX MENU PLANNER *for fussy eaters*

(Transitioning your child off processed sweet food)

	MON	TUES	WED	THURS	FRI
MID MORNING SNACK	Lunch Box-Friendly Muesli Bar. Veggie sticks.	Sweet Potato Pancakes. Veggie sticks.	Strawberry Pancakes. Veggie sticks.	Vanilla Muffin with Cauliflower. Veggie sticks.	Pita Bread with Chia Raspberry Jam. Veggie sticks.
LUNCH	Sweet Potato Pizza. Assorted veggies.	Roast Chicken in Marinade, shredded. Pita Bread. Assorted veggies.	Gluten-Free Yogurt Bread with Healthy Chocolate Spread. Assorted veggies.	Chicken Nuggets in a thermos with Homemade Ketchup on the side. Assorted veggies.	Savory Cheese Scrolls. Assorted veggies.
MID AFTERNOON SNACK	Teff & Parmesan Crackers with grated cheese or sunflower butter. Veggie sticks.	Banana & Cinnamon Scroll. Veggie sticks.	Rich Chocolate Black Bean Brownie. Veggie sticks.	Naan Bread with a boiled egg. Veggie sticks.	Chocolate Zucchini Muffin. Veggie sticks.

Menu Planners

HOW TO PREPARE FOR THE BUSY WEEK AHEAD *A practical guide for busy parents*

WEEK 1	MON	TUES	WED	THURS	FRI	SAT	SUN
BREAKFAST	Paleo Granola with homemade Almond Milk and raspberries.	Leftover vegetable omelette.	Omega-3 Smoothie (freeze leftovers into popsicle molds).	Quinoa Blueberry Porridge.	Mango Chia Pudding.	Shakshuka with Quinoa & Greens and strawberries.	Almond Coconut Waffles.
SNACK	Flaxseed Crackers with Basic Hummus or dip of choice. Veggie sticks.	Banana bread. Veggie sticks.	Lunch Box Friendly Muesli Bar (or muesli bar of choice). Veggie sticks.	Beetroot Berry Smoothie (freeze leftovers in popsicle molds). Handful mixed nuts. Veggie sticks.	Natural yogurt with Quick Homemade Granola. Veggie sticks.	Vegetable Muffins. Veggie sticks.	Leftover omega-3 smoothie popsicle. Veggie sticks.
LUNCH	Mini Salmon Quiche with Tzatziki Dip and raw veggies (freeze leftover salmon quiches).	Leftover koftas with Homemade Ketchup, lettuce and grated carrot in Pita bread.	Leftover fish curry with brown rice and veggies (thermos).	Rice paper wraps with leftover miso chicken (shredded), pesto, lettuce and raw veggies.	Leftover spaghetti bolognaise (thermos) and garden salad.	Leftover lentil and vegetable soup with natural yogurt. Assorted raw vegetables.	Fish Sticks with French fries and ketchup with sliced cucumber and carrot.
SNACK	Lunch Box Friendly Muesli Bar (or muesli bar of choice). Veggie sticks.	Flaxseed Crackers with leftover hummus or dip of choice. Veggie sticks.	Banana Bread. Veggie sticks.	Tropical Turmeric Smoothie. Veggie sticks.	Vegetable Muffins. Veggie sticks.	Chocolate Almond Cake (freeze leftover cake for following weekend).	Choc Chia Pop. Veggie sticks.
DINNER	Lamb Koftas with sweet potato wedges and veggies (save leftover veggies for following day breakfast).	Easy Fish Curry with brown rice (cook double amount for following day) and steamed veggies.	Miso Chicken with Vegetables and quinoa (cook double amount of quinoa for porridge next day).	Supercharged Spaghetti Bolognaise and garden salad.	Lentil & Vegetable Soup served with 1 slice of Gluten-Free Yogurt Bread.	Chicken Drumstick Casserole with baked vegetables and raw veggies.	Adzuki Bean Stew with brown rice.

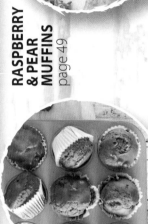

MINI SALMON QUICHES page 253

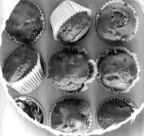

RASPBERRY & PEAR MUFFINS page 49

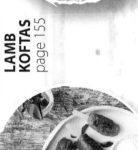

LAMB KOFTAS page 155

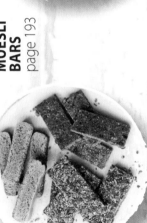

MUESLI BARS page 193

HOW TO PREPARE FOR THE BUSY WEEK AHEAD *A practical guide for busy parents*

WEEK 2	MON	TUES	WED	THURS	FRI	SAT	SUN
BREAKFAST	Strawberry Pancakes.	Quick Homemade Granola with natural yogurt and grated apple.	Pumpkin Porridge.	Avocado Chocolate Smoothie (freeze leftovers in popsicle molds).	Almond & Buckwheat Pancakes.	Quinoa Blueberry Porridge with crushed almonds.	Wholesome Kamut Tortilla Wraps with scrambled egg, spinach, mushrooms, and tomatoes.
SNACK	Beetroot Bliss Ball. Veggie sticks.	Mini Savory Cheese Scroll. Veggie sticks.	Teff & Parmesan Crackers with Roast Garlic Guacamole. Veggie sticks.	Leftover mini salmon quiche. Veggie sticks.	Natural yogurt with Quick Homemade Granola. Veggie sticks.	Leftover almond & buckwheat pancakes. Veggie sticks.	Choc Chia Pop. Veggie sticks.
LUNCH	Leftover adzuki bean stew served in Wholesome Kamut Tortilla Wraps with lettuce and shredded raw veggies.	Leftover hamburger patties with Homemade Ketchup and Sweet Potato Salad.	Leftover salmon rissoles with Tzatziki Dip and garden salad.	Leftover chicken casserole and veggies.	Leftover meatballs in a Gluten-free Hamburger Bun with vegetables.	Leftover lasagne with garden salad.	Leftover falafels with Basic Hummus, Pita Bread and assorted vegetables.
SNACK	Teff & Parmesan Crackers with Roast Garlic Guacamole. Veggie sticks.	Leftover strawberry Pancakes. Veggie sticks.	Mini Savory Cheese Scroll. Veggie sticks.	Beetroot Bliss Ball. Veggie sticks.	Leftover avocado and chocolate popsicle. Veggie sticks.	Leftover chocolate almond cake. Veggie sticks.	Berry and Pineapple Popsicle. Veggie sticks.
DINNER	Hamburger Patties with mashed sweet potato and steamed veggies.	Salmon & Millet Rissoles with Tzatziki Dip and steamed veggies (cook extra pumpkin for breakfast).	Chicken Drumstick Casserole with quinoa/brown rice and steamed veggies.	Beef & Veggie Meatballs with cauliflower and potato mash.	Tuna, Vegetables & Chia Lasagne with steamed veggies.	Cheesy Cauliflower Falafel Patties with brown rice and baked vegetables.	Roast Chicken in Marinade with roast pumpkin, potato and beans.

SUNDAY COOK-UP FOR THE WEEK AHEAD

Prepare ahead by making some of the following to accompany the above menu planner:

BASICS
- Paleo Granola
- Homemade Ketchup/Tzatziki Dip/Basic Hummus/Roasted Garlic Guacamole
- Jelly/Compote
- Homemade almond or coconut milk

SIDES
- Quinoa/Brown rice
- Roast/grilled/steamed vegetables

(Recipes available on the website: www.wholesomechild.com.au)

SWEET AND SAVORY SNACKS
- Choc Chia Pops/Beetroot Bliss Balls
- Savory Scrolls/Banana Scrolls/Veggie Muffins
- Banana Bread/Kamut Wraps/Gluten-Free Yogurt Bread
- Chocolate Almond Cake/Rich Chocolate Black Bean Brownies/Muesli Bars

MAINS (EASY AND FREEZABLE)
- Supercharged Spaghetti Bolognaise
- Lamb Koftas
- Hamburger Patties/Salmon Rissoles
- Stews
- Chicken Drumstick Casserole
- Tuna, Vegetables & Chia Lasagne

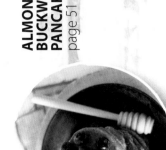

ALMOND & BUCKWHEAT PANCAKES page 51

SALMON & MILLET RISSOLES page 167

289

Menu Planners

PARTY MENU PLANNER *All recipes below can be found in this book*

SWEET	SAVORY
1. Watermelon Cake	1. Healthy Sausage Rolls with Homemade Ketchup
2. Banana Cinnamon Scrolls	2. Vegetarian Sausage Rolls
3. Rich Chocolate Black Bean Brownies	3. Sweet Potato Pizza cut into mini slices
4. Chocolate Zucchini Muffins	4. Lamb Koftas on a stick
5. Vanilla Muffins With Cauliflower & Decadent Chocolate Ganache	5. Mini Hamburger Patties on Gluten-Free Hamburger Buns
6. Chocolate Spelt Cookies	6. Veggie platter with Basic Hummus/Roasted Garlic Guacamole/ Basil & Pine Nut Pesto/Tzatziki Dip
7. Chocolate Almond Cake with Choc Date Frosting	7. Cheesy Cauliflower Falafel Patties
8. Natural Rainbow Cake with Coconut Cream Frosting	8. Savory Scrolls with cheese and tomato
9. Choc Chia Pops	9. Asparagus & Cheese Tart
10. Chocolate Quinoa Treats	10. Flaxseed Crackers/Teff & Parmesan Crackers and Watercress & Cashew Pesto

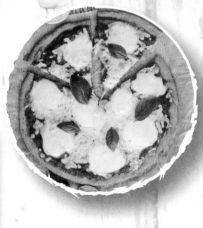

SWEET POTATO PIZZA
page 131

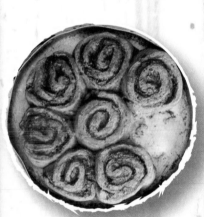

MINI HAMBURGER PATTIES ON GLUTEN-FREE BUNS
pages 159 + 51

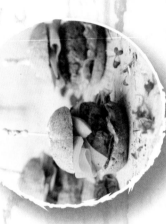

BANANA CINNAMON SCROLLS
page 85

WATERMELON CAKE
page 219

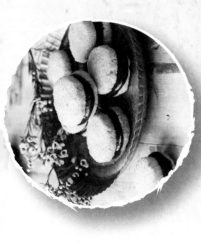

HEALTHY SANDWICH FILLINGS

My favorite lunch boxes are eco-friendly bento-style stainless steel lunch boxes, such as Planet Box or Lunchbots, which have great compartments for little hands. Safe, durable, reusable and recyclable, they are good for the planet and they last for years. For warm weather, ensure you have a well-insulated lunch box and send an ice-pack (simply pop some ice in a reusable bag) or purchase a lunch box cooler bag to ensure food stays fresh.

1. Mashed-up Beef & Veggie Meatballs or Lamb Koftas with Homemade Ketchup.
2. Shredded chicken and lettuce with Basil & Pine Nut Pesto.
3. Mashed egg with Cauliflower and Vegan Mayonnaise, grated carrot and a touch of sweet paprika.
4. Salmon & Millet Rissoles or Cheesy Cauliflower Falafel Patties and Tzatziki Dip (these are great in a wholegrain wrap).
5. Ricotta cheese or sheep's milk cheese with cinnamon and sliced banana.
6. Chia Raspberry Jam on a thin layer of unsalted butter (replacement for conventional jam; start by mixing half/half).
7. Sloppy Joes—Supercharged Bolognaise as a filling in a Pita Bread, sourdough rolls or wrap.
8. Tuna, grated cheese, carrot and corn—use a natural yogurt dressing in place of mayonnaise: 1 tbs natural yogurt, 1 tsp Dijon mustard, 1 tsp balsamic vinegar, 1 tbs extra virgin olive oil.
9. Grilled and flaked salmon or cod (or similar) with lettuce and cherry tomatoes.
10. Sunflower butter with a thin layer of raw honey or maple syrup.
11. Miso paste and mixed sunflower seed butter.
12. Avocado and ricotta cheese.
13. Wholesome cheese toastie with added veggies. Spread bread with sweet potato or pumpkin puree before toasting. You can also add nutritional yeast to the mix.
14. Homemade Chocolate Spread and a sprinkle of chia seeds.
15. Quark cheese or sliced bocconcini cheese, unsalted butter, baby spinach, tomato, and pepper.
16. Tuna or salmon mixed with quark cheese, extra virgin olive oil, lettuce, shredded carrot, and diced cucumber.

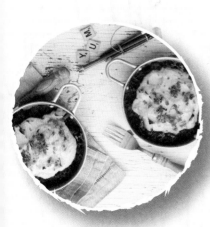

SHEPHERD'S PIE
page 169

TOP 10 THERMOS MEALS

Purchase a good quality thermos that will keep food warm for five or more hours and follow instructions on how to use to prevent food from spoiling.

1. Shepherd's Pie
2. Supercharged Spaghetti Bolognaise
3. Beef & Veggie Meatballs
4. Mac 'n' Cheese
5. Lentil & Vegetable Soup
6. Quinoa Fried Rice
7. Chicken Drumstick Casserole
8. Tuna, Vegetable & Chia Lasagne
9. Adzuki Bean Stew
10. Easy Fish Curry

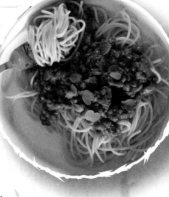

SUPERCHARGED SPAGHETTI BOLOGNAISE
page 123

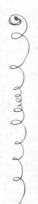

COCONUT MACAROONS
page 199

DESSERT: SHOULD I OR SHOULDN'T I?

Many families like to end their evening meal with something sweet. Fresh fruit is always a good idea. Choose low-sugar versions such as kiwi fruit, raspberries or strawberries and serve with plain yogurt or almond butter. However, for special occasions, fruit may not be enough, so try these delicious and nutritious options:

1. Half a cup of frozen fruit (banana, mango or berries). Add a handful of soaked cashew nuts for an extra creamy taste. Puree in a high-speed blender and eat straight away for a delicious, slushy dessert. Or try our homemade ice creams on page 227.
2. Frozen popsicles made with pure fruit and yogurt. See our homemade versions on page 217.
3. Homemade Coconut Custard (see page 257).
4. Mini Apple Pies (see page 215) with a scoop of natural yogurt or homemade ice cream.
5. Banana Split Trio (see page 227).
6. No-Bake Cheesecake (see page 245).
7. Coconut Macaroons (see page 199).
8. Rich Chocolate Black Bean Brownies (see page 119).
9. Vanilla Muffins with Cauliflower (see page 127).
10. Raw Caramel Chocolate Square (see page 87).

BIBLIOGRAPHY AND RESOURCES

American Academy of Pediatrics **www.aap.org**

American Cancer Society **www.cancer.org**

American Diabetes Association **www.diabetes.org**

American Heart Association **www.heart.org**

Australian Bureau of Statistics **www.abs.gov.au**

Better Health Channel **www.betterhealth.vic.gov.au**

Cancer Council NSW **www.cancercouncil.com.au**

Center for Science in the Public Interest **www.cspinet.org**

CluckAR app (free) **www.choice.com.au**

Chris Kresser **www.chriskresser.com**

Commonwealth Scientific and Industrial Research Organisation (CSIRO) **www.csiro.au**

Dietitians Association of Australia (DAA) **www.daa.asn.au**

Dr. Joseph Mercola **www.mercola.com**

Environmental Working Group **www.ewg.org**

Food Standards Australia and New Zealand **www.foodstandards.govt.nz**

Greenpeace **www.greenpeace.org**

Hyperactive Children's Support Group **www.hacsg.org.uk**

Infant & Toddler Forum **www.infantandtoddlerforum.org**

Madge Australia **www.madge.org.au**

MEND **www.healthyweightpartnership.org**

Mindd Foundation **www.mindd.org**

National Institute of Diabetes and Digestive and Kidney Diseases **www.niddk.nih.gov**

Nutrient Reference Values for Australia and New Zealand (Australian Government, Department of National Health and Ageing; National Health and Medical Research Council; New Zealand Ministry of Health) **www.nhmrc.gov.au/_files_NHMRC/publications/attachments/n35.pdf**

Parents Magazine **www.parents.com**

SOS Approach to Feeding **www.sosapproach-conferences.com**

Star Institute for Sensory Processing Disorder **www.spdstar.org**

United States Department of Agriculture **www.usda.gov**

United States Food and Drug Administration **www.fda.gov**

US National Library of Medicine National Institutes of Health **www.pubmed.gov**

World Health Organization (WHO) **www.who.int**

INDEX

Entries beginning with a capital letter are recipes; lower case entries refer to topics

INDEX